T0259386

Patient and Family Experience in the ICU

Editor

JUDY E. DAVIDSON

CRITICAL CARE NURSING CLINICS OF NORTH AMERICA

www.ccnursing.theclinics.com

Consulting Editor
CYNTHIA BAUTISTA

June 2020 • Volume 32 • Number 2

ELSEVIER

1600 John F. Kennedy Boulevard ● Suite 1800 ● Philadelphia, Pennsylvania, 19103-2899

http://www.theclinics.com

CRITICAL CARE NURSING CLINICS OF NORTH AMERICA Volume 32, Number 2
June 2020 ISSN 0899-5885, ISBN-13: 978-0-323-73354-0

Editor: Kerry Holland
Developmental Editor: Laura Fisher

Critical Care Nursing Clinics of North America (ISSN 0899-5885) is published quarterly by Elsevier Inc., 360 Park Avenue South, New York, NY 10010-1710. Months of issue are March, June, September, and December. Business and Editorial Offices: 1600 John F. Kennedy Blvd., Suite 1800, Philadelphia, PA 19103-2899. Periodicals postage paid at New York, NY and additional mailing offices. Subscription prices are $160.00 per year for US individuals, $428.00 per year for US institutions, $100.00 per year for US students and residents, $206.00 per year for Canadian individuals, $538.00 per year for Canadian institutions, $230.00 per year for international individuals, $538.00 per year for international institutions, $115.00 per year for international students/residents and $100.00 per year for Canadian students/residents. To receive student/resident rate, orders must be accompanied by name of affiliated institution, data of term, and the *signature* of program/residency coordinator on institution letterhead. Orders will be billed at individual rate until proof of status is received. Foreign air speed delivery is included in all *Clinics* subscription prices. All prices are subject to change without notice. **POSTMASTER:** Send address changes to *Critical Care Nursing Clinics of North America*, Elsevier Health Sciences Division, Subscription Customer Service, 3251 Riverport Lane, Maryland Heights, MO 63043. **Customer Service: 1-800-654-2452 (US and Canada); 314-447-8871 (outside US and Canada). Fax: 314-447-8029. E-mail:** JournalsCustomerService-usa@elsevier.com **(for print support)** and JournalsOnlineSupport-usa@elsevier.com **(for online support).**

Reprints. For copies of 100 or more of articles in this publication, please contact the Commercial Reprints Department, Elsevier Inc., 360 Park Avenue South, New York, New York, 10010-1710; Tel.: 212-633-3874, Fax: 212-633-3820, and E-mail: reprints@elsevier.com.

Critical Care Nursing Clinics of North America is covered in *MEDLINE/PubMed (Index Medicus), International Nursing Index, Nursing Citation Index, Cumulative Index to Nursing and Allied Health Literature,* and *RNdex Top 100.*

Contributors

CONSULTING EDITOR

CYNTHIA BAUTISTA, PhD, APRN, FNCS, FCNS
Associate Professor, Egan School of Nursing and Health Studies, Fairfield University, Fairfield, Connecticut, USA

EDITOR

JUDY E. DAVIDSON, DNP, RN, MCCM, FAAN
Nurse Scientist, University of California, San Diego Health, La Jolla, California, USA

AUTHORS

HEATHER ABRAHIM, MSN, MPA, RN, CCRN
University of California, San Diego Health, San Diego, California, USA

DENISE BARCHAS, RN, MSN, CCRN
University of California, San Francisco Medical Center, San Francisco, California, USA

ERIC BARCHAS, DVM
San Bruno Pet Hospital, San Bruno, California, USA

LEANNE M. BOEHM, PhD, RN, ACNS-BC
Assistant Professor, Vanderbilt University School of Nursing, Tennessee Valley Healthcare System, Nashville Veterans Affairs Hospital, Critical Illness, Brain Dysfunction, and Survivorship Center at Vanderbilt, Nashville, Tennessee, USA

ALEXANDRA BOYLAN, BSN, CCRN
Staff Nurse, CMICU, Ochsner Medical Center, New Orleans, Louisiana, USA

LORI BRIEN, DNP, ACNP-BC
Adult Gerontology Acute Care Nurse Practitioner Program, Georgetown University School of Nursing & Health Studies, Washington, DC, USA; Cardiovascular and Thoracic Surgery, Virginia Hospital Center, Arlington, Virginia, USA

JOSÉ MANUEL VELASCO BUENO, RN
Hospital Virgen de la Victoria, Málaga, Spain; Training manager of the International Research Project for the Humanization of Intensive Care Units (Proyecto HU-CI)

APRIL BUFFO, BSN, RN
Co-Manager, Critical Care Nurse Communicator Program, UW Health, Madison, Wisconsin, USA

TOBY C. CAMPBELL, MD, MS
Associate Professor and Chief of Palliative Care, Division of Hem/Onc/Pall Care, The Ellen and Peter O. Johnson Endowed Chair in Palliative Care, University of Wisconsin-Madison School of Medicine and School of Nursing, Madison, Wisconsin, USA

ELISE CHRISTOFERSON, BA
Accelerated BSN Student, Duke University School of Nursing, Durham, North Carolina, USA

CHRISTOPHER JAMES DOIG, MD, MSc, FRCPC
Professor, Departments of Critical Care Medicine, and Community Health Sciences, Cumming School of Medicine, University of Calgary, Foothills Medical Centre, McCaig Tower, ICU Administration, Calgary, Alberta, Canada

LAUREN F. DOIG, BSc (Hons)
Foothills Medical Centre, McCaig Tower, ICU Administration, Calgary, Alberta, Canada; Graduate Student, Department of Occupational Therapy, Faculty of Rehabilitation Medicine, University of Alberta, Edmonton, Alberta, Canada

KELLY DRUMRIGHT, MSN, CNL, CCRN-CMC, CSC
Clinical Nurse Leader, Tennessee Valley Healthcare System, Nashville Veterans Affairs Hospital, Nashville, Tennessee, USA

WILLIAM J. EHLENBACH, MD, MSc
Assistant Professor of Medicine, Pulmonary and Critical Care, University of Wisconsin-Madison School of Medicine and Public Health, Madison, Wisconsin, USA

ALYSSA ERIKSON, RN, PhD
Associate Professor, Department of Nursing, California State University Monterey Bay, Seaside, California, USA

JOANNA EVERSON, MN, NP
Foothills Medical Centre, McCaig Tower, ICU Administration, Nurse Practitioner, Department of Critical Care Medicine. University of Calgary, Calgary, Alberta, Canada

KIRSTEN M. FIEST, PhD
Assistant Professor, Departments of Critical Care Medicine, Community Health Sciences, and Psychiatry, Cumming School of Medicine, University of Calgary, Calgary, Canada

NADINE FOSTER, BN, RN
Patient and Family Advisor, Department of Critical Care, Alberta Health Services, Foothills Medical Centre, McCaig Tower, ICU Administration, Calgary, Alberta, Canada

LINDA S. FRANCK, RN, PhD
Department of Family Health Care Nursing, School of Nursing, University of California, San Francisco, San Francisco, California, USA

RALPH GERVASIO
ICU Survivor, Tennessee Valley Healthcare System, Nashville Veterans Affairs Hospital, Nashville, Tennessee, USA

CHRISTOPHER J. GRANT, MD, FRCPC
Clinical Assistant Professor, Departments of Critical Care Medicine, and Clinical Neurosciences, Cumming School of Medicine, University of Calgary, Foothills Medical Centre, McCaig Tower, ICU Administration, Calgary, Alberta, Canada

MARY BETH HAPP, PhD, RN, FAAN, FGSA
Nursing Distinguished Professor of Critical Care Research, Associate Dean for Research and Innovation, The Ohio State University College of Nursing, Columbus, Ohio, USA

CHRISTOPHER HILL, MDiv
Chaplain, Tennessee Valley Healthcare System, Nashville Veterans Affairs Hospital, Nashville, Tennessee, USA

CARRIE ANNE HUDSON
Executive Administrative Assistant, University of California, San Diego Health, La Jolla, California, USA

KATHLEEN KERBER, MSN, APRN- CNS, CCRN, CNRN
Clinical Nurse Specialist, The MetroHealth System, Cleveland, Ohio, USA

GABRIEL HERAS LA CALLE, MD, PhD cand
Intensive Care Unit, Hospital Universitario de Torrejón, Madrid, Spain; Founder of the International Research Project for the Humanization of Intensive Care Units (Proyecto HU-CI), Universidad Francisco de Vitoria, Madrid, Spain

KARLA LeBLANC-LUCAS, BSN, RN, CPAN
ICU Unit, Director, New Orleans, Louisiana, USA

JENNIFER McADAM, RN, PhD
Associate Professor, School of Nursing, Samuel Merritt University, Oakland, California, USA

ERICA McCARTNEY, BSN, RN, CCRN-CMC
Clinical Supervisor, Critical Care Services, Swedish Edmonds Medical Center, Edmonds, Washington, USA

MARY GRACE McMURRAY, BA
Accelerated BSN Student, Duke University School of Nursing, Durham, North Carolina, USA

MOLLY McNETT, PhD, RN, CNRN, FNCS, FAAN
Professor, Clinical Nursing, Assistant Director, Implementation Science Core, Helene Fuld Health Trust National Institute for Evidence-Based Practice in Nursing and Healthcare, College of Nursing, The Ohio State University, Columbus, Ohio, USA

MELISSA MELARAGNI, RN, BSN, CCRN
University of California, San Francisco Medical Center, San Francisco, California, USA

KAREL O'BRIEN, MD
Department of Paediatrics, Sinai Health System, University of Toronto, Toronto, Ontario, Canada

ANDREW O'DONNELL, DNP, RN, AGPCNP-BC
Interim Co-Manager, Trauma Life Support Center, UW Health, Madison, Wisconsin, USA

PETER OXLAND, BASc
Family Advisor, Alberta Health Services, Critical Care, Patient and Community Engagement Researcher (PaCER), Department of Critical Care Medicine, University of Calgary, Calgary, Canada

KATHRYN A. POLLARD, MD
Assistant Professor of Clinical Medicine, Critical Care and Emergency Medicine, Indiana University Health Methodist Hospital, Indianapolis, Indiana, USA

NANCY REED, LCSW
Social Worker, Tennessee Valley Healthcare System, Nashville Veterans Affairs Hospital, Nashville, Tennessee, USA

KARIN REUTER-RICE, PhD, NP, FCCM, FAAN
Department of Pediatrics, Division of Pediatric Critical Care, Associate Professor, Duke University School of Nursing, Duke University School of Medicine, Duke Institute for Brain Sciences Durham, North Carolina, USA

MARILYN SCHALLOM, RN, PhD, CCNS, FCCM
Director, Department of Research for Patient Care Services, Barnes Jewish Hospital, St Louis, Missouri, USA

ANNE SCHRUPP, RN, BSN, CCRN
Registered Nurse, Surgical/Burn/Trauma ICU, Barnes Jewish Hospital, St Louis, Missouri, USA

JI WON SHIN, PhD, RN
Adjunct Instructor - Research, The Ohio State University College of Nursing, Columbus, Ohio, USA

YOANNA SKROBIK, MD, FRCP(c), MSc, FCCM
Professor, Department of Medicine, McGill University, Montreal, Quebec, Canada

CARRIE SONA, RN, MSN, CCRN, CCNS, ACNS-BC, FCCM
Clinical Nurse Specialist, Surgical/Burn/Trauma ICU, Barnes Jewish Hospital, St Louis, Missouri, USA

JUDITH A. TATE, PhD, RN
Assistant Professor, The Ohio State University College of Nursing, Columbus, Ohio, USA

KELLY A. THOMPSON-BRAZILL, DNP, ACNP-BC, CCRN-CSC, FCCM
Adult Gerontology Acute Care Nurse Practitioner Program, Georgetown University School of Nursing & Health Studies, Washington, DC, USA

CATHERINE C. TIERNEY, DNP, ACNP-BC
Adult Gerontology Acute Care Nurse Practitioner Program, Georgetown University School of Nursing & Health Studies, Washington, DC, USA; Cardiovascular and Thoracic Surgery, Virginia Hospital Center, Arlington, Virginia, USA

CHANDRA WADDINGTON, RN, MSN
School of Nursing, University of British Columbia, Vancouver, British Columbia, Canada

BRIAN T. WESSMAN, MD, FACEP, FCCM
Associate Professor of Anesthesiology and Emergency Medicine, Division Chief, EM/CCM, Departments of Anesthesiology and Emergency Medicine, Washington University in Saint Louis, School of Medicine, St Louis, Missouri, USA

BROOKE WIGGINS, BSN, RN
Vidant Medical Center, Greenville, North Carolina, USA

JUDSON B. WILLIAMS, MD, MHS
Cardiovascular and Thoracic Surgery, WakeMed Health & Hospitals, Raleigh, North Carolina, USA

JEREMY W. WININGER, MSN, AGACNP-BC
Adult Gerontology Acute Care Nurse Practitioner Program, Georgetown University School of Nursing & Health Studies, Washington, DC, USA; Pulmonology and Critical Care Medicine, WakeMed Health & Hospitals, Raleigh, North Carolina, USA

CHRIS WINKELMAN, PhD, ACNP, CCRN, FCCM, FAANP
Associate Professor, Frances Payne Bolton School of Nursing, Case Western Reserve University, Cleveland, Ohio, USA

FIONA A. WINTERBOTTOM, DNP, MSN, APRN, ACNS-BC, ACHPN, CCRN
Clinical Nurse Specialist, Critical Care Medicine, Ochsner Medical Center, New Orleans, Louisiana, USA

HALEY YEAGER, BSN, RN
Indiana University Health Methodist Hospital, Indianapolis, Indiana, USA

JESSICA ZANGMEISTER, BSN, RN
Clinical Nurse, Medical Intensive Care Unit, The MetroHealth System, Cleveland, Ohio, USA

Contents

and discharging home from a hospital, are important milestones, but they represent only the beginning of recovery and healing after a critical illness. Recognizing that these challenges exist both for patients and families is important to improve critical illness outcomes.

Carrie Sona, Kathryn A. Pollard, Marilyn Schallom, Anne Schrupp, and Brian T. Wessman

During critical illness, active discussions about a person's preferences are linked with better patient outcomes. Our intensive care unit implemented an evidence-based standardized communication bundle that included education to providers on effective family communication, focused patient/family discussions to identify Durable Power of Attorney/surrogate decision maker and obtaining advanced directive documents, and documenting conversations in the electronic medical record and appropriately updating the patient's code status. The aim of the bundle was to increase compliance with conducting and documenting family discussions, clearly identifying and documenting surrogate decisions makers, and to improve patient/family satisfaction and caregiver satisfaction.

Chris Winkelman, Kathleen Kerber, Jessica Zangmeister, and Molly McNett

Integration of flexible visitation into a large health system requires concentrated effort. Evaluating impact on patient, family, and staff outcomes is important to facilitate changes and ensure visiting policy success. The medical intensive care unit staff participated in a collaborative quality improvement effort to encourage flexible visitation. The integration of flexible visitation spanned an 18-month period, timed to accompany a transition to a new setting with rooms designed to support visitor presence. This article details these efforts, outcomes, and important gaps for future work evaluating integration of flexible visitation in critical care.

Andrew O'Donnell, April Buffo, Toby C. Campbell, and William J. Ehlenbach

Twenty percent of Americans die in an intensive care unit (ICU), often incapacitated or requiring assisted decision making. Surrogates are often required to make urgent, complex, high-stakes decisions. Communication among patients, families, and clinicians is often delayed and inefficient with frequent missed opportunities to support the emotional and psychological needs of surrogates, particularly at the end of life. The Critical Care Nurse Communicator program is a nurse-led, primary palliative care intervention designed to improve the quality and consistency of communication in the ICU and address the informational, psychological, and emotional needs of surrogate decision-makers through the shared decision-making process.

Ji Won Shin, Judith A. Tate, and Mary Beth Happ

Family caregivers of intensive care unit (ICU) patients are at high risk for adverse psychological outcomes. Communication difficulty due to mechanical ventilation may induce or worsen adverse psychological outcomes. The Facilitated Sensemaking Model (FSM) is the first model to guide nursing interventions to help ICU family caregivers overcome and prevent adverse psychological outcomes. We address an understudied phenomenon, communication between patients and family caregivers during mechanical ventilation. The FSM guides supportive interventions for critical care nurses to improve patient-family communication in the ICU. We provide an example of communication intervention, an electronic communication app, within the preexisting FSM.

CRITICAL CARE NURSING
CLINICS OF NORTH AMERICA

SERIES OF RELATED INTEREST

Nursing Clinics of North America
http://www.nursing.theclinics.com

THE CLINICS ARE AVAILABLE ONLINE!
Access your subscription at:
www.theclinics.com

Preface

Family-Centered Care: A Reflection

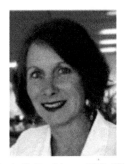
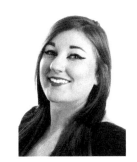

Judy E. Davidson, DNP, RN, MCCM, FAAN, *Editor*

Carrie Anne Hudson, *Executive Administrative Assistant*

Best practices based upon evidence from inspirational leaders around the globe have shaped family-centered care recommendations in national guidelines.[1] However, operationalizing these recommendations is not without challenge. We can learn as much from the challenges as successes; so, in this issue of *Critical Care Nursing Clinics of North America*, both successful and disappointing attempts at optimizing family-centered care are shared for our collective learning.

Molter[2] and Leske[3,4] catapulted the focus to family-centered care nearly 40 years ago with the development of the Critical Care Family Needs Inventory (CCFNI), cited by over 1000 and used by scores of researchers over time to learn more about what the families in intensive care units (ICU) need and desire while in our care. In my own doctoral project, I used the CCFNI (with permission) to not only measure the importance of the 45 family need items on the list but also measure whether those needs were being met. From there I created a weighted index of important needs that were not being met in the unit where the study was conducted. The end result of this process was a list of priorities that a particular department could focus on for improving family-centered care strategies.[5] The process of conducting a needs assessment using the CCFNI would be applicable for use with minor modification to update terminology even today.

At that time, I was testing a strategy of family care in the form of a midrange theory entitled Facilitated Sensemaking.[5–7] Information about Facilitated Sensemaking and other nurse theories may be found at nursology.net. To my delight, one of the articles submitted for this issue proposes an evolved intervention to be added to the theory: expanding ways to improve patient-family communication. The challenge of communicating with mechanically ventilated patients has evolved from using a grip over a lead pencil[5] to the unique approach described herein by Shin and colleagues.

Another early leader to focus on family needs was Dr Ruth Kleinpell. I remember reading her work with interest while in graduate school and developing an interest in the topic myself.[8,9] Dr Kleinpell later became president of the Society of Critical Care Medicine (SCCM) and led a grant-funded 63-site study testing many different interventions related to family-centered care with the goal of measuring improved outcomes.[10] Several of the sites within that project report their results in this issue of *Critical Care Nursing Clinics of North America*.

Structured family conferences have been recommended nationally for many years.[11] However, those who try to standardize the process have certainly had challenges finding a way to time conferences when both families and physicians can be present.[12] Though we know that conferences delivered in a thoughtful organized manner can improve family outcomes,[1] organizing a consistent approach to care conferences is not easy. In this issue we hear from 2 different groups. In the first, Sona describes the challenges they were not able to overcome to improve outcomes as anticipated. In the second, O'Donnell presents a successful, though at first glance costly, solution to the problem. Two full-time nurses dedicated to facilitating communication with families measured marked improvements in all aspects measured. Given what has been reported in the past, as well as within these 2 documents, nurse leaders now have the opportunity to use the O'Donnell report to justify the up-front cost of personnel to decrease resource utilization and improve satisfaction.

One of the issues not explored in the current national guidelines is the topic of pet visitation. The reason pet visitation has not been previously endorsed is not because of harm or potential harm, but simply because there is not yet enough evidence in the ICU-specific literature to overcome naysayers. In this issue, Barchas and colleagues do a splendid job of integrating the literature on all forms of animal presence in the hospital: animal-assisted therapy, service animals, companion animals, and patients' own pets. They had to reach outside of the ICU walls to gather the data on the healing properties of animal interventions. It is our goal to stimulate more research in the ICU setting around this important aspect of family-centered care. One of the biggest concerns raised by the "what-iffers" of our time (those who haven't tried something because they what-if it to death) is that animals will spread infection. My own belief, albeit untested hypothesis, is that health care workers spread more infection than animals. Another untested hypothesis has been that a patient's own pet would likely have less chance of infecting the patient than a strange animal therapy dog the patient has never met. There is evidence that humans and their pets share microbiomes over time living together.[13] This evidence has made me wonder if the immune system is attenuated to what both species are living with, making disease transmission less likely. Others feel the opposite, that because the microbiomes merge, it might be more likely to transmit disease. It would be lovely if someone would test these hypotheses and others like them. If the data bore results supporting the fact that a patient is protected from their own pet's flora, we would be more likely to see standardized pet-welcome policies. In 2018, I conducted a very casual survey with colleagues who were coauthors of the SCCM family-centered care guidelines and found that informally around the world (Canada, United States, United Kingdom, Australia, France, The Netherlands, but NOT Israel) ICU nurses were "sneaking in" pets in the absence of or against policy. In this issue, a sample policy is provided for those who would like to standardize the process of the patient's own pet visitation. We do need more research to study whether it is truly necessary to bathe animal therapy dogs prior to visits. These animals are likely being bathed more than is recommended for the health of their own skin. Also, studies are needed to identify whether it is really necessary to see veterinarian documents rather than simply ask for an attestation of whether the pet is healthy. The rules some put in place surrounding the practice of pet visitation are not built on evidence, but instead on conjecture based upon worry, and warrant further investigation. In any case, it strikes me as odd that many nurses seem more likely to sneak in a pet than to encourage family presence, bringing us to the next topic of family presence.

What compendium of family-centered care literature could be complete without a project related to open-flexible family presence? Family presence and engagement are recommended worldwide because of the evidence that meeting the family's needs for presence improves family outcomes and does not harm the patient.[1] Nonetheless, family presence has been a topic of great dispute throughout time. One of the oldest studies published describing how nurses frequently ignore policies, even when they exist, denying families access was published by Carlson and colleagues.[14] Despite the evidence supporting family presence, nurses often resist family presence, reporting that the process of tending to the needs of the families is a burden. Believe it or not, all of these years later, Winkleman presents a report in this issue describing the very same challenges of overcoming resistance toward engaging families in care.

Reuter-Rice and colleagues present a thorough and informative review of the importance of sleep in the ICU. It is amazing to learn the association between sleep and other physiologically important functions, such as preserving the function of the immune system. To complement this article, one of the most creative strategies presented in this issue of *Critical Care Nursing Clinics of North America* is the sleep and sunshine article presented by Winterbottom and colleagues. This team actually created a volunteer group to come in and do the hard work of taking long-term critical care patients outside to see the sunshine. I remember working with an ICU team to bring a patient outside only once in my career, and writing a short story about it because of the impact the process had on us all. I had entitled it, "The very best death," because we had allowed the patient to be extubated and die outside with his family and dog according to his expressed wishes. This team, however, has gone much further and created a sustained process for providing sunshine to patients to literally brighten their days, using sunshine as a therapeutic intervention.

Guidelines for family-centered care are meant to serve all age groups from neonatal to older adults. In this issue, Franck and colleagues explore quite deeply the interventions used in the neonatal intensive care. Nurses who care for adults and pediatrics will surely find this information quite applicable to their work as well.

Through the years, I have learned a great deal by listening to survivors of critical illness and their families. In the beginning, it was just to get advice on how to perform a research project or change a policy in the ICU.[7] Then, with the national guidelines, survivors and families provided feedback on whether we were focusing on important issues, or defining family properly.[1] As years went on, I knew that we could learn just as much from survivors and families as we could from each other. I began an intention to coauthor with these teachers instead of using them as "case studies" in "text-box 1."[15–17] It was a struggle at first because editors were not accustomed to this approach. However, holding firm to the vision, we pushed through the glass ceiling, and now the clinician/survivor/family authorship teams are becoming more common. In this issue, there are 3 articles with survivor/family authors. Boehm and colleagues describe a post-ICU clinic designed in a Veterans Administration ICU. Doig and colleagues present the outcomes from a qualitative study conducted in partnership with a survivor and family member as members of the research team. Oxland and colleagues report on the various ways that survivors and families can partner in advancing practice. I believe you will agree that their direct testimony informs us in a way that we dilute when speaking for them or about them. These articles describing the work of humanizing the ICU by involving survivors and families demonstrate in action the ideals proposed in the article by Bueno and La Calle from their international movement to humanize the ICU. Their prescribed approach turning from technology to caring as a health-promoting intervention provides guidance to all those who would like to optimize family-centered care.

At this time, I turn this preface over to Carrie Anne Hudson, health care Executive Administrative Assistant. She presents her artwork for us entitled, *Matters of the Heart* (**Fig. 1**), closing this reflection on family-centered care.

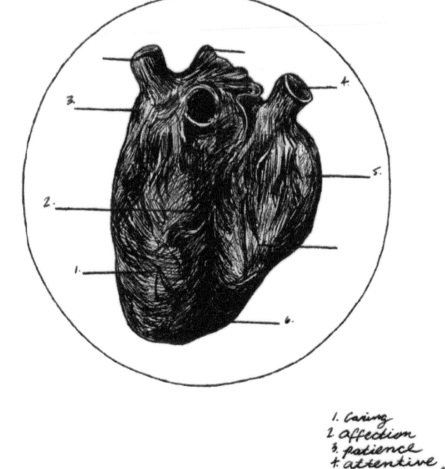

1. Caring
2. affection
3. patience
4. attentive
5. professional
6. needed

Fig. 1. Carrie Anne Hudson's ink drawing, *Matters of the Heart.* (*Courtesy of* Carrie Anne Hudson, University of California, San Diego Health, La Jolla, CA.)

As Philip Reeve writes, "Sometimes, on our way through the world, we meet someone who touches our heart in a way others don't."[18]

Once a year, artists at our organization are invited to translate research findings into art to exhibit at the yearly Nursing Research/Evidence-Based Practice Conference. This piece, exhibited in 2017, was inspired by the findings from a qualitative research study conducted to gain understanding of the meaning "to feel cared for." In this study, our Chief Nurse Officer, Margarita Baggett, MSN, RN, asked patients and family members to comment on a time when they felt cared for during hospitalization.[19]

Through this ink illustration, Matters of the Heart, I wanted to pay homage to the classic medical and anatomy illustrations as those done by artists such as DaVinci and Vesalius. The intention was to create something that represented nursing and medical professions, while portraying the connections between patients and their providers. What do we need from our providers? What do we strive to be as a healer? These are the matters of the heart.

I chose to depict the human heart because of its beauty, its importance, and its varied meaning for every individual. However, instead of traditional medical terminology to specify areas of the human heart, I chose words that were repeated and used most by patients and their families when they reflected on positive experiences during their hospital stay. Surrounding the heart, you will find: caring, affection, patience, attentive, professional, and needed.

In summary, this collection of family-centered care articles helps to inform us of new strategies and approaches, while reminding us of challenges in operationalizing best practices that we still need to overcome. Much more translational research is needed to determine the best approach to implement the recommendations for family-centered care known to improve patient and family outcomes.

Judy E. Davidson, DNP, RN, MCCM, FAAN
University of California
San Diego Health
Health Sciences Drive MCM1
Room 135
La Jolla, CA 92037, USA

Carrie Anne Hudson
University of California
San Diego Health
La Jolla, CA 92037, USA

E-mail addresses:
jdavidson@health.ucsd.edu (J.E. Davidson)
c4hudson@health.ucsd.edu (C.A. Hudson)

REFERENCES

1. Davidson JE, Aslakson RA, Long AC, et al. Guidelines for family-centered care in the neonatal, pediatric, and adult ICU. Crit Care Med 2017;45(1):103–28.

2. Molter NC. Needs of relatives of critically ill patients: a descriptive study. Heart Lung 1979;8(2):332–9.

3. Molter NC, Leske JS. Critical care family needs inventory (CCFNI). Milwaukee (WI): University of Wisconsin–Milwaukee; 1995. Jane S. Leske, PhD, RN, Associate Professor, School of Nursing.
4. Molter N, Leske J. Critical care family needs inventory (CCFNI). Milwaukee (WI): University of Wisconsin–Milwaukee; 1983.
5. Davidson JE, Daly BJ, Agan D, et al. Facilitated sensemaking: testing of a mid-range theory of family support. Commun Nurs Res 2009;42:353.
6. Davidson JE, Zisook S. Implementing family-centered care through facilitated sensemaking. AACN Adv Crit Care 2017;28(2):200–9.
7. Davidson JE, Daly BJ, Agan D, et al. Facilitated sensemaking: a feasibility study for the provision of a family support program in the intensive care unit. Crit Care Nurs Q 2010;33(2):177–89.
8. Daly K, Kleinpell RM, Lawinger S, et al. The effect of two nursing interventions on families of ICU patients. Clin Nurs Res 1994;3(4):414–22.
9. Kleinpell RM. Needs of families of critically ill patients: a literature review. Crit Care Nurse 1991;11(8):34, 38–40.
10. Kleinpell R, Zimmerman J, Vermoch KL, et al. Promoting family engagement in the ICU: experience from a national collaborative of 63 ICUs. Crit Care Med 2019;47(12):1692–8.
11. Davidson JE, Powers K, Hedayat KM, et al. Clinical practice guidelines for support of the family in the patient-centered intensive care unit: American College of Critical Care Medicine Task Force 2004-2005. Crit Care Med 2007;35(2):605–22.
12. Douglas SL, Daly BJ, Lipson AR. Neglect of quality-of-life considerations in intensive care unit family meetings for long-stay intensive care unit patients. Crit Care Med 2012;40(2):461–7.
13. Song SJ, Lauber C, Costello EK, et al. Cohabiting family members share microbiota with one another and with their dogs. Elife 2013;2:e00458.
14. Carlson B, Riegel B, Thomason T. Visitation: policy versus practice. Dimens Crit Care Nurs 1998;17(1):40–7.
15. Elliott D, Davidson JE, Harvey MA, et al. Exploring the scope of post-intensive care syndrome therapy and care: engagement of non-critical care providers and survivors in a second stakeholders meeting. Crit Care Med 2014.
16. Davidson JE, Harvey M, Schuller J, et al. Post-intensive care syndrome: what it is and how to help prevent it. Am Nurs Today 2013;8(5):32–7.
17. Strathdee SA, Hellyar M, Montesa C, et al. The power of family engagement in rounds: an exemplar with global outcomes. Crit Care Nurse 2019;39(5):14–20.
18. Philip Reeve quotes. Available at: https://www.goodreads.com/author/quotes/27379.Philip_Reeve. Accessed December 20, 2019.
19. Davidson J, Baggett M, Giambattista L, et al. Exploring the human emotion of feeling cared for during hospitalization. Int J Car Sci 2017;10(1):1.

Humanizing Intensive Care
From Theory to Practice

José Manuel Velasco Bueno, RN[a,b],
Gabriel Heras La Calle, MD, PhD cand[b,c,d],*

KEYWORDS

- Dignity • Human-centered care model • Patients • Families • Family-centered care

KEY POINTS

- The International Research Project for the Humanization of Intensive Care Units (Proyecto HU-CI) looks for changing the current paradigm toward a human-centered care model.
- The gold standard of humanization is respecting the dignity of every person.
- The main factors that influence the dehumanization of care are technolatry, the complex social–public health world, inadequate working conditions, macroexperts in microtopics, and commercialism in health care management. Redesigning the intensive care unit (ICU) requires active listening of patient needs, families, and professionals.
- Compliance with the 160 good practices in humanization would spread and standardize ICU humanization around the world.

The word, *humanization*, is being used with increasing frequency to describe taking a more person-centered approach to health care, albeit not without debate.[1] The debates arising around this term produce advocates and opponents who brandish different arguments. Some claim that humanizing should be considered implicit in all actions done by humans and aimed at caring for other humans. The authors believe that humanizing requires a thoughtful planned approach to make notable improvements for all those involved in care processes. The purpose of this article is to define and describe optimal humanization of care and present an 8-element tested model for optimizing intensive care unit (ICU) care delivery.

WHAT IS HUMANIZATION?

As Bermejo states,[2] "Speaking of humanization asserts the intrinsic dignity of all human beings and the rights stemming from this fact. And this makes it a need of vital

[a] Hospital Virgen de la Victoria, Málaga, Spain; [b] International Research Project for the Humanization of Intensive Care Units (Proyecto HU-CI); [c] Intensive Care Unit, Hospital Universitario de Torrejón, Madrid, Spain; [d] Universidad Francisco de Vitoria, Madrid, Spain
* Corresponding author.
E-mail address: gabi@proyectohuci.com

Crit Care Nurs Clin N Am 32 (2020) 135–147
https://doi.org/10.1016/j.cnc.2020.02.001
0899-5885/20/© 2020 Elsevier Inc. All rights reserved.

importance and transcendence." From this point of view, humanization is related to what has been defined as the affective-effective model, inspired by the thought and values of Albert Jovell[3]: "It is the method for caring for and curing patients as people, based on scientific evidence, incorporating the aspect of patients' dignity and humanity, establishing care based on trust and empathy, and contributing to their wellbeing and to the best possible health results."

Humanizing the relationship between professionals and ill people, who are in a complex biographic time that directly affects their integrity, always has been a health care challenge. Care frequently has shifted away from the human and instead toward the disease, intervention, or technology. Humanize, from its meaning, is "to act with gentleness, calm and kindness,"[4] making us reengage with our own relationship to people's suffering, speaking to us of understanding and compassion, things that have nothing to do with pity or mercy. Human beings are designed to feel and it is through full attention and feelings that they can detect suffering, understand it, embrace it, and, most importantly, want to do something to alleviate those experiencing it.[5]

Daily experiences affect us both personally and professionally. For this reason, it is necessary to become aware of and implement the suitable and timely measures that facilitate establishing a relationship to help those who ask this of us.

This article reviews some of the causes that may contribute to the dehumanization of health care and considers the associated damages caused to all parties involved—patients, family members, and professionals. The analysis of these situations has favored attracted from different entities and organizations. One such organization is the International Research Project for the Humanization of Intensive Care Units (Proyecto HU-CI), from which interesting ideas have arisen with a vision of friendlier and more human-centered health care, regardless of the person's role, for more personalized care that truly listens to what patients and their families need. To balance the equation of caring, humanizing also means understanding and accepting that professionals are fallible and vulnerable and also need to be heard, given that they are the basic capital for humanizing the health care system.

Patients and families increasingly are better informed and call for more active participation in all areas. They want greater consideration of their autonomy instead of the classic paternalism present in the clinic-patient relationship.[6]

FACTORS THAT INFLUENCE THE DEHUMANIZATION OF CARE

Within this section factors are discussed that influence the dehumanization of care.

Technolatry

When people require health care, they do so with the conviction that they will find suitable resources, equipment, and facilities that will provide a solution to their problems. They also expect to find professionals with the knowledge and skills necessary to facilitate their recovery with these resources. Hospital admission, however, frequently involves a complex situation which, because of the pain and discomfort caused by the illness itself, at times requires unpleasant invasive techniques.

Scientific advances clearly have contributed to considerable improvements in health care outcomes, owing to technological innovations, stronger research, and greater become more objective in making clinical decisions. Consequently, cure and life expectancy rates for health issues also have improved significantly. The use of better technological resources, pharmacologic treatments, and surgical procedures has had a clear impact, requiring significant economic and knowledge-based invest-ments while increasing the complexity of care management.

Without denying the importance of these advances, the authors observe nonethe-less that excessive emphasis on technolatry may have contributed to an orientation toward clinical practices that are more centered on the disease itself and curing it than on the sick person. In the technologically laden health care system, the actual hu-man beings frequently are lost and fade into the background, becoming no more than diseases to fight, professionals in the actual health care system forget the history behind their existence, their feelings, and their values. Today's care models contribute to an objectification of patients in which their personal and individual personality traits are neglected.[7] Technical euphoria can lead to forget the true focus of the human con-dition, which is fallible, finite, and mortal.

In recent decades, there have been some publications that focus on patient-centered and family-centered care.[8] Unfortunately, the conclusions set out in the literature have not been transferred into real and widespread practice. The authors posit that this dictatorship of technolatry[9] is a key factor in dehumanizing care de-livery. Future research is warranted on how to balance technological care with caring.

The Complex Social–Public Health World

All the stakeholders (patients, families and professionals) also are part of a complex social–public health world in which relationships are established at very different levels. On the one hand, there are working relations between professionals to consider and, on the other, clinician relationships with patients and family members. Both rela-tional frameworks are dealt with in different ways that lead to adopting different roles in different encounters. All the stakeholders (patients, families and professionals) are part of a structure with its own life, which often turns its back on the people who comprise it. The established dynamics that end up forming part of the organizational culture, which has great room for improvement, are discussed.

Inadequate working conditions
Relationships are affected by different factors, such as excessive pressure in the pub-lic health arena, unsuitable working conditions, precarious occupational security, lack of resources, and little margin for error. These social determinants easily can contribute to depersonalized care, in which users of health care feel that their suffering and pain are not considered. This lack of personalization during care becomes rele-vant particularly if considering the negative effect it has on establishing trust, which is so essential in a care-giving assistance relationship.[10] Depersonalization, along with emotional exhaustion and low self-fulfillment, also contributes to the construct defined as burnout syndrome.[11]

Macroexperts in microtopics
Another factor that could influence the provision of dehumanized care may be related to the high degree of specialization in health care professionals fields. Medicine ad-vances leads to being highly trained in extremely specific and mutually exclusive areas, which makes comprehensive and complete care of patients difficult. This has produced macroexperts on microtopics that leads to compartmentalizing patients.

Commercialism in health care management
To the factors, discussed previously, can be added the current health care manage-ment models, in which commercial criteria are commercial criteria seems to be the most important issue, centered on achieving targets and obtaining results in which

economic and business issues are the priorities. In the face of this panorama, it is worth asking if it is even possible to humanize health care. One of 2 events need to occur to humanize health care in this commercially centered model of care. In the first, administrators need to see humanization as a way to capitalize on market share. In the second, commercialism would cease to exist, and humanized health care would be a right for all.

PROYECTO HU-CI: A TESTED SOLUTION

The humanization of intensive care movement was launched in Spain in February 2014 with the Proyecto HU-CI. A group of professionals came together who had been working on these issues related to humanization, albeit without being previously connected. This union, along with the integration of patients and families, has resulted in the global concept of humanization of intensive care which has spread throughout the world and is now considered a priority. There is no magic formula that can be applied universally, but it is worthwhile to establish basic premises as a starting point necessary for providing humanized care:

- First, respect for the fact that every person is unique and incomparable and, therefore, responds differently to life crises
- Second, acknowledging that patients and family members must take center stage in care processes, which requires having clear and precise information to understand their situations and to be well informed of their therapeutic options, assuming responsibility for actively collaborating in restoring their health

Humanized health care is centered on the person, as a multidisciplinary, incomparable, and unique being, considering the person's dignity and respecting the person's values and freedom of choice. From this perspective, all the stakeholders (patients, families and professionals) must slow down and evaluate each concrete reality, reconsidering and rethinking the current model and outlining other paths that would lead to better care and service for users, patients, and families and for professionals. Stopping to reflect makes it compulsory to rethink the organization to adapt it to human-centered care. Acting on reflective practice also requires taking measures that will affect management and the adaptation of structures and clinical practice as well as training professionals in nontechnical skills, such as communication and caring.[12] Logically, the application of some of these measures requires specific investments and budgetary allocations to be carried out but also requires thought and introspection on what the foundations and basis of care really are. Care requires competence, individuality, emotion, solidarity, sensitivity, and ethics. Care requires extensive skill in communicating and relating: empathy, active listening, respect, and compassion. These qualities must be assessed, taught, and cultivated.[13]

This change of paradigm obliges considering the concept of the patient experience, which transcends mere satisfaction[14] and can be defined as the sum of the interactions that take place at any organization and that influence a patient's perception over the course of all care received.[15] Some categories tagged as key components of influence in a humanized patient experience include communication, pain management, care continuity, proper information, cleanliness, and noise.[16]

In specialty units, like the ICU, other issues that worsen the situation must be considered, like patients' extreme feeling of vulnerability, dependence on machines, loss of autonomy and mobility, inability to communicate, loss of identity, and lack of information. These issues tend to be relegated to the background due to the seriousness of a clinical situation.

The Proyecto HU-CI was started in this context, which proposes a technical stop to re-think and re-design the care provided, placing human beings at the center and redesigning public health care with the person's dignity as a non-negotiable premise.[17]

Proyecto HU-CI arose as a multidisciplinary research group that planned to evaluate different areas and then implement the pertinent improvement actions, via participative and network-based research.[18] In this Proyecto HU-CI model, care is approached from a 3-fold perspective, considering patients, their family members and loved ones, and the professionals attending to them.

Critical patients are especially vulnerable both from a physical perspective, due to their serious illness and due to the stressing factors they are subjected to during their admission.[19] Faced with these situations, patients expect to be cured but also expect well-being. At times, cure is impossible and, thus, their well-being must be understood as the main objective.

Family members and loved ones also suffer the consequences[20] and their physical and emotional needs far too often are not optimally addressed.[21] Family members have needs centering on the psychosocial parcel of care that so often is alluded to during training yet often neglected while focusing on the disease. From an excessively biological perspective, this psychosocial aspect is set aside. Even though it is known that the presence of family support can have an impact on decreasing time spent in the ICU,[22] family members tend to be the eternally forgotten parties in the process of treatment of a critical illness.

On their part, professionals caring for a patient are exposed to many factors that can lead to interpersonal conflicts and psychological and emotional alterations that interfere with their work. These conflicts have an impact on them both personally and professionally and are liable to influence results with their patients.[23]

Proposing and contributing measures that improve the care of everyone involved—patients, families and professionals—are the main objective of Proyecto HU-CI. This focus on humanizing care arises from a scientific outlook that integrates the research results, along with the preferences of patients and family members, bearing in mind the experiences of professionals and, finally, adapting to each environment. Planning care in this manner transcends a mere declaration of wishes that sounds good, obliging reviewing the relationship model established between the team and the patients and family members.

The Proyecto HU-CI model of care proposes concrete measures along different working lines that can be implemented in practice and evaluated at a later time.[24] These suggestions have been tested in the clinical environment, optimizing practices, unit culture, and physical structure and reorganization of spaces. The tested interventions also have been collected and integrated into humanization plans, such as the one produced by the Community of Madrid,[25] with the purpose of dissemination to the highest number of units possible.

Proyecto HU-CI centers its work on promoting a new model for ICUs. Its strategic lines define the main working priorities, which are set out in **Fig. 1**. Each element of the model is described.

Field of research 1 and 4: Open Intensive Care Unit Visiting Policies and Presence and Participation of Relatives in Intensive Care Units

Despite clear recommendations to the contrary, most current policies on family members visiting patients admitted to the ICU continue to be restrictive.[26] This practice is not based on research results but instead because it makes professionals' jobs easier.

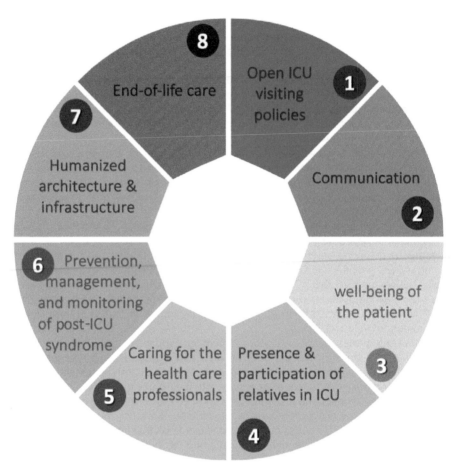

Fig. 1. Care design: the humanizing (H) evolution of ICUs. (Source: The International Research Project for the Humanization of the Intensive Care Units (Proyecto HU-CI) NEJM Catalyst (catalyst.nejm.org) © Massachusetts Medical Society.)

In reality, this limitation is based mainly on custom, on the lack of critical thought on its disadvantages,[27] and on planning centered more on professionals' needs than the needs of patients and families. This occurs despite the fact that family members and loved ones clamor for more time and the possibility of planning their visits with their personal and work obligations. The experience of some units encourages advances in the possibility of considering other models.[28] At present, the evidence available points to the fact that making visiting times more flexible and having open doors at the ICU are indeed possible and beneficial for patients, families, and professionals.[29]

The barriers in place to undertake changes in this direction are related to the physical structure of units and the mental structure of professionals. Moving forward with opening up ICUs requires understanding the positive experiences implemented, having the participation of professionals, training in attitudes and habits and subsequent changes in this area, and adaptation to the particularities of each unit. Progress requires going beyond the concept of visit to take up a vision of partners in care.

Moreover, if clinical conditions thus permit, while present, families who wish to do so could collaborate with different basic care functions (personal hygiene, feeding, and rehabilitation), under the training and supervision of health care professionals. Giving families the chance to contribute to a patient's recovery can have positive effects on the patient, on the actual family members, and on professionals, by reducing emotional stress and contributing to the closeness and communication between everyone involved in care.

The presence of family members, even during specific procedures, is accompanied by professionals' changing their outlooks with respect to privacy, dignity, and pain management during the procedures. This also helps the families, who are more satisfied, accept the situation better helping the mourning process.[30] The presence and participation of family members on daily rounds also contribute to improvement in communication and provide opportunities to ask questions and clarify information, increasing their satisfaction.[31]

2: Communication

Communication between professionals
Communication in the ICU has decisive importance, both between professionals and with patients and families. Effective communication (complete, clear, timely, and concise) among professionals prevents mistakes and promotes consensus about patients' treatments and care.[32] Communication between professionals also entails, in addition to exchange of information, a shifting of responsibility. The use of tools for structuring communication or briefings contributes to multidisciplinary participation and makes processes more effective and safer. These are our keys for improving communication.[33]

The cohesion of teams may be stimulated by support strategies and the acquisition of nontechnical skills (human tools) that minimize the conflicts related to communication problems. These conflicts affect a team and directly influence patient well-being and that of the family, causing professional burnout and having an impact on results.[34] Burnout syndrome is a disorder that encompasses a range of different issues: emotional exhaustion, depersonalization, and feelings of low professional self-esteem.[35]

Communication with patients and families
Information is one of the main needs requested by patients and families in the ICU.[36] Faced with the frequent situation of critical patients deemed incompetent to take decisions, the right to information transfers to family members in these cases. Providing suitable information during situations that are highly emotional requires communication skills, for which many professionals simply have not received specific training. Proper communication with patients and families contributes to promoting a climate of trust and respect and facilitates making joint decisions. Consensus on the content of this information decreases uncertainty and confusion among family members, who frequently notice inconsistencies among the different professionals involved. The participation of nurses in providing information generally is insufficient and is not clearly defined, despite the fundamental role they play in caring for critical patients and their family members.[37]

The use of augmentative and alternative communication systems turns out to be extremely useful as tools that facilitate communication with those patients with communication difficulties, placing technology at the service of people.

3: Patient Well-Being

An illness or disease already causes patients discomfort and pain and, if adding the surgeries and procedures conducted on them, many are quite painful; it is evident that this malaise is only increased. Planning for patients' well-being should be an objective as important as planning their cure, even more so when the latter is not possible.

There are many factors that cause critical patients to suffer and feel discomfort: pain, thirst, cold and heat, and difficulty resting due to too much noise and light[38] as well as having limited mobility, often due to the use of unnecessary constraints.[39] Pain assessment and control, dynamic sedation suitable to each patient's condition, and preventing and handling acute delirium all are essential factors to improving patients' level of comfort.[40]

In addition to physical causes, psychological and emotional suffering can be high. Patients experience feelings of loneliness, isolation, fear, loss of identity, intimacy and dignity, dependence, doubts due to lack of information, and incomprehension, among others. Evaluating and supporting these needs must be considered as core areas in health care quality.[41] Ensuring that professionals are properly trained and promoting measures aimed at handling and mitigating these problems to ensure patient well-being represent the main objectives in caring for critically ill patients.

5: Caring for the Health Care Professionals

Health care professionals' work provides great satisfaction when their expectations are met, when their jobs are done with quality and patients improve, when they prevent suffering, when they enjoy deserved recognition, and so forth. When things do not go well, however, emotional fatigue is considerable and, when this is added to not taking care of their own health and well-being, burnout syndrome appears. This problem affects them both personally and professionally and can even lead to posttraumatic stress disorder and other serious psychological disorders, even suicide. The presence of these problems influences the quality of care, results with patients, and their satisfaction and is related to professionals' lack of involvement in the organizations.[42]

Caring for the caretakers should become a moral duty and an ethical imperative for all organizations, for which a series of objectives should be defined, aimed at executing preventive and therapeutic actions. Demanding that health care workers have empathy, actively listen, provide emotional support, and have an understanding of the emotional factors that accompany patients' disease and families' anguish and fear simply cannot be approached without first and in parallel caring for professionals' well-being.[43]

Different scientific societies have tried to disseminate and make this problem visible by offering recommendations to reduce its appearance and mitigate its consequences. These include establishing specific strategies to suitably provide a response for intensive care professionals' physical, emotional, and psychological needs, stemming from their dedication to and hard work employed in their jobs.[44]

6: Post–Intensive Care Syndrome

After time spent in the ICU, several physical problems may continue or arise to appear (persistent pain, weakness acquired during hospitalization, malnutrition, bed sores, sleep alterations, and dependence on devices), neuropsychological problems (cognitive deficits, memory and/or attention loss, and mental processing speed), and emotional problems (anxiety, depression, and posttraumatic stress). These problems affect a significant number of patients (30%–50%) and have been termed post–intensive care syndrome (PICS).[45] Their medium-term and long-term consequences affect the quality of life of patients and their families.

Minimizing of PICS requires preventive initiatives as well as the proper handling and monitoring of known alterations.[46] This necessitates sensitized and educated multidisciplinary teams who start their work during admission to the unit and continue it after they leave.

Family members and loved ones can be an essential part of handling PICS by participating in patient care and helping patients keep their bearings. Caretakers also can be affected by feelings of worry and confusion that can lead to them neglecting their own health.[47] The health care team must be aware of this in order to recognize and also provide support to family members who need it.

7: Humanized Infrastructure

The architecture of ICUs is one of the main factors that makes the provision of humanized care difficult. There continue to be units with open common areas in which several patients are located, separated by screens or curtains. These spaces make it difficult for families to spend time there, make admitted patients' privacy extremely difficult and making patients feel exposed at times of great weakness and vulnerability. Moreover, these layouts do not contribute to establishing personal relationships between the professionals and the patients they care for.

Along these lines, the creation of spaces is proposed and promoted in which technical efficacy is linked to care quality and the comfort of all users. There are recommendations focused on reducing stress and maximizing comfort by centering on architectural and structural improvements to ICUs. These changes consider suitable locations as well as adaptation to users and work flows in environmental conditions with suitable light, temperature, noise, materials and finishes, furniture, and décor.[48] Adding artificial windows where there is no natural light and adding decorative items and other pieces that contribute to patients' time-space awareness all require minimal investment and can increase the comfort of everyone involved considerably. These modifications can have a positive influence on feelings and emotions, creating more human spaces adapted to the functionality of the units. These concepts are equally applicable to waiting rooms, which should be redesigned so that they are more like living rooms, offering greater comfort and functionality to families. Working areas and break rooms for staff also should be redesigned.

8: End-of-Life Care

Sometimes it is impossible to restore patients' previous health and cure them. In these situations, professionals must be able to reconsider the objectives to focus them on reducing suffering and providing the best care possible, especially for end of life. This permits deaths that are free from agitation and suffering for both patients and family members.[49] It further ensures that their deaths occur in accordance with their wishes and with clinical, cultural, and ethical standards. This is another of the objectives of the Provecto HU-CI Project, starting from the idea that palliative care and intensive care are not mutually exclusive options but instead should coexist throughout the care process of the critically ill.[50]

Limiting life support, frequent in critically ill patients, must be done by following the guidelines and recommendations established by scientific communities.[51,52] When life support is limited, this is done as part of an overall palliative care plan that is multidisciplinary, with the aim of meeting the needs—physical, psychosocial and spiritual—of patients and family members.[53] The existence of specific protocols and the regular evaluation of the care provided should be considered basic requirements.

End-of-life decision making often results in conflict between health care professionals and between them and family members. Professionals should have the competencies and tools necessary to resolve these conflicts, adding open and constructive discussion to these situations as coping strategies to reduce the emotional burden they create.[54]

The fruit of the work of the members of each of the Provecto HU-CI project's work groups was the good practices manual to humanize ICUs, in November 2017, which was later revised in May 2019.[55] The manual contains 160 recommendations, structured for each field of research, which sets out guidelines for those who are on the road or planning to embark on the road to transform their environments toward a more humanized ICU. Numerous units already have begun the humanization process, using the manual after self-evaluating their current situations, based on whether or not they comply with the good practices detailed in the manual.

In parallel with providing a toolkit for humanization, a process to certify good practices in humanizing ICUs was developed, which establishes several levels in accordance with the degree of fulfilment of each of the suggested standards. Dozens of units have expressed interest in the certification process by the Spanish Association for Standardization and Certification (AENOR) International[56] and Proyecto HU-CI, and some already have started it. This process also looks for outlining a map of humanization, from an objective evaluation of complying with the good practices set out in the manual.

Another of the main objectives of Proyecto HU-CI is to make training more widespread on nontechnical or human issues as well as contributing to areas for active reflection among the professional groups that want to undertake a change process aimed at a more humanized care model. After some time has passed, the consequences of the changes suggested and implemented, both to structures and to thoughts of professionals' who are caring for critical patients, will be able to be analyzed.

In conclusion, the members of Proyecto HU-CI have a vision of and commitment to a humanizing revolution, a humanizing evolution that will return caring professionals to the original reasons that made them enter health care and return them to the roles for which they once trained: people helping people. The Proyecto HU-CI model is replicable, and support from the international collective of interested professionals makes the possibility of transformation possible.

DISCLOSURE

The authors have nothing to disclose.

REFERENCES

1. Arias-Rivera S, Sánchez-Sánchez MM. Do Spanish intensive care units need to be "humanised"? Enferm Intensiva 2017;28:1–3.
2. Bermejo JC. Humanizar la asistencia sanitaria. Ed. Desclée De Brouwer. Bilbao; 2014.
3. Jovell AJ. Medicina basada en la afectividad. Med Clin (Barc) 1999;113(5): 173–5.
4. Diccionario de la Real Academia de la lengua española. Available at: http://www.rae.es/. Accessed March 9, 2019.
5. Trzeciak S, Mazzarelli A. Compassionomics: the revolutionary scientific evidence that caring makes a difference. Studer Group; 2019.
6. Probst MA, Noseworthy PA, Brito JP, et al. Shared decision-making as the future of emergency cardiology. Can J Cardiol 2018;34(2):117–24.
7. Todres L, Galvin KT, Holloway I. The humanization of healthcare: a value framework for qualitative research. Int J Qual Stud Health Well-being 2009;4:68–77.

8. Latour JM, Coombs M. Family-centred care in the intensive care unit: more than just flexible visiting hours. Intensive Crit Care Nurs 2019;50:1–2.

9. Sitges-Serra A. Tecnología o tecnolatría: ¿a dónde van los cirujanos? Arch Esp Urol 2012;65(5):519–27.

10. Juárez G, et al. Personalización de cuidados hospitalarios y su efecto sobre la relación de confianza enfermera-paciente. Enferm Clin 2013;23(6):243–51.

11. Rotenstein LS, Torre M, Ramos MA, et al. Prevalence of burnout among physicians: a systematic review. JAMA 2018;320(11):1131–50.

12. Velasco JM, Segovia C, Gálvez M, et al. Human tools: formación en habilidades no técnicas para profesionales sanitarios. In: Gabriel Heras y Miembros del Proyecto HU-CI, editor. Humanizando los Cuidados Intensivos. Presente y futuro centrado en las personas. Bogotá (Colombia): Distribuna Editorial; 2017. p. 297–324.

13. Chochinov HM. Dignity in care: time to take action. J Pain Symptom Manage 2013;46(5):756–9.

14. Romero-García M, de la Cueva-Ariza L, Jover-Sancho C, et al. La percepción del paciente crítico sobre los cuidados enfermeros: una aproximación al concepto de satisfacción. Enferm Intensiva 2013;24:51–62.

15. Wolf JA, Niederhauser V, Marshburn D, et al. Defining patient experience. Patient Exp J 2014;(1):1. Article 3. Available at: http://pxjournal.org/journal/vol1/iss1/3. Accessed March 9, 2019.

16. Cutler LR, Hayter M, Ryan T. A critical review and synthesis of qualitative research on patient experiences of critical illness. Intensive Crit Care Nurs 2013;29(3): 147–57.

17. Davidson JE, Aslakson RA, Long AC, et al. Guidelines for family-centred care in the neonatal, pediatric and adult ICU. Crit Care Med 2017;45(1):103–28.

18. Heras La Calle G, Zaforteza C. HUCI is written with H as in Human. Enferm Intensiva 2014;25(4):123–4.

19. Carrese J, Forbes L, Branyon E, et al. Observations of respect and dignity in the intensive care unit. Narrat Inq Bioeth 2015;5:43–53.

20. Kiwanuka F, Imanipour M, Akhavan Rad S, et al. Family members' experiences in adult intensive care units: a systematic review. Scand J Caring Sci 2019. https://doi.org/10.1111/scs.12675.

21. Pardavila Belio MI, Vivar CG. Necesidades de la familia en las unidades de cuidados intensivos. Revisión de la literatura. Enferm Intensiva 2012;23:51–67.

22. Lee HW, Park Y, Jang EJ, et al. Intensive care unit length of stay is reduced by protocolized family support intervention: a systematic review and meta-analysis. Intensive Care Med 2019. https://doi.org/10.1007/s00134-019-05681-3.

23. Fassier T, Azoulay E. Conflicts and communication gaps in the intensive care unit. Curr Opin Crit Care 2010;16(6):654–65.

24. Heras G, Alonso A, Gómez V. A plan for improving the humanisation of intensive care units. Intensive Care Med 2017;43:547–9.

25. Health Ministry of the community of Madrid: 'plan de Humanización de la Asistencia Sanitaria 2016-2019'. Available at: http://www.madrid.org/bvirtual/BVCM017902.pdf. Accessed March 9, 2019.

26. Escudero D, Martín L, Viña L, et al. Política de visitas, diseño y confortabilidad en las unidades de cuidados intensivos española. Rev Calid Asist 2015;30:243–50.

27. Riley BH, White J, Graham S, et al. 'Traditional/restrictive vs patient-centered intensive care unit visitation: perceptions of patients' family members, physicians, and nurses'. Am J Crit Care 2014;23(4):316–24.

28. Meert KL, Clark J, Eggly S. Family-centered care in the pediatric intensive care unit. Pediatr Clin North Am 2013;60(3):761–72.

29. Nassar Junior AP, Besen BAMP, Robinson CC, et al. Flexible versus restrictive visiting policies in ICUs: a systematic review and meta-analysis. Crit Care Med 2018;46(7):1175–80.

30. Jabre P, Belpomme V, Azoulay E, et al. Family presence during cardiopulmonary resuscitation. N Engl J Med 2013;368(11):1008–18.

31. Au SS, Roze des Ordons A, Soo A, et al. Family participation in intensive care unit rounds: comparing family and provider perspectives. J Crit Care 2017;38:132–6.

32. Curtis JR, Cook DJ, Wall RJ, et al. Intensive care unit quality improvement: a "how-to" guide for the interdisciplinary team. Crit Care Med 2006;34(1):211–8.

33. Abraham J, Kannampallil TG, Almoosa KF, et al. Comparative evaluation of the content and structure of communication using two handoff tools: implications for patient safety. J Crit Care 2014;29(2):311, 1-7.

34. Azoulay E, Timsit JF, Sprung CL, et al, Conflicus Study Investigators and for the Ethics Section of the European Society of Intensive Care Medicine. Prevalence and factors of intensive care unit conflicts: the conflicus study. Am J Respir Crit Care Med 2009;180(9):853–60.

35. Silva JL, Soares RS, Costa FS, et al. Psychosocial factors and prevalence of burnout syndrome among nursing workers in intensive care units. Rev Bras Ter Intensiva 2015;27(2):125–33.

36. Alonso-Ovies A, Álvarez J, Velayos C, et al. Expectativas de los familiares de pacientes críticos respecto a la información médica. Estudio de investigación cualitativa. Rev Calid Asist 2014;29(6):325–33.

37. Velasco Bueno J, Alonso-Ovies A, Heras La Calle G, et al. Main information requests of family members of patients in intensive care units. Med Intensiva 2018;42(6):337–45.

38. Alonso-Ovies Á, Heras La Calle G. ICU: a branch of hell? Intensive Care Med 2016;42(4):591–2.

39. Acevedo-Nuevo M, González-Gil MT, Solís-Muñoz M, et al. Therapeutic restraint management in Intensive Care Units: phenomenological approach to nursing reality. Enferm Intensiva 2016;27(2):67–74.

40. Barr J, Fraser GL, Puntillo K, et al, American College of Critical Care Medicine. Clinical practice guidelines for the management of pain, agitation, and delirium in adult patients in the Intensive Care Unit: executive summary. Am J Health Syst Pharm 2013;70(1):53–8.

41. Vincent JL, Shehabi Y, Walsh TS, et al. Comfort and patient-centred care without excessive sedation: the eCASH concept. Intensive Care Med 2016;42(6):962–71.

42. Van Mol MM, Kompanje EJ, Benoit DD, et al. The prevalence of compassion fatigue and burnout among healthcare professionals in intensive care units: a systematic review. PLoS One 2015;10(8):e0136955.

43. Gálvez Herrer M, Gómez García JM, Martín Delgado MC, et al, members of the HU-CI Project. Humanización de la Sanidad y Salud Laboral: implicaciones, estado de la cuestión y propuesta del Proyecto HU-CI. Med Segur Trab (Madr) 2017;63(247):103–19.

44. Moss M, Good VS, Gozal D, et al. An official critical care societies collaborative statement-burnout syndrome in critical care health-care professionals: a call for action. Chest 2016;150(1):17–26.

45. Stollings JL, Caylor MM. Postintensive care syndrome and the role of a follow-up clinic. Am J Health Syst Pharm 2015;72(15):1315–23.

46. Needham DM, Davidson J, Cohen H, et al. Improving long-term outcomes after discharge from intensive care unit: report from stakeholders'conference. Crit Care Med 2012;40(2):502–9.

47. Johnson CC, Suchyta MR, Darowski ES, et al. Psychological sequelae in family caregivers of critically III intensive care unit patients: a systematic review. Ann Am Thorac Soc 2019;16(7):894–909.

48. Ferrero M, Gómez-Tello V, Escudero D. Arquitectura e infraestructura humanizada. In: Gabriel Heras y Miembros del Proyecto HU-CI, editor. Humanizando los Cuidados Intensivos. Presente y futuro centrado en las personas. Bogotá (Colombia): Distribuna Editorial; 2017. p. 249–75.

49. Velasco Sanz TR. Últimas Voluntades: Su importancia en pacientes ingresados en cuidados intensivos. Saarbrücken (Germany): Editorial Académica Española; 2016.

50. Aslakson RA, Curtis JR, Nelson JE. The changing role of palliative care in the ICU. Crit Care Med 2014;42(11):2418–28.

51. Estella Á, et al. Puesta al día y recomendaciones en la toma de decisiones de limitación de tratamientos de soporte vital. Med Intensiva 2019. Available at: https://www.medintensiva.org/es-puesta-al-dia-recomendaciones-toma-articulo-S0210569119301858. Accessed March 9, 2019.

52. Truog RD, Campbell ML, Curtis JR, et al, American Academy of Critical Care Medicine. Recommendations for end-of-life care in the intensive care unit: a consensus statement by the American College of Critical Care Medicine. Crit Care Med 2008;36(3):953–63.

53. Cook D, Rocker G. Dying with dignity in the intensive care unit. N Engl J Med 2014;370(26):2506–14.

54. Bosslet GT, Pope TM, Rubenfeld GD, et al. An official ATS/AACN/ACCP/ESICM/SCCM policy statement: responding to requests for potentially inappropriate treatments in intensive care units. Am J Respir Crit Care Med 2015;191(11):1318–30.

55. Certification working group for the HU-CI Project. Manual de buenas prácticas de humanización en Unidades de Cuidados Intensivos. Madrid: Proyecto HU-CI; 2019. Available at: https://humanizandoloscuidadosintensivos.com/wp-content/uploads/2019/05/Manual_BP_HUCI_rev2019_web.pdf. Accessed March 9, 2019.

56. AENOR international. Available at: https://www.aenor.com/. Accessed March 9, 2019.

Family Integrated Care for Preterm Infants

Linda S. Franck, RN, PhD[a],*, Chandra Waddington, RN, MSN[b], Karel O'Brien, MD[c,d]

KEYWORDS

- Preterm infant • Parent • Neonatal intensive care unit • Family-centered care
- Family integrated care

KEY POINTS

- Family Integrated Care (FICare) is a model of care for neonatal intensive care units (NICU) that promotes parental empowerment, learning, shared decision making, and positive parent-infant caregiving experiences.
- FICare addresses the hospital and NICU-level structures, processes, and parent support needs.
- FICare requires strong nursing leadership, and expertise for successful implementation.

Each year, 15 million preterm infants worldwide require admission to a neonatal intensive care unit (NICU).[1] It is routine, in most health care settings, for parents to be separated from their infant when their infant requires admission to the NICU, regardless of the reason for admission.[2,3] Parent-infant separation is a major source of stress for parents and their infants. Parent-infant separation often leads to parents feeling powerless and overwhelmed while in hospital and infants receiving little parent support and interaction.[4] At discharge, parents report feeling unprepared to care for their infants at home.[5] Moreover, long-term parent well-being, specifically, parent mental health, and infant developmental outcomes are closely intertwined.[6]

PROGRESS IN PARENTAL INVOLVEMENT IN THE CARE OF PRETERM INFANTS

The critical importance of early involvement and ongoing minimal separation between parents and preterm infants to the health outcomes of the preterm infants and their families is now well recognized.[7,8] Greater attention is being given in NICUs to reduce parent-infant separation and support the mutually dependent parent-infant dyad with

[a] Department of Family Health Care Nursing, School of Nursing, University of California, San Francisco, Box 0606, San Francisco, CA 94143, USA; [b] School of Nursing, University of British Columbia, T201-2211 Wesbrook Mall, Vancouver, British Columbia V6T1Z7, Canada; [c] Department of Pediatrics, Sinai Health System, Toronto, Ontario, Canada; [d] Department of Paediatrics, University of Toronto, 19-231A -600 University Avenue, Toronto, Ontario M5G 1X5, Canada
* Corresponding author.
E-mail address: linda.franck@ucsf.edu

Crit Care Nurs Clin N Am 32 (2020) 149–165
https://doi.org/10.1016/j.cnc.2020.01.001
0899-5885/20/© 2020 Elsevier Inc. All rights reserved.
ccnursing.theclinics.com

methods such as parent-infant skin-to-skin contact (also known as kangaroo mother care).[9,10] Many NICUs have adopted the principles of family-centered care and aim to provide care that promotes respect and dignity, information sharing, participation, and collaboration between the clinical care team and parents.[11,12] There remains a lack of coherence and consistency in the delivery of recommended parental support and involvement.[13]

Fig. 1 shows the range of parent-focused NICU interventions and the parent-partnered care models for which there is evidence of improved outcomes for NICU families.[14] Of the few models of care that have been subject to research, family integrated care (FICare)[15] is the most comprehensive because it specifically addresses the hospital and NICU-level structures and processes as well as the parent support needs. It is also flexible and potentially scalable across other critical care settings, regardless of the age or condition of the patient population. In this article, the authors describe the FICare model and emerging evidence regarding outcomes of FICare for infants and families. They also discuss challenges and opportunities in implementing and maintaining high-quality FICare and explore future directions for FICare research and practice, including application of the model to other critical care settings.

FAMILY INTEGRATED CARE MODEL DEVELOPMENT

FICare is based on the concept of Humane Neonatal Care whereby parents become primary caregivers for their infants in the NICU.[16] Developed in an Estonian NICU experiencing a profound shortage of nurses, mothers were provided with education and support to become primary caregivers for their infant, with the exception of intravenous care, respiratory support, and medication administration. Implementation of the Humane Neonatal Care model was associated with improved infant weight gain and was acceptable to nurses and mothers. Based on these promising results, and the strong evidence for parental support and involvement in preterm infant care, the Canadian FICare model was codeveloped by parents and the multidisciplinary

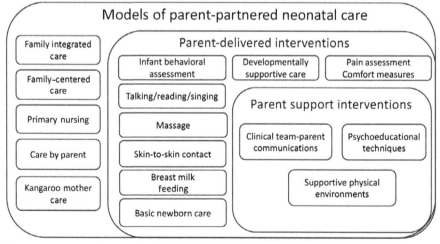

Fig. 1. Taxonomy of parent-focused NICU interventions and parent-partnered care models. (*From* Franck LS, O'Brien K. The evolution of family-centered care: From supporting parent-delivered interventions to a model of family integrated care. Birth Defects Res. 2019;111(15):104459; with permission.)

NICU team in the NICU at Mount Sinai Hospital in Toronto.[17] FICare has 4 main "pillars": NICU environment, NICU team education and support, parent education, and parent support. **Table 1** shows the 4 pillars and the essential and suggested components.

During the development and pilot evaluation of FICare, parents were asked to commit to spending 8 hours per day in the NICU at least 5 days a week to participate in their infant's care and support activities.[17,18] Since that time, there has been a softening of this requirement because it was a barrier for some parents. Parents were asked to commit to 6 hours in a subsequent trial,[15] and following further qualitative analysis,[19] the absolute time commitment has been dropped, and NICUs are encouraged to tailor support to individual family needs. Feedback from parents suggests that to become comfortable in providing care for their infant and to feel like part of their infant's team require that they be present for at least 4 hours per day.

FAMILY INTEGRATED CARE EVIDENCE

Following a promising single-site pilot study,[18] a 25-site multicountry cluster randomized clinical trial[15] demonstrated that stable preterm infants in the FICare NICUs had significantly improved 21-day weight gain (primary outcome), and a greater proportion of them received breast milk at discharge compared with infants in usual care sites. There was also significantly lower maternal stress and anxiety in the FICare NICU participants.[20] A subsequent prospective multisite case-control study of FICare in China found increased breastfeeding rates, breastfeeding duration, enteral nutrition duration, and weight gain at discharge and higher scores on the mental development index and psychomotor development index at 18 months for infants in the FICare NICUs compared with the usual care NICUs.[21]

Qualitative analyses have suggested improved parent confidence, parent-parent, and parent-nurse communication.[17,19] Quality improvement evaluations in the United Kingdom also suggest improved breast feeding rates,[22] increased parental involvement in infant caregiving and positive feelings about their role in their infant's care,[23] reduced overall lengths of stay and special care days, and shortened time to full oral feeding.[24] Given the strong theoretic and research foundations and absence of adverse effects, FICare is a promising intervention for improving parental partnership in the care of NICU infants and providing effective parental support.

IMPLEMENTING FAMILY INTEGRATED CARE

The FICare program uses a strengths-based, family-centered care approach to promote increased parental empowerment, learning, shared decision making, and positive parent-infant caregiving experiences, leading to increased self-efficacy upon discharge and improved parent-infant relationships and infant developmental outcomes.

Components of the Family Integrated Care Intervention Bundle

The FICare model includes interventions that address 4 pillars (see **Table 1**) in a comprehensive intervention bundle with the following components.

Neonatal intensive care unit team educational support

A NICU team education program about the importance of family involvement in infant care; nurses' specific skills and responsibilities for mentoring, coaching; and supporting parents, is the essential first step to implementing FICare. The education program should be adjusted to the team's prior knowledge and knowledge gaps. The education

Table 1
Family integrated care pillars essential and suggested components

Environment	NICU Team Education and Support	Parent Education/Psychological Support	Active Participation/Partnership
Essential			
• Comfortable, semireclining chairs at bedside to support prolonged parent presence and skin-to-skin contact • Dedicated parent room for respite away from but nearby NICU • Food storage and preparation area for parents • Place for parents to store coats and personal belongings • 24-h NICU open access for parents to be with their babies • NICU and hospital policies and services that welcome and support parents • FICare steering committee comprising parent and multidisciplinary NICU team members	• NICU leadership support • FICare nurse champions • Education on FICare for all team members • Additional education for nurses emphasizing their role as teacher and coach with parents • FICare education included in orientation and annual skills updates	• Regularly scheduled parent group classes • Individual teaching and skills building at bedside • Opportunities for peer-peer support with parent mentors	• Parent participation in baby's direct caregiving; parent active involvement in medical rounds and daily care planning • Parent tracking progress (baby, their own)
Suggested			

• Dedicated space for families in patient care area
• Single-family room NICU
• Discounted or subsidized food, parking, and transportation between home and hospital
• Onsite child care
• Extended paid parental leave for parents of NICU infants
	• Enhanced education on:
	  o Developmentally supportive care
	  o Trauma-informed care
	  o Communication skills
	• Parent teaching, coaching, and communication included in NICU team core competencies and performance reviews
		• Parent classes offered evenings and weekends
		• NICU Family Advisory Council
		• Stipends or other honoraria for parent mentors
		• Paid parent liaison position
		• Technology support for parent education
			• Technology support for remote participation in rounds and care planning
			• Technology support for tracking

Note. All components are adapted to local conditions and codesigned and implemented by the multidisciplinary team in partnership with former NICU families, with ongoing feedback from current NICU families.

program may be accomplished with a combination of in-person and online education formats. Key topics include understanding the role of nursing and other members of the team in supporting parent-infant attachment, parent mental health, and parent role development; infant neurodevelopment and developmentally supportive care; review of family-centered care principles and best practices; parent-team communication and relationship development; shared-decision making; and the role of parents on medical rounds.

Environment
A physical and interpersonal environment that welcomes and encourages parents to spend as much time as they are able to be involved in their baby's care is an essential component of the FICare program. A welcoming and comfortable physical environment includes items such as semireclining chairs for skin-to-skin care, access to a refrigerator and parent lounge for meals and relaxation, designated safe space for parents to store their belongings, and access to breast pumps and a private place for breast-milk pumping. The NICU policies must also be supportive and welcoming, enabling 24-hour access for parents to their baby without restriction, visitation for other family members, parent orientation to the NICU and NICU staff roles, and support services for parents' mental health and well-being.

Parent education and support
Parent education and support is a core component of the FICare program. It is imperative that parents receive information about the NICU model of FICare, their important role in their infant's care, and the supports they will receive as soon as possible after admission to the NICU. This information will need to be reinforced often. A parent education program, providing parents an opportunity to learn about their infant's care and their own self-care, is also critical. The most successful parent education programs take place near the NICU, on a regular basis, ideally 3 days per week or more, are facilitated by a range of care team members, and offer parents the opportunity for group learning and support with other NICU parents (**Fig. 2**). Some NICUs include additional ways of providing parental education for families who cannot be present for in-person group sessions, using Web or mobile app resources.[24,25] Parent education is continued at the infant's bedside, with nurses working individually with parents to help them apply what they have learned to the care of their own infant. Resources and templates for parent education plans are available at: http://familyintegratedcare.com/ (**Table 2**).

As part of the FICare model, parents are also offered the opportunity to receive individual peer support from parents who previously had an infant in the NICU. The peer support may be provided in person, or remotely through text, e-mail, or telephone. Parent mentors (also known as veteran parents) are screened and approved by the hospital and receive training and ongoing coaching in peer support techniques.[17] Peer support programs may be locally designed or provided through national NICU peer support programs.

Parent active participation
Parents are respected as critical to their infant's well-being and grow to become their infant's primary caregiver, with nurses as teachers and coaches along that journey. When in the NICU, parents are encouraged to provide as much infant care as they can to include but not limited to bathing, dressing, changing diapers, feeding, weighing, holding skin to skin, and providing comfort during painful procedures, with support from their infant's nurses. Specific guidelines are developed in each NICU

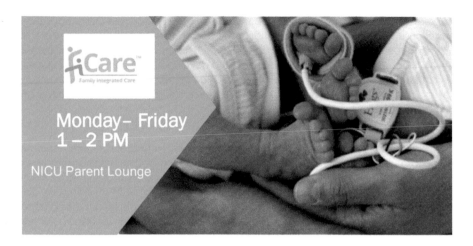

NICU PARENT CLASSES

SEPTEMBER

All PARENTS Welcome!

MON	TUE	WED	THU	FRI
02	**03**	**04**	**05**	**06**
HOLIDAY	Parent Self Care Day!	Medications and your baby	Lung Development and Disease	Helping babies breathe
09	**10**	**11**	**12**	**13**
Rounds – Intro to Who's Who in the ICN	Parenting your baby in the hospital	Parent Wellness: Strategies for Thriving in the NICU	Learning about prematurity and your baby	Finding Resiliency in the NICU
16	**17**	**18**	**19**	**20**
Baby Development	Pain management and comforting your baby	Decreasing risk of infection	Breastmilk and breastfeeding your baby in the hospital	Interacting with your baby part 1
23	**24**	**25**	**26**	**27**
Interacting with your baby part 2	Parent Wellness:	Feeding your baby	Planning for life at home with your baby	Skin-to-Skin: Benefits and How-to
30				
Infant Massage				

Come join our one-hour classes to discuss the topic of the day and learn from each other's experiences

Fig. 2. Sample parent education calendar. (© Regents of the University of California, mobile-enhanced Family Integrated Care Program, reprinted with permission.)

regarding the specific roles and responsibilities of nurses and parents, and what training parents must undertake to handle equipment or participate in the specific clinical caregiving, for example, assisting with positioning, feeding tubes, or respiratory support (**Table 3**).

As partners in care, parents are also encouraged and supported to participate in daily medical rounds either in-person or remotely. By participating in rounds, parents' importance in their infant's care is formally recognized and encouraged. Parent

Table 2
Sample parent education plan (http://familyintegratedcare.com/)

Feeding Your Baby in the NICU	Understanding the role of the dietitian Learning all about the nutrition, feeding, and growth of your baby	• Discussion on the normal feeding stages that a preterm baby goes through from birth to discharge, expected growth, and how breast milk/formula and supplements help your baby to grow • Review feeding your baby, the parent role • Overview of how parents can help to maximize their baby's feeding experiences, skin-to-skin contact, nonnutritive sucking, oral stimulation, breast/bottle • Demonstrations on formula preparation, sterilization, and so forth • Handouts
Medications and Your Baby	Medications given from birth to discharge for the NICU infant Medications and breast feeding	• Discussion of medications used in the NICU and following discharge, their potential benefits, and side effects • Overview of immunizations, respiratory syncytial virus prophylaxis • Taste testing of medications given to infants, for instance, iron • Overview of medications and maternal drug risk in pumping/breastfeeding, community resources • Handouts
Growth & Development	Learning about your premature baby's growth and development in the NICU and following discharge	• Definition of corrected age • Differences in growth and development between full-term and preterm infants • Discussion on promoting normal development in the NICU as well as at home • Overview of principles on positioning, to help soothe, and to organize your baby to re-create the fetal position • Information on activities/positioning and different positions for interaction for infants closer to full term and infants in the crib • Activities and expectations when the infant is at home, community infant programs, neonatal clinic

(continued on next page)

Table 2 (continued)		
		• Examine parent role in promoting development at home, tummy time, head control, equal hand use, head position, flexion, supporting shoulders • Discussion of appropriate baby equipment to promote normal develop, baby books, parental instincts, having fun • Handouts
Discharge Planning	Planning on taking a baby home who has been dependent on medical care	• Discussion of the parent's changing role as the baby moves closer to discharge • Information on getting the house ready, purchasing infant equipment, car seat, crib, playpen, clothing, and so forth • Overview of your baby at home, infection prevention, calling the doctor, SIDS • Discussion on feeding your baby: breast/bottle, sterilization, formula, vitamins • Handouts and videos
Your Baby at Home	Postdischarge care	• Overview of community resources, neonatal clinic, lactation consultants, breast and bottle feeding in the first few months at home, parenting a preterm infant once at home • Discussion of self-care and family relationships
Coping with Your Baby's Hospitalization: Survival Tactics for Parents	Common issues that parents experience Strategies for coping during your baby's hospitalization	• Discussion of supportive strategies, through sharing, baby blues, signs of postpartum depression, and "survival tactics" • Examine process of attachment, learning about your baby, comforting your baby, and paying attention to cues • Discussion of common feelings of disappointment, failure, guilt • Overview of your baby's achievements, watching and learning, bringing you closer to understanding your baby's unique personality and facilitating development • Siblings, isolation, social supports • Handouts and videos
		(continued on next page)

Table 2 (continued)		
Parenting Your Baby	Learning more about developmental care, physical, and social environment	• Overview of being there for your baby in the NICU, your important role, and what does it look like • Review sound, light, and interacting, behavior, and comfort • Discussion on communication, "time-out signals", signs of stress and stability • Examine the importance of state, deep sleep, light sleep, drowsiness, alertness, activity, and crying • Discussion on self-regulation vs immature regulation (being able to self-comfort) • Learn how to recognize your baby's cues as your baby grows and develops • Review of how to recognize and work with your baby's unique temperament • Create a care plan for you and your baby • Learn to interact through touch and holding, soft voice, skin-to-skin contact • Demonstration of handling and touch to decrease stressful, pacing care, flexed position, containment, prevent jerky movements • Discussion of keeping your baby calm, that is, soothing, keep stimulation to a minimum • Demonstration and practice with dolls • Handouts and videos

participation in rounds is a powerful intervention for facilitating transparency and parental understanding of the plan of care and possible outcomes while preparing them for the transition home. Parents' questions are addressed in a more timely manner during the discussion on rounds, improving communication and often reducing the time needed for follow-up communication. In the FICare model, nurses are responsible for working with parents to prepare them for participation in rounds, educating them on what to expect, educating them on role-modeling, practicing with parents to help them increase their skill and confidence, coaching during rounds, and debriefing afterward. Parent participation on rounds is a gradual process that increases over time (**Fig. 3**). With nursing support, most parents become confident in speaking with the multidisciplinary team assembled at their infant's bedside and are able to report standardized data of their infant's status to the rounding care team, ask questions, and reach consensus with the team on the infant's daily plan.

Table 3
Sample roles and responsibilities for nurses and parents involved in infant care in the neonatal intensive care unit (can be adapted to local policy and procedure guidelines)

Task	Nursing Responsibilities	Parent Responsibilities
Orientation to NICU	• Provide orientation • Show layout of the unit • Teach infection control precautions	• Receive orientation • Become familiar with layout of the unit • Follow infection control practices
Nasogastric and oral feeds	• Identify milk in the refrigerator/freezer, check with second nurse • Double check milk with parent • Check volume of milk to be administered with parent • Check position of nasogastric/orogastric tube • Hang drip feed	• Double check milk with nurse • Check volume of milk to be administered with the nurse • Can hold feed
Medications	• Teach indication of routine medications • For approved oral/nasogastric medications check dosage, patient, time, and route • Medications that need independent/double checking, follow unit policy • Supervise administration of medication • Cosign the medication administration record • Specify on record that administration was by parent	• Identify the purpose of routine medication • Administer approved oral medication with nursing supervision
Monitors	• Record vital signs • Ensure upper and lower alarm limits are appropriately set • Adjust alarm limits as appropriate • Ensure proper position of leads and saturation probe • Check tracing on monitor • Silence alarms when necessary	• Have basic understanding of vital signs and alarm limits • Reposition saturation probe and electrocardiogram leads
Oxygen	• Change oxygen concentration as indicated • Document oxygen administration	• Identify concerns with low-flow prongs or oxygen concentration • Adjust low-flow prongs on face
Spells	• Respond to parent calls for apnea, bradycardia, and desaturation, color changes, or additional parent concerns • Assess and provide appropriate assistance	• Recognize signs and symptoms of a spell or distress • Provide stimulation • Call for assistance

Weighing	• Provide supervision and assistance when needed • Document weight changes	• Be familiar with correct weighing procedure • Communicate all changes in weight to infant's nurse • Check with nurse if weight is significantly different
Skin-to-skin contact	• Assist in preparation and position of infant and parent • Secure all tubing • Document skin-to-skin contact by parent (duration, infant and parent response)	• Whenever possible, as much as possible perform skin-to-skin contact with infant
Bathing	• Teach, monitor, and record safe practices • Demonstrate and observe bathing procedures and provides assistance • Document bath, parent involvement, and infant response	• Prepare for and bathe in a consistent manner • Request nurse assistance • Consistently adhere to safe bathing practices • Report baby response and any concerns to nurse after each bath

From http://familyintegratedcare.com/wp-content/uploads/2016/01/FICARE-Sample-NICU-Parent-Info-Binder.pdf; with permission.

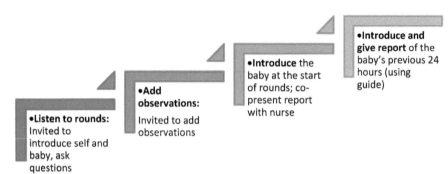

Fig. 3. Stages of parental involvement in daily NICU team rounds. Step 1: Parents begin by listening in on rounds; parents invited by the rounds team leader or their nurse to introduce themselves and their baby to the team and to ask questions at the end of rounds. Step 2: Step 1 plus parents are invited to share an observation about their baby during rounds. Step 3: Parents share report about the baby with their nurse. Parents begin rounds by introducing themselves and their baby to the team, then copresent with their nurse information about the baby's status over the past 24 hours. Step 4: Parents prepare for rounds with their nurse, then introduce themselves and their baby, give report on their baby's status providing some or all of the following information: baby's name, gestational age at birth, current corrected and gestational age, weight, weight change. Parents may also report time spent skin to skin and any barriers, their impression of how their baby is doing, and any concerns they may have Note: Parents will proceed at their own pace, with some advancing immediately to step 4 after initial coaching from nurses and others preferring to participate at step 2 or 3 for several weeks. (© Regents of the University of California, mobile-enhanced Family Integrated Care Program, reprinted with permission.)

Finally, parents participate in documenting their observations of their infant and participation in infant caregiving (eg skin-to-skin care and feeding). They also document their own skills acquisition and are encouraged to keep a journal of their thoughts and feeling throughout the NICU stay.

Planning and Implementing Family Integrated Care

The first step in implementing FICare is to form a planning group that includes members of the NICU multidisciplinary team and parents of former NICU patients. This group will make a thorough assessment of the NICU assets that currently exist to support FICare as well as identify components of FICare that need to be developed. Many NICUs will have implemented at least some of the FICare essential or recommended interventions (see **Table 1**) as part of their current family-centered care approach. Resources for assessing NICU assets for FICare and implementation guidelines and tools are available at www.familyintegratedcare.com. A sample checklist for FICare implementation is shown in **Table 4**.

The second step in implementing FICare is to determine the roles and responsibilities for the different components of the intervention bundle. When FICare is implemented within the context of research, a research coordinator or coordinators may have responsibility for implementing components such as the parent classes or parent mentor program. When FICare is implemented as a NICU initiative or within a quality improvement program, then the roles and responsibilities may be more dispersed. For example, nurse educators may be responsible for leading NICU team education; the medical team may be responsible for the parent participation on rounds protocol; medical social workers may be responsible for the

Table 4
Sample family integrated care implementation checklist (can be adapted to local policy and procedure guidelines)

Nurse Education	Parent Education	Rounds	Peer Support Program
☐ Identify team champions (nurse, medical staff, social work, respiratory therapy)	☐ Identify education materials, current classes, or other parent groups already being held	☐ Evaluate current rounds format	☐ Evaluate if any peer support is already available to parents (online, groups)
☐ Review parent/nurse responsibilities table with bedside nurses and nursing administration for feasibility and buy-in	☐ Review master list of topics and decide which ones are a priority for your population	☐ Determine changes needed to meet FICare rounds requirements	☐ Evaluate if parent volunteers are already engaged in any activities in the NICU, for example, paid parent, advisors, committees
☐ Schedule nurse training (in-person, online, other resources)	☐ Identify how best to provide parent education and potential facilitators for parent classes	☐ Engage with physicians, nurse practitioners, nurses, and other NICU staff to decide how best to implement FICare rounds for participants	☐ Determine how you might support a peer support program
☐ Schedule "road show" for other NICU staff	☐ Decide who on the team is in charge of class logistics (scheduling, and so forth)	☐ Decide how staff can participate to support FICare rounds	☐ Determine requirements for volunteers if applicable
☐ Plan content for trainings and road shows	☐ Decide on the time and location of classes	☐ Determine how to track daily parent presence and participation	☐ Recruit parents (reunion, and so forth)
☐ Conduct trainings and road show	☐ Conduct facilitator training	☐ Draft rounds protocol	☐ Determine what NICU staff will support peer program (eg, social work)
☐ Create reference materials	☐ Schedule first month of classes	☐ *Ongoing*: engage with NICU provider team and parents in a continual feedback loop	☐ Plan peer training
☐ *Ongoing*: engage with FICare nurses and NICU staff in a continual feedback loop	☐ Decide on whether you can provide catering		☐ Plan linkage process, support for mentors, and other logistical pieces
	☐ *Ongoing*: round on unit to invite parents to the classes and communicate with nurses about the classes		☐ *Ongoing*: support for mentors, ongoing recruitment
	☐ Prepare calendar and decide how best to inform families, text messages, announcements, signs, and posters		
	☐ Determine how to track parent participation		
	☐ *Ongoing*: schedule classes at least a month ahead of time		
	☐ *Ongoing*: engage with facilitators, parents, and nurse administration on a continual feedback loop		

parent mentor program. Mature family-centered care or FICare programs may have created a paid part-time or full-time parent liaison position to deliver and coordinate parent support activities.[26]

As the components of FICare are implemented, audit and quality improvement strategies are needed to ensure fidelity of the FICare model and to evaluate the effectiveness. Quality improvement efforts include regular measurement of both the quantity and the quality with which parents receive support and are active in infant caregiving and shared decision making. Infant and parent outcomes at discharge are monitored. NICU team and parent knowledge and attitudes about FICare are also tracked. The specific methods for audit and quality improvement will depend on the FICare component and NICU quality improvement goals.[22–24]

Common Challenges with Family Integrated Care Implementation

As with any major practice model change, FICare can present challenges that could limit the potential benefits. Common challenges can be grouped under 3 main themes: resources and leadership, NICU teamwork, and parent concerns.

Resources and leadership

NICUs may lack physical space and equipment to comfortably and safely accommodate prolonged periods of parental presence and active involvement in their infant's care. There may also be outdated hospital or NICU policies that place restrictions on parental presence in the NICU. Strong and supportive hospital and NICU leadership will be needed to address these structural barriers and obtain needed resources. The mounting and compelling national and international evidence for family-centered and family integration in infant caregiving can be used to make a persuasive case for resources for FICare based on the potential to improve quality, safety, and cost.[24,27]

Neonatal intensive care unit teamwork

Teamwork concerns may also impede FICare implementation. Misunderstanding or concerns among the NICU team can create resistance and block progress to FICare implementation, if they are not addressed early on, and can negatively affect ongoing collaboration between parents and the NICU team. For some NICUs, full implementation of FICare may uncover perhaps unconscious biases about information sharing as well as about parents' role in health care decision making for their infant.[28] Myths, such as "parents are not ready to help with care because they are too stressed" or "it is not safe for parents to provide care for acutely ill infant," persist despite decades of research on a wide range of NICU caregiving activities that can be safely and effectively performed by parents.[14] The process of changing the model of care may also reveal teamwork challenges within the NICU team,[28] or limitations in the scope of practice for nurses that then impedes their ability to support parents, such as being restricted from participating in patient rounds.[29]

Open dialogue among members of the NICU team as well as education and supportive leadership is essential to overcoming the underlying communication and attitudinal challenges exposed during FICare implementation.[14,17,18] For nurses, skills in teaching and coaching parents and integrating them earlier and more fully into the infant's caregiving workflow is a skill that will need practice and experience, just as precepting a new nurse requires confidence in one's own expertise and application of adult learning principles.[17,30] Additional work on communication, conflict resolution, team building, and resilience may be needed before FICare can be implemented effectively.[31]

Parent concerns

Even with all of the environmental and programmatic supports provided by the FICare model, parents may face personal and family challenges that present barriers to their full involvement in their infant's care. Common challenges for parents include physical or mental health challenges, competing family responsibilities, and financial challenges (eg, need to return to employment too soon, transportation, accommodation near the hospital, and so forth). Parents should be connected as soon as possible, ideally within the first 48 to 72 hours, with a specialist NICU medical social worker to assess their support needs and link them to resources. Nursing and peer support provided by FICare, especially if it can be flexibly offered to engage parents outside the NICU as well, can help build parental confidence, competence, and resilience. Some families may be facing significant financial or social crises as a result of, or in addition to, their current situation of the birth of a preterm infant. NICU teams and hospital leaders need to recognize these challenges and engage with policy makers to address the social concerns that place additional strain on parents of preterm infants and prevent their full involvement in FICare.[1]

FUTURE DIRECTIONS OF FAMILY INTEGRATED CARE: RESEARCH AND PRACTICE OPPORTUNITIES

The research and quality improvement evidence for the effectiveness of the FICare model to improve outcomes for preterm infants and their families are compelling. Research on the effectiveness of FICare in level II NICUs and in the US health care context is currently underway.[32,33] Because most FICare research has been focused on preterm infants, further research on the FICare model in other populations, such as neonates with surgical or other conditions, is needed. Further research is also needed to determine the minimally necessary "dose" of the individual FICare components and the bundle as a whole. Longitudinal studies comparing child and family outcomes after discharge from the NICU are also needed. FICare effects on the NICU team also need further investigation.

The FICare pillars and underlying foundational principles of family-centered care suggest that the FICare model could be adapted to other areas of hospital care. There are many patient care areas of an acute care hospital where patients are dependent and not able to fully participate as partners in their care, such as geriatric or adult intensive care units, where family or significant others act as surrogates and are actively encouraged to be involved in their loved one's care.[12] In these settings, age, condition, and setting-specific content could be developed for each of the 4 FICare pillars. Feasibility and acceptability would need to be established and then efficacy would need to be determined in randomized clinical trials.

SUMMARY

FICare is a theory-driven, evidence-based model of NICU care for preterm infants and their families. The model is strongly dependent on nursing expertise and leadership for successful implementation and has the potential to positively transform the NICU culture and partnership with families. As the worldwide adoption of FICare and ongoing evaluation continues, new knowledge will be applied to further refine and adapt the model with a goal of further improving outcomes for infants and families. Application of the model to other hospitalized patient groups is a potential new frontier for nursing research and practice.

DISCLOSURE

The authors have nothing to disclose.

REFERENCES

1. Survive and thrive: transforming care for every small and sick newborn. 2019. Available at: https://www.healthynewbornnetwork.org/hnn-content/uploads/Survive-and-Thrive_Final.pdf. Accessed March 6, 2020.
2. Pierrat V, Coquelin A, Cuttini M, et al. Translating neurodevelopmental care policies into practice: the experience of neonatal ICUs in France-The EPIPAGE-2 cohort study. Pediatr Crit Care Med 2016;17(10):957–67.
3. Franck L, McNulty A, Alderdice F. The perinatal-neonatal care journey for parents of preterm infants. J Perinat Neonatal Nurs 2017;31(3):244–55.
4. Beck CT, Woynar J. Posttraumatic stress in mothers while their preterm infants are in the newborn intensive care unit: a mixed research synthesis. ANS Adv Nurs Sci 2017;40(4):337–55.
5. Sneath N. Discharge teaching in the NICU: are parents prepared? An integrative review of parents' perceptions. Neonatal Netw 2009;28(4):237–46.
6. Kommers D, Oei G, Chen W, et al. Suboptimal bonding impairs hormonal, epigenetic and neuronal development in preterm infants, but these impairments can be reversed. Acta Paediatr 2016;105(7):738–51.
7. Gooding JS, Cooper LG, Blaine AI, et al. Family support and family-centered care in the neonatal intensive care unit: origins, advances, impact. Semin Perinatol 2011;35(1):20–8.
8. Klawetter S, Greenfield JC, Speer SR, et al. An integrative review: maternal engagement in the neonatal intensive care unit and health outcomes for U.S.-born preterm infants and their parents. AIMS Public Health 2019;6(2):160–83.
9. Bergman NJ, Ludwig RJ, Westrup B, et al. Nurturescience versus neuroscience: a case for rethinking perinatal mother-infant behaviors and relationship. Birth Defects Res 2019;111(15):1110–27.
10. Milette I, Martel M-J, Ribeiro da Silva M, et al. Guidelines for the institutional implementation of developmental neuroprotective care in the neonatal intensive care unit. Part A: background and rationale. A Joint Position Statement from the CANN, CAPWHN, NANN, and COINN. Can J Nurs Res 2017;49(2):46–62.
11. Committee on Hospital Care, Institute For Patient- and Family-Centered Care. Patient- and family-centered care and the pediatrician's role. Pediatrics 2012; 129(2):394–404.
12. Davidson JE, Aslakson RA, Long AC, et al. Guidelines for family-centered care in the neonatal, pediatric, and adult ICU. Crit Care Med 2017;45(1):103–28.
13. Treyvaud K, Spittle A, Anderson PJ, et al. A multilayered approach is needed in the NICU to support parents after the preterm birth of their infant. Early Hum Dev 2019;139:104838.
14. Franck LS, O'Brien K. The evolution of family-centered care: from supporting parent-delivered interventions to a model of family integrated care. Birth Defects Res 2019;111(15):1044–59.
15. O'Brien K, Robson K, Bracht M, et al. Effectiveness of Family Integrated Care in neonatal intensive care units on infant and parent outcomes: a multicentre, multinational, cluster-randomised controlled trial. Lancet Child Adolesc Health 2018; 2(4):245–54.
16. Levin A. The mother-infant unit at Tallinn Children's Hospital, Estonia: a truly baby-friendly unit. Birth 1994;21(1):39–44 [discussion: 45–6].

17. Bracht M, O'Leary L, Lee SK, et al. Implementing family-integrated care in the NICU: a parent education and support program. Adv Neonatal Care 2013; 13(2):115–26.
18. O'Brien K, Bracht M, Macdonell K, et al. A pilot cohort analytic study of Family Integrated Care in a Canadian neonatal intensive care unit. BMC Pregnancy Childbirth 2013;13(Suppl 1):S12.
19. Broom M, Parsons G, Carlisle H, et al. Exploring parental and staff perceptions of the family-integrated care model: a qualitative focus group study. Adv Neonatal Care 2017;17(6):E12–9.
20. Cheng C, Franck LS, Ye XY, et al. Evaluating the effect of Family Integrated Care on maternal stress and anxiety in neonatal intensive care units. J Reprod Infant Psychol 2019;1–14.
21. He S, Xiong Y, Zhu L, et al. Impact of family integrated care on infants' clinical outcomes in two children's hospitals in China: a pre-post intervention study. Ital J Pediatr 2018;44(1):65.
22. Young A, McKechnie L, Harrison CM. Family integrated care: what's all the fuss about? Arch Dis Child Fetal Neonatal Ed 2019;104(2):F118–9.
23. Patel N, Ballantyne A, Bowker G, et al. Family integrated care: changing the culture in the neonatal unit. Arch Dis Child 2018;103(5):415–9.
24. Banerjee J, Aloysius A, Mitchell K, et al. Improving infant outcomes through implementation of a family integrated care bundle including a parent supporting mobile application. Arch Dis Child Fetal Neonatal Ed 2020;105:172–7.
25. Franck LS, Kriz RM, Bisgaard R, et al. Protocol for the improving preterm infant outcomes with Family Integrated Care and mobile technology trial. Rev 2019.
26. Bourque CJ, Dahan S, Mantha G, et al. Improving neonatal care with the help of veteran resource parents: an overview of current practices. Semin Fetal Neonatal Med 2018;23(1):44–51.
27. Cox ED, Jacobsohn GC, Rajamanickam VP, et al. A family-centered rounds checklist, family engagement, and patient safety: a randomized trial. Pediatrics 2017;139(5):e20161688.
28. Profit J, Sharek PJ, Cui X, et al. The correlation between neonatal intensive care unit safety culture and quality of care. J Patient Saf 2018. [Epub ahead of print].
29. Gormley DK, Costanzo AJ, Goetz J, et al. Impact of nurse-led interprofessional rounding on patient experience. Nurs Clin North Am 2019;54(1):115–26.
30. Shinners J, Franqueiro T. Preceptor skills and characteristics: considerations for preceptor education. J Contin Educ Nurs 2015;46:233–6.
31. Tawfik DS, Sexton JB, Adair KC, et al. Context in quality of care: improving teamwork and resilience. Clin Perinatol 2017;44(3):541–52.
32. Benzies KM, Shah V, Aziz K, et al. Family integrated care (FICare) in level II neonatal intensive care units: study protocol for a cluster randomized controlled trial. Trials 2017;18:467.
33. Franck LS, Kriz RM, Bisgaard R, et al. Protocol for the improving preterm infant outcomes with family integrated care and mobile technology trial. BMC Pediatrics 2019;19(1):469.

The Best Medicine
Personal Pets and Therapy Animals in the Hospital Setting

Denise Barchas, RN, MSN, CCRN[a],*, Melissa Melaragni, RN, BSN, CCRN[a],
Heather Abrahim, MSN, MPA, RN, CCRN[b], Eric Barchas, DVM[c]

KEYWORDS

- Patient-centered and family-centered care • Alternative therapies • Pet therapy
- Animal-assisted intervention • Program implementation • Zoonosis

KEY POINTS

- Hospitals are increasingly allowing personal pets to visit patients. These visits can improve patient well-being and decrease anxiety, loneliness, and depression.
- Animal-assisted interventions (AAIs) with therapy animals provide benefits to hospitalized patients, including decreased pain, blood pressure, stress, depression, and anxiety.
- Personal pet visitation and AAIs carry few risks. AAI programs should include specific polices and guidelines to reduce potential risks.

PERSONAL PET VISITATION
The Human–Companion Animal Relationship

The relationship between humans and animals has developed over thousands of years. Domestication of many species of animals occurred throughout the world as humans and animals found ways to take advantage of their mutual need for food, shelter, and protection.[1] As human culture evolved, so did the relationship with domesticated animals. In modern times, the role of the companion animal has flourished.[1,2] More Americans than ever are sharing their homes with pets. Sixty-seven percent of American households, 84.9 million homes, have pets. Americans spent almost $73 billion on their pets in 2018, and it is estimated that 2019 expenditures increased to approximately $75.4 billion.[3]

Funding: None.
[a] University of California San Francisco Medical Center, 505 Parnassus Avenue M902R, San Francisco, CA 94117, USA; [b] University of California San Diego Health, Jacobs Medical Center, 5H mail code 7306, 9300 Campus Point Dr, La Jolla, CA 92037, USA; [c] San Bruno Pet Hospital, 1111 El Camino Real, San Bruno, CA 94066, USA
* Corresponding author.
E-mail address: denise.barchas@ucsf.edu

As companion animals have become more important in the lives of Americans, interest in the human-animal connection has grown.[4] In 1987, the National Institutes of Health held the workshop The Health Benefits of Pets. It provided a synthesis and examination of the current knowledge and identified areas for future research. In the 3 decades since the call for research, a large body of knowledge has developed regarding the benefits of the human-animal bond.[1,4] Studies have shown that interaction with animals can improve cardiovascular health, help manage stress, increase physical activity, help retain health and mobility with aging, encourage engagement with new people, and strengthen communities.[5] Most studies have focused on animal-assisted interventions (AAIs); this article discussing therapy animals provides a review of the current literature on AAIs. Few studies have explored the benefits of personal pet ownership; this area is ripe for future inquiry. Although limited, the few published studies have shown that personal pets do offer health benefits to their owners.

Health Benefits of Companion Animals

Pet ownership, and the responsibilities associated with it, can improve health and help community-dwelling adults manage chronic health conditions more effectively. Several studies have shown a link between pet ownership, increased physical activity, and perceived social support among older adults living in the community.[6–14] Levine and colleagues,[14] Kramer and colleagues,[15] and Chowdhury and colleagues[16] found that pet ownership improved survival in patients with known cardiovascular disease. In their qualitative study of 17 stroke survivors, Johansson and colleagues[17] found that pets help give meaning to life as well as provide physical and psychosocial aid in the stroke recovery process.

Pet ownership in itself has not been found to be effective to help manage chronic pain. Characteristics of the companion animal and its relationship with the owner weigh heavily on the impact.[18,19] Bradley and Bennett[18] found that simply owning and caring for a pet was not enough to decrease chronic pain levels reported by adults living in the community compared with those of nonowners. However, pet owners who actively used human-animal interaction as a pain management strategy reported less pain than owners who did not. Chur-Hansen and colleagues[19] conducted a comprehensive survey of peer-reviewed literature on the role of companion animals in hospice and palliative care. Only 5 published empirical studies on the role of companion animals in hospice care were identified. Although there is not a robust base of empirical evidence to support the role of companion animals at the end of life, there exists a larger body of peripheral literature, anecdotal evidence, case studies, descriptions, and opinion pieces to support the "conviction within the health care professions, academia, and the community in general that animals, as social supports, provide benefits to humans."[19(p672)] Such strong beliefs held by many with little supportive empirical evidence is a powerful call for further research into the importance of companion animals at the end of life.

Personal Pets as Family Members

Pets often are considered to be integral members of the family.[1,4,20–22] In their qualitative study, Maharaj and Haney[23] examined the significance of the human-canine relationship. One of the primary themes they identified is the dog as a family member. "Dog owners frequently referred to their dogs as their baby, kid, child, or grandchild.[23(p1180)] Muraco and colleagues[13] studied the role of pets in the lives of older lesbian, gay, bisexual, and transgender adults. Participants in their study often identified their pets as kin, characterizing them as family or children. One participant said, "I talk to them like they were kids. I tell them when I'm coming back, or be [sic] a little longer. I apologize if I haven't done something."[13(p869)]

The aforementioned study participant is not alone: according to cognitive scientist Dr Alexandra Horowitz, people talk to their dogs a lot. They speak to them in much the same way as they speak to children: they simplify their language, raise their pitch, and use a sing-song intonation. People have a running commentary with their pets that is both a result of and an expression of their intimate relationship with them.[21]

Cole[24] explored this intimate relationship in a 2019 qualitative study examining the nature and meaning of older adults' relationships with their dogs. Cole[24] observed strong and deep emotional ties between seniors and their animals. "Seniors, who have deep attachment to their dogs, think of their dogs as cherished family members rather than as animals with benefits."[24(p238)] The participant's own words help describe the strong bond between the older adults and their dogs. One participant referred to his dog as an integral part of the family. Another stated, "Teddy is like sunshine to me. He brightens every day. He means the world to me."[(p240)]

Personal Pet Visitation in the Hospital Setting

Patient-centered and family-centered care revolves around the 4 principles of respect and dignity, participation, sharing information, and collaboration.[25] Both the tenets of patient-centered and family-centered care and the Joint Commission patient-centered communication standards compel health care providers to respect that family can be whoever or whatever a patient chooses.[25,26] As collaborators in care, clinicians respect their patients' definition of family and understand the role a pet can play in an individual's health and well-being. Therefore, the paradigm of patient-centered and family-centered care needs to evolve to incorporate opportunities for personal pet visitation during patients' hospitalizations (**Fig. 1**).[22]

Personal pet visitation during hospitalization has been shown to improve the well-being of patients. In a survey of patients after pet visits, Sehr and colleagues[27] reported that patients whose personal pets visited during a hospitalization described feeling "less anxiety, sadness, loneliness, isolation, and depression."[27(p58)] Personal pet visits can also help staff provide more personalized, patient-centered care. In a 2018 multimethod qualitative study of a personal pet hospital visitation program in a southern US city, Yamasaki[22] observed visits and interviewed program volunteers. The researcher found that the visits "facilitate storied conversations, foster healing relationships, and offer alternative ways of knowing that can promote … more personalized care and improved well-being."[22(p830)]

Reverend Susan Roy, Director of the Department of Pastoral Care Services at the University of Maryland Medical Center, identified that patients having their own pets visit during hospitalization is akin to having family visits[28]: "I often say that it's great that we have … therapy pets … and we also have animal-assisted therapy. However, if I am hospitalized – and I think many people who have pets would echo the same feeling – I am likely going to want to see my pet."

Current Personal Pet Visitation Practice in United States and Canada

With a focus on patient-centered and family-centered care and an appreciation for the impact of a personal pet on an individual's health and well-being, many hospitals allow personal pets to visit inpatients.[22,24,28–49] Note that personal pet visitation policies are different from policies regarding service animals in hospitals. Service animal accessibility in hospitals is governed by the Americans with Disabilities Act, which requires service animals be allowed to accompany people with disabilities in all areas of the facility where the public is normally allowed to go. **Table 1** provides a summary of the

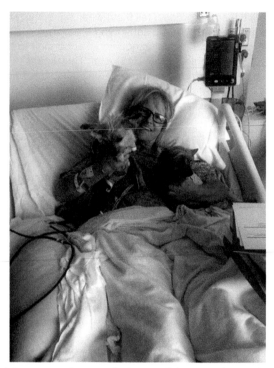

Fig. 1. Patient with her personal pets. "I feel so much better today just being able to see my dogs ... I think it's the best medicine you can give somebody."

legal standing of and differences between service animals, therapy animals, and personal pets.

Health care facilities are promoting personal pet visitation policies to the public online. More than 20 hospital and hospital system Web pages that provide patients and families with guidelines and/or policies for arranging a personal pet visit were reviewed. Each hospital or hospital system had its own policy or guidelines, some more stringent than others (**Fig. 2, Table 2**). Policies and guidelines frequently prohibit pet visitation in the intensive care unit (ICU). This broad-sweeping, one-size-fits-all policy is not in the best interests of patients, nor is it congruent with the goals of patient-centered and family-centered care. The organization Pets Are Wonderful Support (PAWS) Houston has overcome this prejudice against pet visitation in the critical care setting. PAWS Houston is a nonprofit organization whose volunteers facilitate personal pet visits to inpatients at area hospitals. The organization has patient pet visitation agreements with every major hospital in Houston. These agreements allow PAWS visits in all areas of the hospital except for the Bone Marrow Transplant Unit. Most of the visits facilitated are to ICUs.[51] The authors posit that, considering the significant potential benefits, hospitals should consider personal pet visitation in the critical care setting on a case-by-case basis rather than categorically prohibiting it.

THERAPY ANIMALS: THE HEALING POWER OF MAN'S BEST FRIEND
Therapy Animals and Animal-Assisted Interventions

Because of length of travel, hospital pet restrictions, or other circumstances, it may be unattainable for personal pet visitation. Fortunately, hospitals around the world are

Table 1
Comparisons between service animals, therapy animals, and personal pets

	Service Animal	Therapy Animal	Personal Pet
Training required?	Extensively trained to perform specific tasks to assist disabled handlers	Should be screened for temperament and obedience trained	None required
Where allowed?	Any place the public is allowed per the ADA. In a hospital, it would be inappropriate to exclude a service animal from areas such as patient rooms, clinics, cafeterias, or examination rooms. However, it may be appropriate to exclude a service animal from operating rooms or burn units where the animal's presence may compromise a sterile environment[50]	Only allowed in non–pet-friendly venues with special permission	Only allowed in non–pet–friendly venues with special permission
What types of animals?	Only dogs are included in the definition of service animal, but some provisions in the ADA for miniature horses	Any type	Any type
Certification required?	None	Usually yes, but depends on the hosting venue's requirements	NA
Licensing and vaccination required?	Subject to locality's normal requirements	Subject to locality's normal requirements	Subject to locality's normal requirements
Are they pets?	No	Yes	Yes

Abbreviations: ADA, Americans with Disabilities Act; NA, not applicable.

welcoming therapy animals and developing AAI programs as a therapeutic intervention for patients and families. Therapy animals and their handlers are trained and evaluated to safely interact with patients and staff. Organizations such as Pet Partners, Therapy Dogs International, and Alliance of Therapy Dogs offer handler and animal training and temperament evaluations, and require veterinary health screening evaluations and vaccinations.[52–54]

Nursing is focused on the holistic care of patients and strives to look beyond the illness-cure model of medicine. Integrating animals as part of the holistic care plan supports the psychological needs of patients and families.[55] AAI serves as a valuable intervention that can mitigate the need for pharmacologic interventions, which come

UC San Diego Health

Planning a Pet Visit

There is a growing amount of research to support the healing power of animals. Animals may help in coping with illness. Benefits to pet visits may include reduced: anxiety, agitation, heart rate, respiratory rate, blood pressure, pain, depression, social isolation, social withdrawal, and fear.

About Pet Visits

- ☐ Dogs or cats are permitted as pet visitors. Other animals are not permitted due to increased risk of infection. This handout is not about service animals or therapy animals.
- ☐ Pet visits may be discouraged when patients are in isolation. The doctor will determine whether it is safe for the pet to visit in these cases.
- ☐ The visit is planned in advance with the nurse.
- ☐ If able, the patient will confirm that a visit is desired. If the patient is unable to confirm, a family member may work with the hospital team to arrange the visit.

Guidelines for Pet Visits:

- ✓ The pet is current on immunizations.
- ✓ The pet has no fleas, diarrhea or signs of illness.
- ✓ The pet is not aggressive.
- ✓ The pet must be bathed and brushed before the start of visits to decrease dander.
- ✓ You will bring the pet in on a leash or in a carrier.
- ✓ You agree to stay with the pet during the entire visit
- ✓ You will toilet the animal before entering the facility and when needed.
- ✓ You will put pet waste in a bag and throw away in the trash.
- ✓ You agree to inform staff if the pet has an 'accident' so that the area can be cleaned.

Note: No paperwork is required.

Thank you for helping us with healing. We look forward to meeting your furry friend!

Fig. 2. Example of pet visitation guidelines for patients/families.

with a host of negative side effects. In addition, AAI is cost-effective, feasible to implement, and has been shown to increase both patient and family satisfaction.[56–60]

Three main topics on AAI are discussed to guide clinicians on implementation and identification of stakeholders for an AAI program. A literature review explores the

Table 2	
Personal pet visitation requirements	
Common Personal Pet Visitation Requirements	**Less-Common Additional Personal Pet Visitation Requirements**

• Pet must:
  ○ Be current on vaccinations
  ○ Be groomed or bathed before visit
  ○ Be well behaved
  ○ Be accompanied by a handler (not the patient) who is responsible for the pet while in the hospital
  ○ Be leashed or crated
• Only dogs or cats may visit
• Visitation not allowed in isolation rooms, with immunocompromised patients, or in ICUs
• Coordination with unit nursing staff
	• Physician order for visitation
	• Certificate of health from veterinarian
	• Minimum age of pet
	• Time-limited visits
	• Only dogs may visit

Abbreviation: ICUs, intensive care units.

benefits and challenges of AAI to patients and families in the hospital setting. In addition, zoonosis risks are examined and steps to mitigate these risks are outlined.

Animal-Assisted Interventions and Animal-Assisted Therapy Defined

Many definitions have been used to describe AAI and animal-assisted therapy (AAT). The American Veterinary Medical Association defines AAIs as interventions that use various species of animals in diverse manners to benefit humans.[61] The International Association of Human-Animal Interaction Organizations (IAHAIO) defines AAIs as goal-oriented and structured interventions that incorporate animals in health, education, and human services for the therapeutic gain of humans.[62] Similarly, AAT is a goal oriented, planned, and structured therapeutic intervention directed and/or delivered by health, education, and human service professionals. Interactions focus on enhancing the physical, cognitive, behavioral, and/or social-emotional functions of the particular human client.[62] This article uses the accepted AAI term as an umbrella term for AAT, AAI, animal-assisted activities, and animal-assisted education. Canines are generally used during AAI and are the primary term used in this article.

Animal-Assisted Interventions Literature Review

The use of AAIs in health care was investigated using 19 articles compiled through the use of computerized databases: PubMed, Science Direct, EBSCOhost, and CINAHL. Keywords included AAT*, animal-assisted therapy*, animal-assisted intervention*, and animal-assisted activity*. A total of 53 articles were reviewed. Inclusion criteria included (1) articles pertaining to AAI that did not involve the patient's own pet, (2) validated measures were used to evaluate data, (3) canine species (therapy dogs) for meaningful comparison, and (4) institutional review board approval was obtained. Patient ages ranged from 2 to 88 years. No negative outcomes or adverse effects were reported in any study. All studies excluded subjects who were allergic and/or afraid of animals.

AAI has been shown to benefit the young and the old, in both inpatient and outpatient settings, with medical conditions both acute and chronic. AAI studies have shown physiologic and psychological reductions in pain, blood pressure, stress, depression, and anxiety.[58,63–65] Furthermore, feelings of well-being, self-esteem, self-efficacy and, social interactions are increased.[55,57,58,65,66] AAI improves the hospital experience by increasing patient satisfaction and may also lead to a decrease in hospital costs because most AAI is volunteer based. Studies have shown that short sessions (5–20 minutes) have been just as effective as longer sessions (>20 minutes).[57,65,66]

Pain reduction and well-being

Studies have shown that AAI reduces pain and increases feelings of well-being.[55,57,58,64–71] Procedural pain is experienced by hospitalized patients, especially in the ICU.[72] Pharmacologic pain management can lead to delirium, respiratory depression, gastrointestinal bleeding, constipation, nausea, and dependence, among other undesirable side effects.[73] AAI is a cost-effective strategy without these drawbacks and potential negative outcomes. Marcus and colleagues[58] evaluated 235 patients within a chronic pain clinic waiting room where pain, fatigue, and emotional distress were scored before and after dog visits. Significant improvements in pain and emotional well-being were noted in those who received AAI. Similar studies reported significant pain reductions postoperatively after total hip replacement and total knee replacement surgeries.[57] Bolden and colleagues[70] found that 21 patients with spinal cord injuries reported less pain after occupational therapy (OT) when AAI was provided. These results show that AAI has the potential to allow decreased pharmacologic pain medication use and increased mobility in the immediate postoperative period.

Furthermore, hospitalized patients with varying degrees of acuity have been shown to benefit from AAI. Pain, anxiety, and fatigue were significantly decreased during a before/after intervention study in 128 hospitalized patients across multiple ICUs and surgical, neurologic, oncological, and rehabilitation units.[64] The average intervention was 5 to 10 minutes, making it possible to provide AAI to a large number of patients in a short period of time. Braun and colleagues[69] showed a reduction in pain by 4-fold in 57 children who received AAI compared with a control group within an acute care setting. Waite and colleagues[65] conducted a meta-analysis of 22 quantitative studies (13 child and 18 adult) and found significant improvements in pain, anxiety, and distress. They postulated that these results may be from social interventions in general. Thus, it cannot be said that similar social interventions would not yield similar results.

Mobilization

Mobilization of patients improves patient outcomes and decreases hospital length of stay.[74,75] AAI results in increased motivation and ability to work with physical therapy (PT) and OT.[57,66,70] Abate and colleagues[66] studied patients with chronic heart failure (CHF) and found they were more compliant in walking and ambulated twice as far compared with the historical baseline when accompanied by a therapy dog. All the participants enjoyed the opportunity to walk with the therapy dog and the presence of the dog influenced their decision to walk. Similarly, postoperative orthopedic patients who walked with a dog experienced statistically significant reductions in pain with PT and OT with their first ambulation postoperatively compared with the control group.[57] These studies show how pain reduction with AAI could also serve as a motivating factor in postoperative ambulation.

Palliative

AAI addresses the physical, emotional, and spiritual components that require care during palliative illness. Participants of an inpatient palliative care unit reported increased positive feelings, reduced pain, increased relaxation, improved coping, and improved quality of life.[55,76] Fifty-two inpatients receiving palliative care for terminal diagnosis discovered that sessions with a therapy dog improved relaxation, pleasure, and patients' contact with positively rewarding activities.[55] Increased fatigue was noted in some patients, but these patients found AAI so appealing that they wished to continue even when fatigue was reached. Patients are more communicative when AAI is applied; they may express feelings that they could/would not otherwise express with staff.[77] The comfort of a dog is a powerful tool which nurses can use that allows access to their patients' emotions and decreases the suffering involved with illness.[77]

Psychological

Approximately one-third of hospitalized patients experience depression.[76] Depressed patients have poorer outcomes, are less likely to comply with medical treatments and follow-ups, have increased length of stay, and are more likely to be readmitted.[76] This problem increases the cost of health care as well as overall suffering.

AAI has also been shown to reduce depression, anxiety, and stress, and improve self-efficacy and mood, as well as encouraging increased socialization with staff and families.[58,63–65,67,68,77–80] In multiple before/after intervention studies, significant reductions in depression and anxiety were noted among hospitalized patients in acute psychological distress during an acute or chronic illness.[67,68,81] Nepps and colleagues[67] found significant changes in depression and anxiety in 1-hour group sessions of AAI versus a 1-hour group stress management program among 218 participants. In a similar study, significant improvements in anger and fatigue in one-on-one 10-minute sessions with a therapy dog were noted.[68] Thirty hospitalized psychiatric patients with a known history of schizophrenia reported significant increases in self-esteem, self-determination, and positive psychiatric symptoms after 50-minute weekly sessions with a therapy dog.[78]

Children who are hospitalized experience stress and the hospitalization may affect their development.[80] AAI provides an outlet through which children can express feelings, reduce anxiety, and have an active role in their treatment that increases self-efficacy and self-esteem.[80] A study of 70 hospitalized children compared child-life activities with AAI and found both groups yielded improved mood in the children.[80] This finding signifies that AAI can be as beneficial as child-life activities with the added benefit of direct contact that most children lack in the inpatient setting.[80]

Physiologic

There are mixed results on the physiologic changes of AAI. Odendaal[79] studied how the interactions within AAI affected the physiology of its participants. In the end, 18 dogs and 18 patients experienced decreases in blood pressure and changes in neurohormones within 5 to 24 minutes of AAI.[79] Affiliation behaviors (necessary, mutually beneficial social interactions) are thought to result in a release of these same neurohormones as well as a decrease in blood pressure.[79] Specifically, the neurohormones beta-endorphin, oxytocin, prolactin, dopamine, and phenylacetic acid are known to be released with positive interpersonal experiences.[79] Odendaal[79] found a statistically significant increase in levels of all 5 of these neurohormones in both the humans and the dogs after AAI.[79] This finding could biologically account for some of the increased feelings of well-being noted in previously discussed studies.[58,63–65,67,68,77–80]

Cole and colleagues[63] also found significant decreases in neurohormone (epinephrine and norepinephrine) levels as well as multiple cardiopulmonary pressures in 76 patients with CHF. In contrast, other studies did not find significant changes in blood pressure.[67,80,82] No significant changes in heart rate were noted in any adult studies.[63,67,79,80,82] However, 2 studies involving children with AAI dogs did show significant increases in heart rate during and after the sessions.[80,82] Anticipatory excitement may account for these increases because they resolved within several minutes after AAI.[80]

Adult and child studies examined the possible endocrinological changes of salivary cortisol levels before and after AAI with no significant results.[67,80,82] Calcaterra and colleagues[82] found significant increases in beta waves within electroencephalograms of 40 postoperative children between the ages of 3 and 17 years after AAI. The changes are associated with wakefulness and attention and may reduce recovery time after anesthesia. Similarly, a study used near-infrared spectroscopy on adults to examine brain functioning and found significantly higher activation in the prefrontal cortex (PFT) after a dog was placed in the patients' laps.[83] It is noteworthy that those who experience mood disorders and depression have been found to have low activation within the PFT. This low activation may be the physiologic manifestation of the psychological impacts noted previously.

Limitations

There is a dearth of rigorous, peer-reviewed studies that involve the research of AAI within inpatient environments. Further research is necessary to replicate the results. In addition, the delivery method (session length, environment, canine breed, target population, interaction with the handler) in AAI varies from study to study. An abundance of AAI research is qualitative and this poses a threat to validity. It is unclear whether pain is diminished through placebo effect and/or the distraction that AAI might present. People who have a fear of or lack of desire for AAI were excluded from all of these studies. Furthermore, nursing and other ancillary staff are not exposed to AAI in their formal training. Despite these limitations, AAI can benefit the physical and emotional well-being of patients and families.[58,63–65,67,68,77–80] Nurses are vital in advocating for the use of AAI as a meaningful addition to holistic, nonpharmacologic treatment methods for their patients.

Animal-Assisted Intervention Program Implementation

Therapy animals provide physical, psychological, and emotional benefits to individuals in many different settings, such as hospitals, assisted living residences, and community programs.[55,57,58,66,84,85] Specifically, in hospital settings, therapy animals provide a unique therapeutic benefit to patients and families.

Despite the growing evidence that supports the benefits for AAI in the hospital setting, implementation of a program may pose a challenge. Barriers to implementation include the potential for infections and adverse events to patients or staff that may include bites, phobias, or allergic reactions. Hospital policies and work flow guidelines must be established among hospital stakeholders to reduce these potential risks. Distinction between therapy animals, emotional support animals, service dogs, and personal pets should be included in these policies.[86]

Collaboration of Stakeholders

Stakeholders from multiple disciplines, departments, and outside agencies/organizations are necessary for implementation of an AAI program.[87] **Table 3** summarizes key stakeholders and their roles in AAI implementation. Involving participants early in the process ensures that concerns and perceived risks can be discussed and addressed in policy and guideline development.

Table 3
Stakeholders and roles for animal-assisted intervention implementation

Stakeholders	Role with AAI
Leadership team	• Provide support for animal visits • Identify specific patient populations to visit (inpatient, outpatient, staff visits, or at specific units) • Determine inclusion/exclusion criteria for visits • Provide financial support
Infection control	• Discuss interventions to reduce infection risks to patients, families, and staff • Discuss need for infection tracking
Risk management	• Examine safety concerns, liability, and insurance
Security	• Determine need for animal badges
Patient relations	• May help to provide support for AAI related to patient/family requests
Frontline staff	• Unit champions to help facilitate program • Educate staff on policy and procedures • Review AAI work flow and staff expectations during visits
Outside agencies	• Provide handler/animal training, evaluation, animal health screening, testing, insurance, and scheduling • Provide policy and procedure guidelines and recommendations
Volunteer services	• Facilitate volunteer handler onboarding (background checks, modules, hospital training, vaccinations) • Coordinate visits with outside agency and or with specific units • Evaluate and update policy and procedures • Track and log visits

Staff Perceptions

Buy-in from staff is essential for a successful AAI program. Studies have shown that staff generally are positive about AAI.[56,59,86,88–90] Moreover, AAI has been shown to decrease stress and anxiety in staff members.[58,59,71] Nurses reported that AAI made their jobs more interesting and created happiness at the workplace.[56,86] Staff even reported missing the therapy dogs when they were not present.[86] Staff reported that AAI animals created an icebreaker between staff and patients and potentially help patients heal.[77,86] Nurses did not think that their workload increased as a consequence of AAI.[56,58,59,84,88] Uglow[91] found that 100% of staff and parents in a children's hospital reported zero concerns regarding safety or sanitation.

Policy and Guideline Development

Although most staff approve of AAI visits, some staff have reported fear and/or concern for infections or harm to patients.[59,90,92] Policies and guidelines help ensure the safety of staff, patients, and families, and safeguard the wellness of animals. At present, consensus on guidelines and policies does not exist for AAI hospital programs. Linder and colleagues[92] conducted a survey of 45 hospitals in the United States and found most hospitals surveyed had policies related to AAI but differences existed between these policies.

Despite lack of consensus, several organizations and agencies provide guidelines for AAI program implementation. Just like hospitals, agencies and organizations offer variances in practices such as handler and animal requirements and testing. **Table 4** summarizes and compares a partial list of key elements and recommendations from leading agencies, organizations, and published journals. Animal Assisted Intervention

International[93] provides a comprehensive standard of practice for organizations interested in implementing a program. In an effort to prevent the transmission of infections, Hardin and colleagues[96] established specific infection control guidelines for AAI programs. These guidelines include specific patient restrictions, hand hygiene before and after visits, and barrier protection (linen disposal or new sheets on bed and removed after visits) during visitations. Hardin and colleagues[96] showed no infection risks to patients following adherence to the developed guidelines during a 16-year program.

In addition to policy and guideline development, the work flow for AAI visits must be discussed before implementation. **Fig. 3** offers guidance on work flow questions to address. Facilities with AAI programs must review policies, guidelines, and work flow to ensure safety. In addition, patient, family, and staff survey tools assist in evaluating the programs and offer suggestions for improvement.

Initial Pilot Programs

Pilot programs evaluate developed workflows, confirm readiness for full implementation, and guide the outcomes of a program. Caprilli and Messeri[97] conducted a 1-year pilot to examine the benefit of an AAT program for pediatric patients. They showed that infection rates did not change and the program had beneficial impact on patients, families, and staff. Similarly, Gagnon and colleagues[98] conducted a 1-year pilot of hospitalized pediatric patients with cancer and showed no infections or allergic harms to patients.

A VETERERINARIAN PERSPECTIVE
Potential Risks to Humans and Animals During Hospital Visitation

AAI generally carries few risks for the human patients participating in a program. However, AAI is not completely risk free, and program designers should include risk mitigation steps in their program designs. Fortunately, most of the risks are easily mitigated, and, in general, healthy animals participating in AAI programs are unlikely to cause harm to the humans with whom they interact.

The risks to human patients can broadly be grouped into 5 categories: phobias, allergies, animals acting as fomites, zoonoses, and traumatic injuries. A brief discussion of each of these categories, and prevention of harms associated with them, follows.

Although the goal of AAI is to provide comfort and a positive experience to patients, some individuals, including staff members, have adverse feelings or fears of certain species of animals. People with animal phobia have an unpleasant experience when visited by a member of that species. Patient selection is the key to preventing these unpleasant experiences. Animals should only visit patients who desire the interaction. Care should be taken to close doors or provide physical or visual barriers between animals and individuals who do not desire contact with them.

Allergies to cats, dogs, and other species can cause symptoms ranging from mild discomfort (sneezing, watery eyes) to severe, life-threatening reactions.[99] Careful patient selection prevents harm to patients with allergies to animal species. Patients should be carefully screened before AAI visits. Program designers should consider that residual dander may linger in the environment for a period of time after animal visits, potentially triggering allergic reactions in especially sensitive individuals.

Fomites spread diseases by physically passing pathogens from one susceptible individual to another. In the context of AAI, nearly perfect environmental conditions and complex variables would need to exist for transmission of disease to occur between an animal and patient. Programs should include measures to prevent fomite transmission of diseases. Basic preventive measures for possible incorporation include (1)

Table 4
Animal, facility, and handler recommendations for hospital visit

Animal Recommendations

Organization	Animal Species	Age	Training from a Formal Program	Vet Medical Evaluation Before Start	Vaccination	Health Screening by Veterinarian	Raw Diets	Routine Screening for Zoonosis
SHEA[100]	Dogs only	At least 1 y	Yes	Yes	Yes	At least once a year	No	No
AJIC[94]	Domesticated	At least 1 y	Yes	—	Yes	At least once a year	No	No
HICPAC[95]	No nonhuman primates	—	—	—	Yes	—	—	—
IAHAIO[62]	Domesticated	—	—	Yes	—	At least once a year	No	—
AVMA[61]	—	At least 6 mo	Socialized and trained	—	Yes	Frequent communication	—	—

Animal and Facility Recommendations

Organization	Hand Hygiene	Develop Policies	Report Any Scratches, Bites, or Inappropriate Behavior	Log Visits	Visit Time (h)	Develop Contact Tracking	Sheet on Bed (Barrier Protection)	Routine Cleaning and Disinfection of Environment Surfaces
SHEA	Before/after	Yes	Yes	Yes	1	Yes	Yes	After
AJIC	Before/after	Yes	Yes	Yes	1	Yes	Yes	After
HICPAC	After	—	Yes	—	—	—	—	After
IAHAIO	—	Yes	—	—	—	—	—	—
AVMA	—	—	—	—	—	—	—	—

Animal Visit Recommendations

Organization	Brush/Bathe Animal Before Visit	Trim Nails	Consent or Consultation from Attending MD	Specific Restricted Areas	Discourage
SHEA	Yes	Yes	Preferably	ICU, isolation rooms, newborn nurseries, areas that may cause distress to animals	No licking, No paw shaking, No treats/feeding
AJIC	Yes	Do not recommend declawing	—	ICU, neonatal nurseries, dialysis, burn units, isolations	No licking, No paw shaking
HICPAC	Yes	—	—	Case by case for immunocompromised patients	—
IAHAIO	—	—	—	Allergies, High-risk patients	—
AVMA	Provide information	Provide information	—	Develop code systems of rooms not to enter	—

Handler Recommendations

Organization	Trained Handlers	Certification by Organization	Training Modules	Escort During Visits	Observe/Training Animal for Wellness	Refrain from Cell Phone Use
SHEA	Yes	Yes	Yes	Yes	Yes	Yes
AJIC	Yes	Yes	Yes	Yes	Yes	Yes
HICPAC	Yes	—	—	—	Yes	—
IAHAIO	Yes	Yes	—	—	Yes	—
AVMA	—	—	—	—	Yes	—

Dash indicates no mention by organization/author.

Abbreviations: AJIC, American Journal of Infection Control; AVMA, American Veterinary Medical Association; HICPAC, Healthcare Infection Control Practices Advisory Committee (guidelines for environmental infection control in health care facilities [Centers for Disease Control And Prevention]); IAHAIO, International Association of Human-Animal Interaction Organization; MD, doctor of medicine; SHEA, The Society for Healthcare Epidemiology of America.

Handler Expectations and Animal Wellness	Animal Visit Work Flow
• Who will escort the handler and animal and will they have a designated meeting location before they enter the facility? • Will the handler log visit times? • Does the facility have a designated area for the animal to urinate/defecate? • Is water available for the animal?	• What type of visits will occur and what is the goal of the visit? Will a visit be for staff wellness, one-on-one visits, or a whole unit? Even if the visit is intended for patients, staff will often want to visit the animal. Consider the size of the animal based on specific population and environmental space • When will the visits occur? Be mindful of meal times with certain animals. Will documentation of visits be required and who will document? Otherwise, tracking the number of visits and keeping in a secure location can be helpful to show the success and needs of a program • Define exclusion criteria for visits, potentially including isolation rooms or roommates that are frightened of or allergic to animals. Staff members may also be frightened of and/or allergic to animals and may need notice prior to visits • Who will determine which patient to visit and how will consent be obtained? Will request be made by staff phoned to a designated department, or will orders go through the electronic health record? Will a list be at the front desk with interested patients/families? • Will MD orders be required for animal visits? Inform departments/primary service of animal visits before implementation to ensure they are on board with AAI. Some MDs/departments may have specific exclusion criteria. If MD orders are required, ensure enough time is made for orders to be written (be mindful of rounding times)
Harm Reduction Measures	
• Establish procedures if harm occurs to a patient, family, or staff member (bite, allergic reaction, etc.) • What infection control practices will be implemented before and after visits? This should include hand hygiene, barrier protection, and disinfestation of environment	
Miscellaneous	
• How will the facility market the new program and provide education to patients, families, and staff? • How will the facility secure initial and future funding costs? • How will feedback and evaluation of the program be conducted?	

Fig. 3. Work flow questions to address before AAI implementation. *Abbreviation*: MD, doctor of medicine.

animals should not visit patients with diagnosed or suspected transmissible disease or patients placed on isolation precautions,[100] (2) barrier protection should be implemented when appropriate,[94,100] (3) no licking or kisses (both to and from the animal),[94,100] and (4) patients should wash or sanitize their hands before and after the interaction.[94,100]

A zoonosis is a disease that can be transmitted to humans from animals.[101] Although most animal diseases are species specific or not contagious to humans, zoonotic diseases are in 4 broad categories: bacteria, parasites, fungi, and viruses. Significant examples of diseases from each category are discussed, as are mitigation measures.

Animals involved in AAI may harbor pathogenic strains of intestinal bacteria. Commonly encountered bacteria include *Escherichia coli*, *Salmonella*, and *Campylobacter*. Dogs and cats have the capacity to be asymptomatic carriers of these bacteria, which may then spread to humans. There are several actions that can be taken to prevent harm from pathogenic intestinal bacteria when planning AAI programs.

- Only healthy animals should participate in AAI programs. Dogs or cats with diarrhea are more likely to shed pathogenic bacteria. They also are more likely to have contamination of their hair coats with bacteria.
- AAI animals should be bathed and groomed before visits.[94,100,95] This action reduces bacterial contamination of the hair coat.
- Animals participating in AAI programs should not be fed raw diets.[94,100,62] Because cooking kills bacteria, animals fed raw diets are more likely to be exposed to, and subsequently shed, pathogenic intestinal bacteria.
- Patients should practice good hygiene. Patients should always wash their hands after interactions, should not kiss the animals, and should avoid contact with the animal's hindquarters.[94,100]

Leptospirosis is a bacterium that can infect the bloodstream, liver, and kidneys of dogs and humans. It is spread through urine, and dogs and humans may contract the disease after coming into contact with water that has been contaminated by the urine of a reservoir species. There is at least a theoretic potential for the disease to spread from dogs to humans.[102] A vaccine for the most common serovars (strains) of *Leptospirosis* is available for dogs, and it is recommended that dogs participating in AAI programs receive the vaccine.

Reports exist of personal pet dogs being colonized (but not infected) with methicillin-resistant *Staphylococcus aureus* (MRSA).[103,104] However, dogs seem to be more susceptible to methicillin-resistant *Staphylococcus pseudintermedius*, which in turn is less common in humans. Dogs with any sort of skin lesion or illness should not participate in AAI programs; however, the likelihood of dogs transmitting MRSA is considered to be low in the AAI setting and reports of transmission do not exist.

Significant Parasitic Zoonoses

The most common intestinal worms of cats and dogs have zoonotic potential. In particular, the common canine and feline roundworm (*Toxocara* spp) is a zoonotic disease in humans.[105–107] Most humans infected with *Toxocara* experience no symptoms or mild symptoms. However, children or immunocompromised individuals in particular may be prone to experiencing visceral, ocular, or cerebral larval migrans with severe consequences. Zoonotic potential from intestinal worms can be dramatically reduced with the following steps:

- Only adult animals (at least 1 year old) should participate in AAI programs.[94,100] Puppies and kittens are dramatically more likely to shed intestinal worm eggs than their adult counterparts.
- Good hygiene practices should be followed. Intestinal worms are spread through fecal-to-oral transmission; good hygiene reduces the likelihood of human infestation.
- Animals participating in AAI programs should be regularly dewormed with products that remove most intestinal worms. Use of broad-spectrum monthly heartworm preventives dramatically reduces the likelihood of intestinal worm transmission.
- Annual or semiannual stool testing with fecal centrifugation and parasite antigen screening should be required for animals participating in AAI programs.

Giardia is commonly encountered in dogs, but its pathogenicity in dogs, as well as its zoonotic potential, is a subject of controversy in veterinary medicine. In dogs, *Giardia* may cause or exacerbate diarrhea but also may be found in clinically healthy individuals. It is recommended that dogs with diarrhea not participate in AAI visits. AAI participants also should undergo regular fecal screening, including testing for *Giardia* antigen.

Fleas and ticks that infest dogs have the potential to feed on humans. These parasites may spread human diseases such as plague, tularemia, bartonellosis, Lyme disease, Rocky Mountain spotted fever, and ehrlichiosis. They are easily prevented by regular use of modern ectoparasite preventives in the isoxazoline class of drugs.

Significant Fungal and Viral Zoonoses

The species of ringworm most common in dogs and cats have the potential to spread to humans.[108] In animal patients, dermatophytes may cause scabbing, crusting, and hair loss. In animals, ringworm can be diagnosed with a combination of fungal culture, with a polymerase chain reaction test available through commercial laboratories. Animals without skin lesions are unlikely to spread ringworm; animals with skin lesions should not participate in AAI programs. Dermatophytes are more likely to be found on juvenile animals; only adult animals should participate in AAT programs.

Note that in developed countries there are very few instances of the spread of viral zoonoses from animals to humans.[108] However, in parts of the developing world, rabies remains a significant threat.

Rabies is the deadliest known transmissible disease of dogs, cats, and humans. In humans, fatality approaches 100% if the patient is not vaccinated before symptoms develop. An estimated 59,000 humans die each year from rabies; most deaths occur in India, Sri Lanka, and sub-Saharan Africa.[109] Most of the people infected with rabies are children who are bitten by rabid dogs. In the United States, 125 human rabies cases were reported between 1960 and 2018.[110] Of these cases, 70% were from bats and 25% came from dog bites outside the United States.

In the developed world, mass vaccination of dogs has dramatically reduced the instance of rabies, and most human exposures are the result of cat or bat bites. The rabies vaccine for cats and dogs is highly effective, and any cat or dog participating in an AAI program should have a current rabies vaccine.

Injury Prevention

Patients participating in AAI programs have the potential to be injured by the visiting animal. Fortunately, most injuries are easily preventable with proper animal selection, proper animal care, and proper handling. Accidental scratches are unlikely to occur if the animal's nails are trimmed before visits and the animal is properly monitored and handled during visits. Other accidental injuries, such as trips/falls and crushing injuries, are unlikely to occur if the animal is properly monitored and handled during visits.

Personal Pet Visitation Program Implementation

In a similar manner to AAT, established policies and guidelines for personal pet visitation are essential to reduce potential risks to staff and patients. Information specific to personal pet visitation is presented here.

Studies have shown several potential benefits that hospitalized patients may derive from visits by their own pets.[22,27] Such benefits include improved mood and increased motivation to get well.[27] Hospitalized patients and their families may therefore request personal pet visitation. Personal pets, unlike AAI animals, are not specially trained nor is temperament screened prior to visits. They also may pose some of the same risks to patients as their AAI counterparts, but no evidence exists that visits cause harm.

- Visits should be scheduled in advance, and should not occur when allergic or phobic individuals may be present.
- Aggressive animals should not be permitted to visit. Any pet that displays fearful or aggressive behavior (growling or hissing, baring teeth, holding ears back, showing dilated pupils) may be more likely to harm a patient, family member, or staff member.
- It is recommended that personal pets be subject to the same rules regarding vaccination, parasite preventives, fecal testing, and evidence of disease as AAI animals. The animals should be current on vaccinations, free of fleas, and free of illness. This status may be obtained by a veterinary professional in writing or attestation.
- Grooming and bathing maintain cleanliness and help minimize allergens. It is not recommended that personal pets be required to bathe before every visit but only when the dog is soiled. Excessive bathing may lead to dry and irritated skin by stripping oils off the animal.

- A designated person should carefully monitor and control the animal at all times and ensure the animal is leashed. The designated person should assume the responsibility to ensure that the animal has access to water and tend to the bathroom needs of the animal.
- Anyone that has contact with the animals should perform hand hygiene before and after visitations.

SUMMARY

Personal pets and therapy animals provide emotional support, add comfort, and aid in the recovery of hospitalized patients. Animal presence in the hospital poses minimal risks to families, patients, and staff. Developing policies and guidelines assists with minimizing these risks and ensures the overall well-being of humans and animals. There are vast opportunities for future research in order to add to the current knowledge on the physiologic and psychological benefits of AAI and personal pet visitation. For instance, it is not yet known whether AAI/personal pet length of visit time (dose response) plays a role in potential patient immune risk. Additional studies should also compare AAI versus personal pet therapy to establish which visits have less risk and which visits provide more benefits to patients. Equally important, tracking of adverse events in all patient populations and settings, particularly infections, should be compiled across programs to gain a better understanding of whether AAT/personal pet visitation causes harm and which patient populations are at higher risk for harm. Research can focus on additional strategies to reduce potential risks to patient, families, and staff. Nursing schools could consider the addition of AAI into their curricula in order for nurses to obtain the exposure and understanding necessary to safely offer AAI.

As more people view companion animals as family members, hospitals have the opportunity to welcome personal pets and therapy animals as an integrative health intervention for patient-centered and family-centered care. Nurses are vital in advocating for the use of companion and therapy animals as a meaningful addition to holistic, nonpharmacologic treatment methods for their patients.

ACKNOWLEDGMENTS

The authors would like to acknowledge and thank Pamela Tecca for her contributions.

DISCLOSURE

The authors have nothing to disclose.

REFERENCES

1. Walsh F. Human-animal bonds I: the relational significance of companion animals. Fam Process 2009;48(4):462–80.
2. Serpell JA. Companion animals. In: Hosey G, Melfi V, editors. Anthrozoology: human-animal interactions in domesticated and wild animals. New York: Oxford University Press; 2018. p. 17–31.
3. Pet industry market size & ownership statistics. American Pet Products Association. Available at: https://www.americanpetproducts.org/press_industrytrends.asp. Accessed August 13, 2019.
4. Fine AH, Beck AM. Understanding our kinship with animals: input for health care professionals interested in the human-animal bond. In: Fine A, editor. Handbook

on animal assisted therapy. 4th edition. San Diego (CA): Academic Press; 2015. p. 3–9.

5. McCune S, Kruger KA, Griffin JA, et al. Evolution of research into the mutual benefits of human-animal interaction. Anim Front 2014;4(3):49–58.

6. Toohey AM, McCormack GR, Doyle-Baker PK, et al. Dog-walking and sense of community in neighborhoods: implications for promoting regular physical activity in adults 50 years and older. Health Place 2013;22:75–81.

7. Curl AL, Bibbo J, Johnson RA. Dog-walking, the human-animal bond, and older adults' physical health. Gerontologist 2017;57(5):930–9.

8. Feng Z, Dibben C, Witham MD, et al. Dog ownership and physical activity in later life: a cross-sectional observational study. Prev Med 2014;66:101–6.

9. Pruncho R, Heid AR, Wilson-Genderson M. Successful aging, social support, and ownership of a companion animal. Anthrozoos 2018;31(1):23–39.

10. Gretebeck KA, Radius K, Black DR, et al. Dog ownership, functional ability, and walking in community-dwelling older adults. J Phys Act Health 2013;10(5): 646–55.

11. Dall PM, Ellis SLH, Ellis BM, et al. The influence of dog ownership on objective measures of free-living physical activity and sedentary behaviour in community-dwelling older adults: a longitudinal case-controlled study. BMC Public Health 2017;17(1):496.

12. Creagan ET, Bauer BA, Thomley BS, et al. Animal-assisted therapy at Mayo Clinic: the time is now. Complement Ther Clin Pract 2015;21(2):101–4.

13. Muraco A, Putney J, Shiu C, et al. Lifesaving in every way: the role of companion animals in the lives of older lesbian, gay, bisexual, and transgender adults age 50 and over. Res Aging 2018;40(9):859–82.

14. Levine GN, Allen K, Braun LT, et al. Pet ownership and cardiovascular risk: a scientific statement from the American Heart Association. Circulation 2013; 127(23):2353–63.

15. Kramer CK, Mehmood S, Suen RS. Dog ownership and survival: a systematic review and meta-analysis. Circ Cardiovasc Qual Outcomes 2019;12(10): e005554.

16. Chowdhury EK, Nelson MR, Jennings GL, et al. Pet ownership and survival in the elderly hypertensive population. J Hypertens 2017;35(4):769–75.

17. Johansson M, Ahlstrom G, Jonsson AC. Living with companion animals after stroke: experiences of older people in community and primary care nursing. Br J Community Nurs 2014;19(12):578–84.

18. Bradley L, Bennett PC. Companion-animals' effectiveness in managing chronic pain in adult community members. Anthrozoos 2015;28(4):635–47.

19. Chur-Hansen A, Zambrano SC, Crawford GB. Furry and feathered family members–a critical review of their role in palliative care. Am J Hosp Palliat Care 2014; 31(6):672–7.

20. Hodgson K, Barton L, Darling M, et al. Pets' impact on your patients' health: leveraging benefits and mitigating risk. J Am Board Fam Med 2015;28(4): 526–34.

21. Horowitz A. Things people say to their dogs. New York Times. Available at: https://www.nytimes.com/2019/08/02/opinion/sunday/talking-dog.html. Accessed August 2, 2019.

22. Yamasaki J. The communicative role of companion pets in patient-centered critical care. Patient Educ Couns 2018;101(5):830–5.

23. Maharaj N, Haney CJ. A qualitative investigation of the significance of companion dogs. West J Nurs Res 2015;37(9):1175–93.

24. Cole A. Grow Old along with me: the Meaning of Dogs in seniors' lives. Int Journal of Com WB 2 2019;235–52. https://doi.org/10.1007/s42413-019-00034-w.

25. Gonzalez E. Impact of pet music therapy. Society of Critical Care Medicine. Project dispatch. Available at: https://www.youtube.com/watch?v=uoxK_APHlZc. Accessed August 30, 2019.

26. Understanding the historical context for visiting policies. Institute for patient- and family-centered care. Available at: https://www.ipfcc.org/bestpractices/Understanding-Historical-Context.pdf. Accessed August 30, 2019.

27. Sehr J, Eisele-Hlubocky L, Junker R, et al. Family pet visitation. Am J Nurs 2013; 113(12):54–9.

28. Pet visitation program frequently asked questions. University of Maryland Medical Center. Available at: https://www.umms.org/ummc/patients-visitors/for-patients/pastoral-care/personal-pet-visitation. Accessed October 19, 2019.

29. Furry friends family pet dog and cat visitation program: a guide for families. University of Iowa Health Care. Available at: https://uihc.org/sites/default/files/family_pet_visitation_brochure.pdf. Accessed December 5, 2017.

30. Pet visitation guide. Floyd medical center. Available at: https://www.floyd.org/patients-visitors/for-patients/Pages/Pet-Visitation-Guide.aspx. Accessed July 27, 2019.

31. Pet visitation policy. University of Pittsburgh medical center. Available at: https://www.upmc.com/patients-visitors/patient-info/during-your-stay#petvisitation. Accessed August 30, 2019.

32. Visitor information & Amenities. Aurora health care. Available at: https://www.aurorahealthcare.org/locations/hospital/aurora-medical-center-in-manitowoc-county/visitor-information-and-amenities. Accessed August 30, 2019.

33. Personal pet visitation. University of Florida Health. Available at: https://ufhealth.org/personal-pet-visitation. Accessed July 27, 2019.

34. Pet Visitation. Northern light eastern Maine Medical center. Available at: https://northernlighthealth.org/Locations/Eastern-Maine-Medical-Center/About-Us/About-Us-For-Visitors/Pet-Visitation. Accessed July 27, 2019.

35. Patient care policy and procedure manual – patient own pet visitation. Lauderdale Community Hospital. Available at: https://urldefense.proofpoint.com/v2/url?u=https-3A__health.ucsd.edu_PATIENTS_YOURHOSPITALSTAY_Pages_default.aspx&d=DwMFAg&c=iORugZls2LIYyCAZRB3XLg&r=TEelOOmXzVaeAYeMimUhgClS8GT0XGyvRQofJ6NiadY&m=c1efEdvkVzl4chUfbovA4Bf6yFl2XI7xFTYKT-fGi9k&s=KKyifmhWrdEmmvpMMoDtCUS08JHwqcxWe_T13svkMD0&e=. Accessed July 25, 2018.

36. Service dog and pet visitation. Dartmouth-Hitchcock. Available at: https://www.dartmouth-hitchcock.org/at-hospital/service-dog-pet-visitation.html. Accessed July 27, 2019.

37. Montana state hospital policy and procedure-visitation with personal pets. Montana State Hospital. Available at: https://dphhs.mt.gov/Portals/85/amdd/documents/MSH/volumeii/treatment/VisitationWithPersonalPets.pdf. Accessed July 27, 2019.

38. Pet visitation guidelines. Texas Rehabilitation Hospital of Fort Worth. Available at: http://texasrehabhospital.com/page/pet. Accessed July 27, 2019.

39. Patient and visitor guide. Spring View Hospital. Available at: https://www.springviewhospital.com/for-patients-and-visitors. Accessed July 27, 2019.

40. Policies-pet visitation. Aspen Valley Hospital. Available at: https://www.qualityhealthnd.org/wp-content/uploads/Aspen-Valley-Hospital-pet-visitation-policy.pdf. Accessed July 27, 2019.

41. Visitation guidelines. North Valley Hospital. Available at: https://www.krh.org/nvh/visitors/visitation-guidelines. Accessed July 27, 2019.
42. Hospital Resources-family pet center. Cincinnati Children's. Available at: https://www.cincinnatichildrens.org/patients/resources/pet-center. Accessed August 30, 2019.
43. Operational directives-pet therapy and pet visitation in acute care facilities. Winnipeg Regional Health Authority. Available at: http://www.wrha.mb.ca/extranet/ipc/files/manuals/acutecare/Rev1111_03.48.pdf. Accessed July 27, 2019.
44. Visiting A patient. Kingston General Hospital. Available at: http://www.kingstonhsc.ca/patients-families-and- visitors/visiting-patient. Accessed July 27, 2019.
45. Animal visitation. Covenant health. Available at: https://kingstonhsc.ca/patients-families-and-visitors/visiting-patient. Accessed July, 27, 2019.
46. Pet therapy and visitation. Interior Health. Available at: https://www.interiorhealth.ca/AboutUs/QualityCare/IPCManual/Pet%20Therapy%20and%20Visitation.pdf. Accessed July 27, 2019.
47. Visitor information. Halton Healthcare. Available at: https://www.haltonhealthcare.on.ca/patients/visitor-information. Accessed July 27, 2019.
48. Perth and smiths falls district hospital policy & procedure: accessibility-service animals, pet visitation and therapy dogs. Perth and Smiths Falls District Hospital. Available at: http://psfdh.on.ca/wp-content/uploads/2010/07/PSFDH-Policy-Procedure-Accessibility-Service-Animals-Pet-Visitation-and-Therapy-Dogs.pdf. Accessed July 27, 2019.
49. Animals at Mount Sinai Hospital. Sinai Health System. Available at: https://www.mountsinai.on.ca/about_us/accessibility/copy3_of_accessibility/Animals-At-Mount-Sinai-Hospital-Policy-Procedure-2016-Revisions_FINAL-aoda.pdf. Accessed July 27, 2019.
50. ADA Requirements: Service Animals. US Dept of Justice. Available at: https://www.ada.gov/service_animals_2010.htm. Accessed October 19, 2019.
51. Volunteer. PAWS Houston. Available at: https://www.pawshouston.org/volunteer.html. Accessed July 27, 2019.
52. Pet partners. Available at: https://petpartners.org. Accessed April 2, 2019.
53. Therapy dogs international. Available at: https://www.tdi-dog.org/default.aspx. Accessed March 2, 2019.
54. Alliance for therapy dogs. Available at: https://www.therapydogs.com. Accessed April 2, 2019.
55. Schmitz A, Beermann M, MacKenzie CR, et al. Animal-assisted therapy at a University Centre for Palliative Medicine - a qualitative content analysis of patient records. BMC Palliat Care 2017;16(1):50.
56. Halm MA. The healing power of the human-animal connection. Am J Crit Care 2008;17(4):373–6.
57. Harper CM, Dong Y, Thornhill TS, et al. Can therapy dogs improve pain and satisfaction after total joint arthroplasty? A randomized controlled trial. Clin Orthop Relat Res 2015;473(1):372–9.
58. Marcus DA, Bernstein CD, Constantin JM, et al. Animal-assisted therapy at an outpatient pain management clinic. Pain Med 2012;13(1):45–57.
59. Nahm N, Lubin J, Lubin J, et al. Therapy dogs in the emergency department. West J Emerg Med 2012;13(4):363–5.
60. McCullough A, Ruehrdanz A, Jenkins MA, et al. Measuring the effects of an animal-assisted intervention for pediatric oncology patients and their parents:

a multisite randomized controlled trial [Formula: see text]. J Pediatr Oncol Nurs 2018;35(3):159–77.

61. American Veterinary Medical Association. Available at: https://www.avma.org/KB/Policies/Pages/Animal- Assisted-Interventions-Definitions.aspx. Accessed March 1, 2019.

62. International Association of Human-Animal Interaction Organization. Available at: https://iahaio.org/wp/wp-content/uploads/2019/01/iahaio_wp_updated-2018-19-final.pdf. Accessed March 1, 2019.

63. Cole KM, Gawlinski A, Steers N, et al. Animal-assisted therapy in patients hospitalized with heart failure. Am J Crit Care 2007;16(6):575–85.

64. Phung A, Joyce C, Ambutas S, et al. Animal-assisted therapy for inpatient adults. Nursing 2017;47(1):63–6.

65. Waite TC, Hamilton L, O'Brien W. A meta-analysis of animal assisted interventions targeting pain, anxiety and distress in medical settings. Complement Ther Clin Pract 2018;33:49–55.

66. Abate SV, Zucconi M, Boxer BA. Impact of canine-assisted ambulation on hospitalized chronic heart failure patients' ambulation outcomes and satisfaction: a pilot study. J Cardiovasc Nurs 2011;26(3):224–30.

67. Nepps P, Stewart CN, Bruckno SR. Animal-assisted activity: effects of a complementary intervention program on psychological and physiological variables. J Evid Based Complementary Altern Med 2014;19(3):211–5.

68. Coakley AB, Mahoney EK. Creating a therapeutic and healing environment with a pet therapy program. Complement Ther Clin Pract 2009;15(3):141–6.

69. Braun C, Stangler T, Narveson J, et al. Animal-assisted therapy as a pain relief intervention for children. Complement Ther Clin Pract 2009;15(2):105–9.

70. Bolden L, Bentley D, Adkins S, et al. The effects of animal assisted therapy on perceived pain in patients with spinal cord injury. Arch Phys Med Rehabil 2017;98(10):679–90.

71. Engelman SR. Palliative care and use of animal-assisted therapy. Omega(Westport) 2013;67(1–2):63–7.

72. Puntillo KA, White C, Morris AB, et al. Patients' perceptions and responses to procedural pain: results from Thunder Project II. Am J Crit Care 2001;10(4):238–51.

73. Portenoy RK, Mehta Z, Ahmed E. Cancer pain management with opioids: optimizing analgesia. Waitham (MA): UpToDate; 2019.

74. Schweickert WD, Pohlman MC, Pohlman AS, et al. Early physical and occupational therapy in mechanically ventilated, critically ill patients: a randomised controlled trial. Lancet 2009;373(9678):1874–82.

75. Schaller SJ, Anstey M, Blobner M, et al. Early, goal-directed mobilisation in the surgical intensive care unit: a randomised controlled trial. Lancet 2016;388(10052):1377–88.

76. IsHak WW, Collison K, Danovitch I, et al. Screening for depression in hospitalized medical patients. J Hosp Med 2017;12(2):118–25.

77. Matuszek S. Animal-facilitated therapy in various patient populations: systematic literature review. Holist Nurs Pract 2010;24(4):187–203.

78. Chu CI, Liu CY, Sun CT, et al. The effect of animal-assisted activity on inpatients with schizophrenia. J Psychosoc Nurs Ment Health Serv 2009;47(12):42–8.

79. Odendaal JS. Animal-assisted therapy - magic or medicine? J Psychosom Res 2000;49(4):275–80.

80. Kaminski M, Pellino T, Wish J. Play and pets: the physical and emotional impact of child-life and pet therapy on hospitalized children. Children's Health Care 2002;31. https://doi.org/10.1207/S15326888CHC3104_5.

81. Hoffman OM, Lee AH, Wertenauer F, et al. Dog-assisted interventions significantly anxiety in hospitalized patients reduces anxiety in hospitalized patients with major depression. Eur J Integr Med 2009;1(3):145–8.

82. Calcaterra V, Veggiotti P, Palestrini C, et al. Post-operative benefits of animal-assisted therapy in pediatric surgery: a randomised study. PLoS One 2015; 10(6):e0125813.

83. Aoki J, Iwahashi K, Ishigooka J, et al. Evaluation of cerebral activity in the prefrontal cortex in mood[affective] disorders during animal-assisted therapy (AAT) by near-infrared spectroscopy (NIRS): a pilot study. Int J Psychiatry Clin Pract 2012;16(3):205–13.

84. Abrahamson K, Cai Y, Richards E, et al. Perceptions of a hospital-based animal assisted intervention program: an exploratory study. Complement Ther Clin Pract 2016;25:150–4.

85. Moretti F, De Ronchi D, Bernabei V, et al. Pet therapy in elderly patients with mental illness. Psychogeriatrics 2011;11(2):125–9.

86. DiSalvo H, Haiduven D, Johnson N, et al. Who let the dogs out? Infection control did: utility of dogs in health care settings and infection control aspects. Am J Infect Control 2006;34(5):301–7.

87. Barba BE. The positive influence of animals: animal-assisted therapy in acute care. Clin Nurse Spec 1995;9(4):199–202.

88. Bibbo J. Staff members' perceptions of an animal-assisted activity. Oncol Nurs Forum 2013;40(4):E320–6.

89. Pinto A, De Santis M, Moretti C, et al. Medical practitioners' attitudes towards animal assisted interventions. An Italian Survey. Complement Ther Med 2017; 33:20–6.

90. Crowley-Robinson, Blackshaw JK. Nursing home staffs' empathy for a missing therapy dog, their attitudes to animal assisted therapy programs and suitable dog breeds. Anthrozoos 1998;11(2):101–4.

91. Uglow LS. The benefits of an animal-assisted intervention service to patients and staff at a children's hospital. Br J Nurs 2019;28(8):509–15.

92. Linder DE, Siebens HC, Mueller MK, et al. Animal-assisted interventions: a national survey of health and safety policies in hospitals, eldercare facilities, and therapy animal organizations. Am J Infect Control 2017;45(8):883–7.

93. Animal assisted intervention international. Available at: https://aai-int.org/wp-content/uploads/2019/02/AAII-Standards-of-Practice.pdf. Accessed September 1, 2019.

94. Lefebvre SL, Golab GC, Christensen E, et al. Guidelines for animal-assisted interventions in health care facilities. Am J Infect Control 2008;36(2):78–85.

95. Centers for Disease Control and Prevention. Guideless for environmental infections control in health care facilities. Available at: https://www.cdc.gov/infectioncontrol/pdf/guidelines/environmental-guidelines-P.pdf. Accessed September 1, 2019.

96. Hardin P, Brown J, Wright ME. Prevention of transmitted infections in a pet therapy program: an exemplar. Am J Infect Control 2016;44(7):846–50.

97. Caprilli S, Messeri A. Animal-assisted activity at A. Meyer Children's Hospital: a pilot study. Evid Based Complement Alternat Med 2006;3(3):379–83.

98. Gagnon J, Bouchard F, Landry M, et al. Implementing a hospital-based animal therapy program for children with cancer: a descriptive study. Can Oncol Nurs J 2004;14(4):217–22.

99. American Academy of Allergy Asthma and Immunology. Available at: https://www.aaaai.org/conditions-and-treatments/allergies/pet-allergy. Accessed September 1, 2019.

100. Murthy R, Bearman G, Brown S, et al. Animals in healthcare facilities: recommendations to minimize potential risks. Infect Control Hosp Epidemiol 2015; 36(5):495–516.

101. Centers for disease control and preventions. Available at: https://www.cdc.gov/onehealth/basics/zoonotic-diseases.html. Accessed September 1, 2019.

102. Schuller S, Francey T, Hartmann K, et al. European consensus statement on leptospirosis in dogs and cats. J Small Anim Pract 2015;56(3):159–79.

103. Hogan PG, Mork RL, Boyle MG, et al. Interplay of personal, pet, and environmental colonization in households affected by community-associated methicillin-resistant Staphylococcus aureus. J Infect 2019;78(3):200–7.

104. Davis MF, Misic AM, Morris DO, et al. Genome sequencing reveals strain dynamics of methicillin-resistant Staphylococcus aureus in the same household in the context of clinical disease in a person and a dog. Vet Microbiol 2015; 180(3–4):304–7.

105. Overgaauw PA, van Knapen F. Veterinary and public health aspects of Toxocara spp. Vet Parasitol 2013;193(4):398–403.

106. Won KY, Kruszon-Moran D, Schantz PM, et al. National seroprevalence and risk factors for Zoonotic Toxocara spp. infection. Am J Trop Med Hyg 2008;79(4): 552–7.

107. Center for Disease Control and Preventions. Available at: https://www.cdc.gov/healthypets/diseases/ringworm.html. Accessed September 1, 2019.

108. Center for Disease Control and Prevention. Available at: https://www.cdc.gov/healthypets/outbreaks.html. Accessed September 1, 2019.

109. World Health Organization. Available at: https://www.who.int/rabies/epidemiology/en. Accessed September 1, 2019.

110. Center for Disease Control and Prevention. Available at: https://www.cdc.gov/rabies/location/usa/index.html. Accessed September 1, 2019.

Sleep in the Intensive Care Unit

Biological, Environmental, and Pharmacologic Implications for Nurses

Karin Reuter-Rice, PhD, NP, FCCM[a],*, Mary Grace McMurray, BA[b],
Elise Christoferson, BA[b], Haley Yeager, BSN, RN[c],
Brooke Wiggins, BSN, RN[d]

KEYWORDS

• Critical illness • Environment • Intensive care unit • Nursing • Sleep

KEY POINTS

- The biology of sleep and dysregulation of hormones such as cortisol and melatonin can negatively affect the quality of sleep.
- Environmental disruptors such as light and sound can greatly impact sleep.
- Pharmacologic interventions also contribute to sleep disruption, including oversedation with benzodiazepines.
- Improving sleep within the intensive care unit can have a positive effect in patient recovery.
- Important implications for nursing practice include assessing sleep disruptors, monitoring the sleep environment, and promoting a multicomponent sleep promoting protocols.

BACKGROUND

Sleep is a critical component of survival and, when disturbed, reduced, or disrupted, results in poorer health outcomes and socioeconomic burden. The United States does not specifically report the cost burden that sleep disruptions and disturbances have on the overall intensive care unit (ICU) cost. However, costs are reported to be as high as $74,144 per ICU hospitalization for mechanically ventilated patients and $33,500 for nonmechanically ventilated patients.[1] Documented ICU hospitalizations average

[a] Department of Pediatrics, Division of Pediatric Critical Care, Duke University School of Nursing, Duke University School of Medicine, Duke Institute for Brain Sciences 307 Trent Drive, Durham, NC 27710, USA; [b] Duke University School of Nursing, 307 Trent Drive, Durham, NC 27701, USA; [c] Indiana University Health Methodist Hospital, 1701 North Senate Avenue, Indianapolis, IN 46202, USA; [d] Vidant Medical Center, 2100 Stantonsburg Road, Greenville, NC 27834, USA
* Corresponding author.
E-mail address: karin.reuter-rice@duke.edu

Crit Care Nurs Clin N Am 32 (2020) 191–201
https://doi.org/10.1016/j.cnc.2020.02.002   **ccnursing.theclinics.com**
0899-5885/20/© 2020 Elsevier Inc. All rights reserved.

30.2 days for patients requiring mechanical ventilation and 19 days for nonmechanical ventilated pateints.[1] Therefore, length and costs of ICU hospitalizations may be greatly impacted by unappreciated sleep disruption, thereby contributing to the cost burden.[2] The potential to decrease health care spending and improve health outcomes in the ICU can be addressed by promoting sleep in the ICU.

Poor sleep is a common complaint as well as a prevalent source of distress for many critically ill patients and their families.[2] A survey conducted with adult ICU patients found that the most common barriers to sleep included light levels, high levels of overnight noise, discomfort and pain, being awoken for procedures, being attached to medical devices, and stress and anxiety.[3] The 2018 published *Clinical Practice Guidelines for the Prevention and Management of Pain, Agitation/Sedation, Delirium, Immobility, and Sleep Disruption in Adult Patients in the ICU* addresses factors unique to ICU patients and their families. The guidelines specifically call out and describe factors that contribute to patient-perceived poor quality sleep.[2] Reported factors that disrupt sleep include physiologic, pathophysiologic, psychological, psychosocial, sensory, environmental, and health care provider related (**Fig. 1, Table 1**). Furthermore, the interaction between critical illness, medications, delirium, and sleep is complex and becoming an increasingly prevalent area of research focus.[2] Sleep disruption has been found to contribute to emotional distress, prolonged duration of mechanical ventilation, ICU delirium, disrupted immune function, and neurocognitive dysfunction.[2] This review examines risk factors associated with disrupted sleep and provide evidence-based nursing approaches that may be used to improve sleep in the ICU.

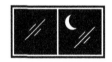

Sensory/Environmental

Physiological/Pathophysiological

Provider-Driven

Psychological/Psychosocial

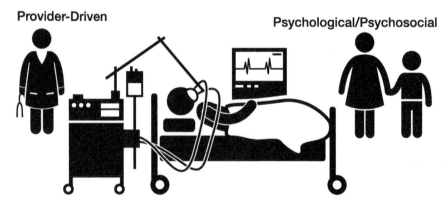

Fig. 1. Patient-reported sleep disruptors in the ICU. This figure illustrates primary categories that contribute to disruptive sleep.

Table 1
Sleep disruptors reported by ICU patients

Environmental	Physiologic and Pathophysiologic
Noise (447, 453, 454, 480, 483–488, 490, 491)	Pain (454, 483–486, 488, 490, 491)
Light (241, 453, 454, 480, 482–484, 486–488)	Discomfort (454, 483, 486, 488, 490)
Comfort of bed (483, 486–488)	Feeling too hot or too cold (484, 486, 488)
Activities at other bedsides (483, 486, 487)	Breathing difficulty (484, 491)
Visitors (clinician or family) (483)	Coughing (484, 491)
Room ventilation system (483)	Thirst (484, 486) and hunger (486, 488)
Hand washing by clinicians (483)	Nausea (484, 488)
Bad odor (486, 488)	Needing to use bedpan/urinal (486, 488)
Care Related	**Psychological**
Nursing care (447, 453, 480, 482–484, 486, 488, 491)	Anxiety/worry/stress (483, 484, 486, 489–491)
Patient procedures (447, 453, 480, 482, 483, 487, 488)	Fear (485, 486, 489)
Vital sign measurement (442, 448, 475, 477, 481, 483)	Unfamiliar environment (485, 488, 491)
Diagnostic tests (447, 453, 480, 483)	Disorientation to time (454, 486)
Medication administration (447, 453, 480, 482)	Loneliness (488, 491)
Restricted mobility from lines/catheters (454, 486, 488)	Lack of privacy (485, 488)
Monitoring equipment (454, 486, 488)	Hospital attire (486, 488)
Oxygen mask (486, 488)	Missing bedtime routine (483)
Endotracheal tube (491)	Not knowing nurses' names (486)
Urinary catheters (486)	Not understanding medical terms (486)

From Devlin JW, Skrobik Y, Gélinas C, et al. Clinical practice guidelines for the prevention and management of pain, agitation/sedation, delirium, immobility, and sleep disruption in adult patients in the ICU. Crit Care Med 2018;46(9):e854; with permission.

THE BIOLOGY OF SLEEP

Sleep disruption is described as changes to baseline sleep such as total sleep time, sleep architecture, and circadian rhythm.[4] The sleep cycle consists of 2 types of sleep: rapid eye movement (REM) and non-REM (NREM).[5] Each cycle helps to aid in recovery from illness.[5,6] REM sleep promotes emotional recovery, brain restoration, and growth, whereas NREM sleep is associated with physical recovery and growth.[5,6] Furthermore, NREM sleep can be described by 3 sequential categories (*N1*, *N2*, and *N3*). The first stage is *N1* sleep, which is typified by physical drowsiness and reduced muscle activity. This stage is followed by *N2*, which makes up the majority of the NREM cycle and is characterized by a decreased level of consciousness; however, individuals can still be easily awakened by noise.[7] The third and last stage is *N3*, which consists of slow-wave activity and is the most restful stage of sleep.[7] In NREM sleep, the body secretes the growth hormone that stimulates the building of proteins needed for cell repair and cell growth.[5] Furthermore, both REM and NREM sleep deprivation are associated with depression, irritability, disorientation, and combativeness.[5,6] More specifically, NREM sleep deprivation is associated with immunosuppression, decreased tissue repair, decreased pain tolerance, and fatigue on the sympathetic nervous system.[2,5]

In a typical circadian rhythm, several hormones are produced or inhibited to promote adequate sleep. First, cortisol decreases throughout the day time hours, with the lowest level typically reached around midnight.[8] Then around 2 to 3 AM, cortisol levels begin to increase again and peak at approximately 9 AM.[8] Chronic exposure to increased levels of cortisol, such as in Cushing's disease, has been shown to lead to reduced slow-wave sleep and shortened REM latency.[9] Similarly, when an ill individual's body is under an extreme amount of stress, such as when fighting an infection, glucocorticoids are elevated, thus negatively impacting sleep.[8] As cortisol levels begin to increase, this causes increases in electroencephalogram frequency, decreases in short-wave sleep, and consequently an increase in light sleep and wakening.[10] Second, melatonin is a naturally occurring hormone released by the pineal gland and, like cortisol, affects sleep regulation.[11] Melatonin provides feedback to the body's circadian rhythm and plays a critical role in sleep wake cycles.[11] Melatonin, regulated primarily through light, will demonstrate peak blood levels during the night and the lowest levels during the day.[11] Although research findings focused on melatonin levels in critically ill patients remain inconsistent, Olofsson and colleagues[12] found that in 7 of 8 critically ill adult ICU patients studied, rhythmicity of melatonin secretion was disturbed and nearly nonexistent.

INTENSIVE CARE UNIT ENVIRONMENT AND SLEEP

Although attempts to regulate the biologic response to illness and to promote sleep are often part of the ICU patient's care plan, independent variables such as light and sound often lack consideration within that plan.[13] The ICU is often described as a chaotic and busy 24-hour care environment.[14] ICU patients, when asked, report that intense lighting and high levels of noise contribute to their disrupted sleep.[14] Freedman and team[15] examined 22 adult medical ICU patients and found that, in a 24-hour period, ICU patients had a mean total sleep time of 8.8 hours, with less than 50% of those sleep hours occurring during the night. When they further examined the sleep patterns they found that patient slept in 15-minutes periods and that environmental noise was responsible for 17% of sleep awakenings.[15] A review conducted by Calandriello and colleagues[16] identified environmental factors (eg, light, noise, intrusive monitoring, and interventions) and medication administration to influence sleep disruption and delirium risk in pediatric ICU (PICU) patients. And in another study, which examined 12 children 13 to 35 months of age who were admitted to a PICU, researchers determined that patients lost up to 54% of their normal expected amount of sleep as a result of both external and physiologic environmental stimuli.[17]

Light

Light is the most important environmental factor that alters the circadian rhythm and melatonin secretion.[18] Continuous exposure to artificial light can disrupt the circadian rhythm and diminish the normal peak in endogenous melatonin secretion at night.[6] More specifically, blue light has a greater tendency to diminish melatonin secretion.[19] Exposure to blue light also alters vital signs by increasing heart rate and temperature.[19] Patients seem to report greater satisfaction when placed in a room with natural light. For example, placing a patient in an ICU in a room with a window was found to result in shorter hospital stays.[20] Furthermore, windows providing an outside view may help to relieve anxiety and stress, improve care, enhance patient comfort, and improve patient orientation.[21] The Guidelines for ICU Design recommend that each patient care space should have at least one window of appropriate size with visual access to the outdoors, other than skylights.[21]

The suppression of melatonin and, therefore, a disrupted circadian rhythm, reduces the immune response.[19] This alteration, in conjunction with poor sleep, places a greater stress on the body and prevents the brain from recovering.[18] Disruption of the normal 24-hour light–dark cycle that influences the circadian rhythm increases morbidity and mortality and is related to fragmented sleep, increased delirium, and delayed recovery from illness.[18]

Sound

High levels of noise are a significant barrier to sleep for patients in the ICU. The World Health Organization recommends that noise levels remain below 35 dB to ensure adequate sleep.[22] However, a PICU study found that the average noise level was greater than 48 dB, with the highest noise level reaching 103 dB.[23] In contrast, a study examining 5 adult ICUs found that the average sound levels across all ICUs consistently exceeded 45 dB and for 50% of the time sound levels exceeded 59 dB.[24] They also appreciated a diurnal variation with sound levels decreasing with overnight to an average minimum of 51 dB at 4 AM.[24] Peaks of greater than 85 dB occurred at all sites up to 16 times per hour overnight and more frequently during the day.[24] More important, these investigators determined that they could only achieve World Health Organization guidelines sound levels by turning off all ICU equipment.[24]

In the ICU, noise levels may escalate depending on the unit's acuity and architectural configuration. A 2008 study in the medical ICU focused on activities attributable to high noise levels and found that the highest noise levels on the unit were associated with footsteps coming from both patient rooms and the hallways (84 dB), staff conversations (74 dB), and vacuum cleaners (64 dB).[25] Adult patients also commented that noise from other patients and noise from recurring alarms were highly disruptive.[25] In another study that included 13 adult ICU patients, 21% of arousals and awakenings were found to be a result of noise peaks on the unit.[26] High noise levels clearly decrease the amount of time a patient sleeps while in the ICU.[26] Furthermore, frequent disruptions in sleep result in a decrease in the time spent in both NREM and REM sleep.[15] With noise levels consistently being well above the recommended levels, it is not surprising that patients in the ICU have disrupted sleep and risk for ICU delirium and post-traumatic stress disorder (PTSD).

MEDICATION EFFECTS ON SLEEP

During the acute phase of an illness or injury, the ICU team's focus is on patient stability and safety, often involving the use of medical devices and sedation and analgesic medications. In addition, the unfamiliar environment as well as the uncomfortable and at times painful medical devices and treatments can result in the need for even more sedation and pain-controlling medications. These medications and the ICU environment together can result in sleep disturbances. Sleep disturbance includes sleep disorders such as initiating and maintaining sleep (eg, insomnia), excessive somnolence, reversal of sleep–wake schedule, and sleep dysfunction (eg, parasomnias). Medications frequently used in the ICU cause decreased slow-wave and REM sleep phases.[27] When these sleep phases are decreased or interrupted, it places the patient at higher risk for sleep disturbance.[28] Examples of medications that decrease slow-wave and REM sleep phases include benzodiazepines, opioids, norepinephrine, and corticosteroids.[27] Bourne and Mills[27] offer insight into approaches that health care providers such as nurses can use to assess for medication interactions affecting sleep and appropriate sedation scoring systems to monitor for withdrawal symptoms. Additionally, daily assessment and evaluation of a patient's medications by nurses allows for advocacy of sleep-promoting agents over sleep-disrupting agents. Wetter and team[29] found that missed opportunities to promote sleep can often occur with patients who are habit-ually regulated to the use of daily stimulants; for example, patients with a history of chronic smoking experienced better sleep when nicotine patches were prescribed. Medication reconciliation is a critical activity that can promote sleep because it de-creases the number of ineffective or discontinued medications that can interact with or reduce sleep.[27] There is a common misconception that benzodiazepines increase the quality of sleep. Conversely, Bourne and Mills[27] explain that, although benzodi-azepines often prolong stage 2 of NREM sleep initially, they make it more difficult for patients to transition into stage 4 NREM, which is the most restful phase of the cycle. Therefore, medication reconciliation, appropriate use of sedation, sedation and pain scoring systems, and sleep tracking can all improve ICU patient sleep.[30]

EFFECTS OF SLEEP DISRUPTION AND DISTURBANCES

Health care systems have yet to fully appreciate the negative impact of sleep disrup-tions on ICU patients and its importance in recovery.[3] Poor sleep quality in the ICU directly and negatively impacts several body systems.[31] For example, decreased sleep has been linked to increased rates of upper airway collapse, which can lead to challenges in the extubation of mechanically ventilated patients.[31] In addition, insuf-ficient sleep has been found to elevate rates of catecholamines, thereby resulting in blood pressure lability and increased risk for myocardial infarction.[31]

Sleep disruption has been associated with pain.[32] By definition, pain is an unpleas-ant sensory and emotional experience associated with actual or potential tissue dam-age and is considered to be whatever the patient says it is.[33,34] Medical interventions, especially those performed in ICU patients, are associated with pain as a side effect, which then contributes to poor sleep.[35] Sleep disruption is a known associate of pain. Longitudinal studies have demonstrated sleep disruption to linearly predict next-day pain reports in patients with depression and older adults.[36,37] Although some ICU pa-tients are unable to self-report their pain, nurses are still encouraged to use validated behavioral pain scales to determine a patient's pain level.[2] Severe pain negatively im-pacts a patient's health status and can contribute to cardiac instability, immunosup-pression, and respiratory compromise.[2] Furthermore, pain can affect a patient's sleep quality in the ICU, thereby leading to risk for poorer ICU outcomes.[2]

Additionally, there are psychological impacts of sleep disruption, including PTSD.[28] The diagnosis of PTSD in ICU patients has been associated with delirium and sleep disruption. Davydow and team[28] reviewed data on the prevalence of PTSD in general ICU survivors, risk factors for post-ICU PTSD and the impact of post-ICU PTSD on health-related quality of life.[28] They included 15 studies in their review and determined that the prevalence of PTSD in ICU survivors was high and that it negatively impacted their health-related quality of life.[28] Specifically, they found that 20% of patients re-ported clinically significant symptoms of PTSD within 1 year of discharge.[28] They also recommended that early recognition of PTSD and ICU delirium could potentially mitigate PTSD.[28]

ICU delirium is a noticeable change in a patient's neurocognitive baseline with an acute disturbance in attention, awareness, and cognition.[38] It is also an alteration in both cogni-tion and arousal.[38] Three delirium subtypes exist among ICU patients: hyperactive, hypoactive, and mixed. Hyperactive delirium is characterized by agitation and aggression.[38] Hypoactive delirium is characterized by a decrease in mental status and lethargy.[38] Mixed delirium, also known as emerging delirium, presents with signs of both hyperactive and hypoactive delirium.[38]

ICU delirium, a severe complication of critical illness, is associated with adverse short-term outcomes.[2,39–41] These outcomes include up to a 3-fold increase in length of hospitalization stay and hospital mortality.[39] In addition, delirium can be disturbing for both affected patients and their families.[2] Delirium is a prevalent problem in both the adult ICU and the PICU. A study of 818 surgical ICU patients reported that 11% were diagnosed ICU delirium,[42] whereas in the PICU, up to 30% of patients were reported to experience ICU delirium.[43]

Sleep disruptions contribute to ICU delirium and vice versa, because they share similar physiologic mechanisms, which include the imbalance in melatonin production and neurotransmitters.[44] Alterations in melatonin secretion were detected in a study that included 41 ICU patients who underwent thoracic esophagectomy.[45] When serum melatonin levels were measured every 6 hours over 4 days, investigators noted that irregular patterns of melatonin secretion were associated with the development of ICU delirium in the 11 patients (26.8%).[45] Although the ICU delirious patients were more likely to have abnormally low melatonin levels when compared with the patients without ICU delirium, the differences were not significant.[45] The study team concluded that this was due to the sample size.[45] Additionally, studies have explored genetic predisposition and patient outcomes in patients with ICU delirium. One study showed a significant association between the apolipoprotein E4 genotype and a longer duration of ICU delirium.[46] Although more studies are required to articulate the physiologic and genomic mechanisms and outside factors that contribute to ICU delirium, it is reasonable to consider that barriers to quality sleep in ICU patients contribute to ICU delirium and should be addressed as a part of ICU care.

IMPLICATIONS FOR NURSING

Increased attention to the role of sleep and ICU delirium have led to interventions to reduce sleep disruption. By identifying patient-reported sleep disruptors in the ICU (see **Fig. 1**, **Table 1**), nurses are better prepared to advocate and provide clustered nursing care. The clustering of care eliminates and minimizes potential disruptors, which can promote a better quality of sleep for the critically ill patient. The 2013 *Clinical Practice Guidelines for Pain, Agitation, and Delirium (PAD) in Adult Patients in the ICU* recommend optimizing patients' environments, using strategies to control light and noise, clustering patient care activities, and decreasing night-time stimuli.[47] Nonpharmacologic ICU interventions include maintaining structure and continuity in the patient's schedule, reduced mid-day lighting during a 2-hour quiet time period, and involving the family members in the patient's care.[43]

Although health care providers can agree that sleep disruption is a problem for ICU patients and their families, 1 global ICU study found many ICUs did not have sleep promotion protocols in place. Of the more than 1223 surveys administered across 24 countries, only 32% of respondents reported having sleep-promoting protocols currently in place.[48] Reasons listed by the study participants included variables that the providers felt were out of their control, such as allowing patients uninterrupted blocks of time for sleep as well as noise control and light regulation.[48] Additionally, units that implemented a sleep protocol indicated they were better able to control lighting conditions and environmental noise levels, assess whether their patients were getting enough sleep, delay nonemergency disturbances to allow their patients to sleep, adhere to a clustered ICU sleep protocol, and create dedicated sleeping conditions for stable patients.[48]

Nurses are posited as leaders in changing sleep disruptive ICU protocols. Nurses spend more minutes of care per patient than any other health care provider.[49] Therefore, nurses are well-positioned to engage in the development of sleep protective multicomponent protocols that will positively impact patient outcomes. Multicomponent protocols have been tested successfully with promising results in non-ICU patients and have been recommended for use in the critically ill.[2,50,51] Sleep-promoting protocols may include earplugs, eyeshades, and/or discouraging the use of sedating medications known to alter sleep that can cause ICU delirium.[2]

Nonpharmacologic interventions have been both recommended and discouraged to improve sleep for critically ill ICU patients. First, using assist-control ventilation at night (vs pressure support ventilation) for critically ill adults on mechanical ventilation has been determined to improve sleep.[2] In contrast, aromatherapy, acupressure, or music at night are not recommended as interventions to improve sleep in critically ill adults.[2] In 2 small randomized control trial studies, no measurable benefit was found by using aromatherapy or acupuncture to improve sleep.[2] Additionally, 1 study raised concern that aromatherapy had a negative impact on the respiratory system.[2] The use of nonpharmacologic interventions to decrease or alleviate pain, such as with holistic pain care approaches (eg, massage, music therapy, cold therapy for procedural pain management, and relaxation techniques related to breathing) have been found to assist with sleep promotion.[2] A study involving patients who complained of sleep disturbances and the use of nonpharmacologic sleep interventions (eg, back rubs, warm drinks, and relaxation tapes), reported the number of interventions provided strongly correlated with increased rates of quality sleep.[50] Although a warm drink may not be feasible for some ICU patients, the others nonpharmacologic interventions may be an option for ICU patients to promote sleep and have a positive clinical impact.[50]

Although sleep disruptions occur in ICU patients, their family members are also impacted. Day and colleagues[52] found that the majority of ICU family members reported moderate to severe sleep disturbances, fatigue, and mild anxiety using validated self-report tools. Additionally, more than 65% of participants in the study reported having difficulty sleeping during their family member's ICU admission.[52] Furthermore, sleep spaces and surfaces for family members within a patient's room in the ICU can be limited, further contributing to sleep deprivation and sleep disturbances.[53] The burden of sleep disturbances and sleep deprivation for family members may have dramatic consequences, specifically because sleep deprivation may interfere with decision-making and care-taking abilities.[52] The Family-Centered Care Guidelines recommend providing sufficient sleep space for family members within any hospital setting.[54] To promote sleep and decrease anxiety, nurses can use bidirectional communication to encourage family and care team awareness as to the patients' status, treatment plan, and level of fatigue of family members. Therapeutic listening as well as strategies to assist families with stress reduction may include relaxation techniques, meditation, visual imagery, or referrals for psychosocial support.[52]

SUMMARY

Studies consistently demonstrate that poor sleep is a problem for critically ill patients. Evidence exists that conditions in the ICU environment play a significant role in a patient's sleep quality. Although ICUs are not a conducive environment that promotes sleep, nurse-led standardized protocols and nonpharmacologic interventions can drastically decrease the incidence of sleep disturbances and delirium in the ICU.

The importance of identifying and mitigating environmental and other factors that disrupt sleep are critical to improving the health outcomes and recovery of critically ill patients. Multicomponent, protocolized, nonpharmacologically focused approaches to improving sleep may offer ICU patients and their families their best opportunity for a higher quality and quantity of sleep.[2] Future research should focus on articulating the linkages between sleep, delirium, PTSD, and potential genetic predispositions in ICU patients. More effective methods for measuring sleep and the ICU environment would allow us to develop intervention strategies and new models for ICU sleep promotion.

ACKNOWLEDGMENTS

The authors thank Keeley Phillips Hall, RN, BSN, Duke University Health System, for her contributions to the article outline; and Karen Judge, Senior Program Coordinator, Duke University School of Nursing, for her contribution of the graphic titled "Patient-Reported Sleep Disruptors in the ICU." HARD Manufacturing – World Federation of Pediatric Intensive and Critical Care Societies (WFPICCS) Pediatric Critical Care Research Grant (2019-2020).

DISCLOSURE

The authors have nothing to disclose.

REFERENCES

1. Dasta JF, McLaughlin TP, Mody SH, et al. Daily cost of an intensive care unit day: the contribution of mechanical ventilation. Crit Care Med 2005;33(6):1266–71.
2. Devlin JW, Skrobik Y, Gélinas C, et al. Clinical practice guidelines for the prevention and management of pain, agitation/sedation, delirium, immobility, and sleep disruption in adult patients in the ICU. Crit Care Med 2018;46(9):e825–73.
3. Stewart JA, Green C, Stewart J, et al. Factors influencing quality of sleep among non-mechanically ventilated patients in the intensive care unit. Aust Crit Care 2017;30(2):85–90.
4. Schieveld JNM, Ista E, Knoester H, et al. Pediatric delirium: a practical approach. In: Rey JM, Martin A, editors. IACAPAP e-textbook of child and adolescent mental health. Geneva (CH): International Association for Child and Adolescent Psychiatry and Allied Professions; 2015. p. 1–17.
5. Ibarra-Coronado EG, Pantaleón-Martinez AM, Velazquéz-Moctezuma J, et al. The bidirectional relationship between sleep and immunity against infections. J Immunol Res 2015;2015:1–14.
6. Kudchakar SR, Barnes S, Anton B, et al. Non-pharmacological interventions for sleep promotion in hospitalized children. Cochrane Database Syst Rev 2017; 12:1–15.
7. Delaney LJ, Haren FV, Lopez V. Sleeping on a problem: the impact of sleep disturbance on intensive care patients - a clinical review. Ann Intensive Care 2015; 5(3):1–10.
8. Carley DW, Farabi SS. Physiology of sleep. Diabetes Spectr 2016;29(1):5–9.
9. Hirotsu C, Tufik S, Andersen ML. Interactions between sleep, stress, and metabolism: from physiological to pathological conditions. Sleep Sci 2015;8(3):143–52.
10. Bush B, Hudson T. The role of cortisol in sleep. Nat Med J 2010;2(6). Available at: https://www.naturalmedicinejournal.com/journal/2010-06/role-cortisol-sleep. Accessed August 22, 2019.

11. Brown GM. Light, melatonin and the sleep-wake cycle. J Psychiatry Neurosci 1994;19(5):345–53.
12. Olofsson K, Alling C, Lundberg D, et al. Abolished circadian rhythm of melatonin secretion in sedated and artificially ventilated intensive care patients. Acta Anaesthesiol Scand 2004;48(6):679–84.
13. Boyko Y, Jennum P, Toft P. Sleep quality and circadian rhythm disruption in the intensive care unit: a review. Nat Sci Sleep 2017;9:277–84.
14. Pulak LM, Jensen L. Sleep in the intensive care unit: a review. J Intensive Care Med 2016;31(1):14–23.
15. Freedman NS, Gazendam J, Levan L, et al. Abnormal sleep/wake cycles and the effect of environmental noise on sleep disruption in the intensive care unit. Am J Respir Crit Care Med 2001;163(2):451–7.
16. Calandriello A, Tylka JC, Patwari PP. Sleep and delirium in pediatric critical illness: what is the relationship? Med Sci (Basel) 2018;6(90):1–17.
17. Corser NC. Sleep of 1-and 2-year old children in intensive care. Issues Compr Pediatr Nurs 1996;19(1):17–31.
18. Durrington HJ, Clark R, Greer R, et al. 'In a dark place, we find ourselves': light intensity in critical care units. Intensive Care Med Exp 2017;5(9):1–5.
19. Castro R, Angus DC, Rosengart MR. The effect of light on critical illness. Crit Care 2011;15(2):218.
20. Kohn R, Harhay MO, Cooney E, et al. Do windows or natural views affect outcomes of cost among patients in ICUs? Crit Care Med 2013;41(7):1645–55.
21. Thompson DR, Hamilton DK, Cadenhead CD, et al. Guidelines for intensive care unit design. Crit Care Med 2012;40(5):1586–600.
22. World Health Organization. Data and statistics. In: WHO health Topics: environment and health: noise. 2009. Available at: http://www.euro.who.int/en/health-topics/environment-and-health/noise/data-and-statistics. Accessed August 21, 2019.
23. Al-Samsam RH, Cullen P. Sleep and adverse environmental factors in sedated mechanically ventilated pediatric intensive care patients. Pediatr Crit Care Med 2005;6(5):562–7.
24. Darbyshire JL, Young JD. An investigation of sound levels on intensive care units with reference to the WHO guidelines. Crit Care 2013;17(5):R187.
25. Akansel N, Kaymakci S. Effects of intensive care unit noise on patients: a study on coronary artery bypass graft surgery patients. J Clin Nurs 2008;17(12):1581–90.
26. Gabor JY, Cooper AB, Crombach SA, et al. Contribution of the intensive care unit environment to sleep disruption in mechanically ventilated patients and healthy subjects. Am J Respir Crit Care Med 2003;167(5):708–15.
27. Bourne RS, Mills GH. Sleep disruption in critically ill patients - pharmacological considerations. Anaesthesia 2004;59(4):374–84.
28. Davydow DS, Gifford JM, Desai SV, et al. Posttraumatic stress disorder in general intensive care unit survivors: a systematic review. Gen Hosp Psychiatry 2008; 30(5):421–34.
29. Wetter DW, Fiore MC, Baker TB, et al. Tobacco withdrawal and nicotine replacement influence objective measures of sleep. J Consult Clin Psychol 1995;63(4):658–67.
30. Medrzycka-Dabrowska W, Lewandowska K, Kwiecień-Jaguś K, et al. Sleep deprivation in intensive care unit – systematic review. Open Med (Wars) 2018; 13:384–93.
31. Kamdar, Needham DM, Collop NA. Sleep deprivation in critical illness: its role in physical and psychological recovery. J Intensive Care Med 2012;27(2):97–111.
32. Finan PH, Goodin BR, Smith MT. The association of sleep and pain: an update and a path forward. J Pain 2013;14(12):1539–52.

33. Loeser JD, Treede RD. The Kyoto protocol of IASP basic pain terminology. Pain 2008;137:473–7.
34. McCaffery M, Alexander AB. Pain: clinical manual for nursing practice. Saint Louis (MO): Mosby; 1994.
35. Doufas AG, Panagiotou OA, Ioannidis JP. Concordance of sleep and pain outcomes of diverse interventions: an umbrella review. PLoS One 2012;7(7):e40891.
36. Chung KF, Tso KC. Relationship between insomnia and pain in major depressive disorder: a sleep diary and actigraphy study. Sleep Med 2010;11:752–8.
37. Dzierzewski JM, Williams JM, Roditi D, et al. Daily variations in objective nighttime sleep and subjective morning pain in older adults with insomnia: evidence of covariation over time. J Am Geriatr Soc 2010;58:925–30.
38. American Psychiatric Association. Diagnostic and statistical manual of mental disorders. 5th edition. Washington, DC: American Psychiatric Association; 2013.
39. Ely EW, Shintani A, Truman B, et al. Delirium as a predictor of mortality in mechanically ventilated patients in the intensive care unit. JAMA 2004;291(14):1753–62.
40. Lin S, Liu C, Wang C, et al. The impact of delirium on the survival of mechanically ventilated patients. Crit Care Med 2004;32(11):2254–9.
41. Pompei P, Foreman M, Rudberg MA, et al. Delirium in hospitalized older persons: outcomes and predictors. J Am Geriatr Soc 1994;42(8):809–15.
42. Aldemir M, Ozen S, Kara IH, et al. Predisposing factors for delirium in the surgical intensive care unit. Crit Care 2001;5(5):265–70.
43. Bettencourt A, Mullen JE. Delirium in children: identification, prevention and management. Crit Care Nurse 2017;37(3):e9–18.
44. Figueroa-Ramos MI, Arroyo-Novoa CM, Lee KA, et al. Sleep and delirium in ICU patients: a review of mechanisms and manifestations. Intensive Care Med 2009; 35(5):781–5.
45. Miyazaki T, Kuwano H, Kato H, et al. Correlation between serum melatonin circadian rhythm and intensive care unit psychosis after thoracic esophagectomy. Surgery 2003;133:662–8.
46. Ely EW, Girard TD, Shintani AK, et al. Apolipoprotein E4 polymorphism as a genetic predisposition to delirium in critically ill patients. Crit Care Med 2007;35:112–7.
47. Barr J, Fraser GL, Puntillo K, et al. Clinical practice guidelines for the management of pain, agitation, and delirium in adult patients in the intensive care unit. Crit Care Med 2013;41(1):263–306.
48. Kamdar BB, Knauert MP, Jones SF, et al. Perceptions and practices regarding sleep in the intensive care unit. A Survey of 1,223 critical care providers. Ann Am Thorac Soc 2016;13(8):1370–7.
49. Butler R, Monsalve M, Thomas GW, et al. Estimating time physicians and other health care workers spend with patients in an intensive care unit using a sensor network. Am J Med 2018;131(8). 972.e9–972.e15.
50. McDowell JA, Mion LC, Lydon TJ, et al. A non-pharmacologic sleep protocol for hospitalized older patients. J Am Geriatr Soc 1998;46(6):700–5.
51. Hu RF, Jiang XY, Chen J, et al. Non-pharmacological interventions for sleep promotion in the intensive care unit. Cochrane Database Syst Rev 2015;10:1–98.
52. Day A, Haj-Bakri S, Lubchansky S, et al. Sleep, anxiety and fatigue in family members of patients admitted to the intensive care unit: a questionnaire study. Crit Care 2013;17(3):1–7.
53. Huynh TG, Owens RL, Davidson JE. Impact of built design on nighttime family presence in the intensive care unit. HERD 2020;13(1):106–13.
54. Davidson JE, Aslakson RA, Long AC, et al. Guidelines for family-centered care in the neonatal, pediatric, and adult ICU. Crit Care Med 2017;45(1):103–28.

Implementation of a Patient and Family-Centered Intensive Care Unit Peer Support Program at a Veterans Affairs Hospital

Leanne M. Boehm, PhD, RN, ACNS-BC[a,b,c,*],
Kelly Drumright, MSN, CNL, CCRN-CMC, CSC[b], Ralph Gervasio[b],
Christopher Hill, MDiv[b], Nancy Reed, LCSW[b]

KEYWORDS

- Critical illness • Intensive care • Post-intensive care syndrome (PICS) • Peer support

KEY POINTS

- Postintensive care syndrome is decidedly prevalent among intensive care unit survivors.
- Peer support programs are a recommended method to alleviate the anxiety, post-traumatic stress disorder, and depressive symptoms associated with postintensive care syndrome.
- Implementation of a peer support program at a Veterans Affairs hospital was well-received by patient and family member participants.

INTRODUCTION

Increasing numbers of survivors of critical illness have also resulted in the recognition of long-term impairments to physical function, mental health, and cognitive function lasting for months to years after a critical illness.[1] This constellation of physical, mental health, and cognitive impairments is referred to as postintensive care syndrome (PICS) with elements prevalent in up to 80% of intensive care unit (ICU) survivors.[2,3] In addition, family members and support persons for ICU survivors experience a cluster of anxiety, post-traumatic stress disorder, and depressive symptoms referred to as PICS-family (PICS-F).[2] Peer support has been recommended as a novel strategy to alleviate PICS for ICU survivors and family members.[4] Peer support programs provide

[a] Vanderbilt University School of Nursing, 461 21st Avenue South, Nashville, TN, USA; [b] TN Valley Healthcare System, Nashville Veterans Affairs Hospital, 1310 24th Avenue South, Nashville, TN, USA; [c] Critical Illness, Brain Dysfunction, and Survivorship Center at Vanderbilt, 2525 West end Avenue, Suite 450, Nashville, TN, USA
* Corresponding author. 461 21st Avenue South, 419 Godchaux Hall, Nashville, TN.
E-mail address: Leanne.boehm@vanderbilt.edu

Crit Care Nurs Clin N Am 32 (2020) 203–210
https://doi.org/10.1016/j.cnc.2020.02.003
0899-5885/20/© 2020 Elsevier Inc. All rights reserved.

a community for the promotion of health and well-being for those suffering from PICS and PICS-F via shared experiences of critical illness and recovery.[4]

The purpose of this project was to implement a peer support program at the Nashville Veterans Affairs Medical Center (VAMC) to build an ICU recovery community and provide counseling, stress management, and coping skill development for patients and family members.

METHODS
Context

The Nashville VAMC is a tertiary hospital providing care to veterans in middle Tennessee and southern Kentucky. Nashville VAMC has both medical and surgical ICUs equaling 20 critical care beds in total. Beginning in October 2016, we have participated in the Society of Critical Care Medicine international THRIVE Peer Support Collaborative bringing together clinicians implementing peer support programs to improve patient and caregiver outcomes after a critical illness.

Intervention

A multidisciplinary team including social work, pastoral care, a clinical nurse leader, nurse management, and a quality improvement specialist was formed in June 2016 to develop the peer support intervention for a veteran population. Multidisciplinary planning occurred from June through October 2016. Peer support groups were implemented late October 2016 after an open house to introduce our initiative goals and needs to the executive leadership, faculty, and hospital staff (both ICU and non-ICU providers and nurses). The final structure for peer support group implementation is as follows.

Meeting location

Factors influencing determination of location of the meeting included transportation options provided by the VAMC, ease of finding location, consistent availability, and promotes comfort and sharing. After discussion of on- and off-site meeting locations it was determined to hold peer support meetings in the medical ICU family consultation room because this was the only comfortable room easily located, consistently available for a standing meeting, and familiar to participants.

Meeting frequency and time

Staff availability, release time for peer support group meetings, and schedules were important factors in determining meeting frequency and time. We also considered unit turnover and our desire to provide counseling, stress management, and coping skill development to as many potential participants as possible. Upon consideration of these factors, it was decided to have a peer support meeting every Monday at 10:30 AM.

Meeting participants

Multiple models of peer support have been reported through the Society of Critical Care Medicine THRIVE Peer Support Collaborative. Some peer support groups include both patients and family members in 1 meeting, whereas others separate patients and family members into different support groups.[5] Additionally, some peer support programs invite only those who have been discharged from the hospital, whereas others include patients and family members who are still in the hospital.[5] Knowing our patient population comes from a large catchment area with difficulty returning to the hospital for peer support meetings, we decided it was most beneficial to offer our peer support group to ICU survivors and family members together in addition to including those patients (if able) and family members currently in the ICU or still in the hospital.

Group facilitation and format

The ICU social worker and chaplain both completed training and had experience facilitating support groups using an open, free-flow format for communication that aims to share and normalize the experiences of group participants. Another beneficial feature of this facilitation format is that experienced participants often end up providing support to new group members.[5] Thus, this facilitation format was chosen for our support group implementation with the aim to eventually recruit ICU survivors and family members to aid in group facilitation alongside the ICU social worker and chaplain. After 1 year of implementation, a patient (RG) returned for peer support group and has since cofacilitated more than 10 meetings with the chaplain and social worker.

It was determined that the presence of a registered nurse at peer support group meetings could be beneficial in helping patients to make sense of ICU memories, answer questions for participants, or provide resources as needed. Finally, 1 to 2 unit providers (eg, nurses, physicians) were invited to attend each peer support meetings to facilitate an understanding of the critical illness and ICU recovery experience.

Advertising and recruitment

Room size and proper facilitation led to the conclusion that a maximum of 6 participants per week is ideal. Flyers were posted in each medical and surgical ICU patient room and large poster boards containing meeting information were placed at the ICU entrance (**Fig. 1**). A meeting announcement was also added to the electronic notification system on television screens located throughout the hospital. To recruit participants, the chaplain and social worker informed patients and family members of the peer support group during 1:1 meetings. As a last step, on Monday mornings the clinical nurse leader for each unit reminds all family members in the ICU about the peer

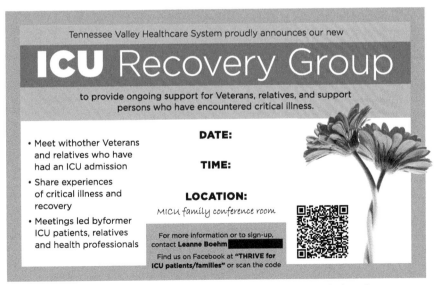

Fig. 1. ICU recovery group flyer. This flyer was developed by the multidisciplinary team and displayed throughout the Nashville VAMC.

support group. Funds were secured to provide coffee and snacks as an additional of-fering to support group participants.

Measures

Support group uptake was measured as the number of participants attending each support group meeting. An 11-item support group evaluation survey informed by the Domestic Violence Evidence Project was developed to assess acceptability and usefulness of our peer support program.[6] (The full survey is available online as Data S1.) Free form comments were invited as the final item on the evaluation survey. The voluntary anonymous surveys were distributed at the conclusion of each peer support group meeting.

Analysis

Descriptive statistical summaries are used to report evaluation survey responses. Statistical summaries were developed using Microsoft Excel (Microsoft Corporation, Redmond, WA). Qualitative feedback from peer support participants were evaluated and verbatim comments supporting survey descriptive summaries are provided.

Ethical Considerations

The project was reviewed by the Nashville VAMC Institutional Review Board and it was agreed that this work was quality improvement and, thus, not subject to ethics approval.

RESULTS

From October 2016 through September 2019, total support group attendance was 268 persons. The median weekly support group attendance was 3 persons (interquartile range, 2–4). The evaluation survey response rate was 40% (n = 106). Of evaluation survey respondents, 6% (n = 6) attended more than 2 peer support meetings (**Fig. 2**). The majority of survey respondents (94%; n = 100; very much) reported attending the peer support group made them feel emotionally supported and helped them to learn

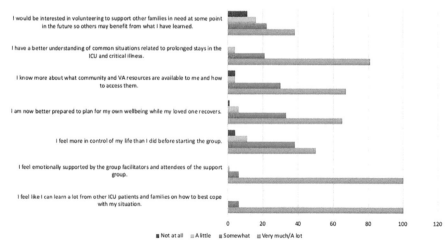

Fig. 2. Peer support group evaluation survey findings (n=106). An 11-item voluntary survey was administered anonymously to peer support group participants.

from other ICU patients and families on how to best cope with the current situation. A lesser proportion (76%; n = 81; very much) reported having a better understanding of common situations related to prolonged stays in the ICU and critical illness. Respondents (61%; n = 65; very much) reported peer support participation helped them to plan for their well-being during recovery and 63% (n = 67; very much) know more about community and VA resources to help with recovery. Fewer than one-half (47%; n = 50; very much) of respondents felt more in control of their life than before starting the peer support group. Last, few survey participants (36%; n = 38) reported very much interest in volunteering to support other families in need at some time point in the future. Most survey respondents (85%; n = 90) would strongly recommend peer support group participation to a friend.

Open-Ended Survey Responses

Participants reported the peer support group as being "wonderful," "very encouraging, brings more of a peace," and "very helpful knowing what to expect." Some participants did not realize they needed the group until attending their first meeting.

The hurt caregivers are in need of more support. There is a lot of help the caregiver does not know until you go to a meeting. A lot of information was given that I feel the caregiver should know.

I was asked to come and now I feel like I really can do it. Enjoyed sharing with the group. I am not alone.

An overwhelming theme of support group participation was feeling supported by knowing you are not alone in your struggles of critical illness and recovery.

It was very helpful and reassuring to know we were not alone with what was going on.

It helps not to feel alone.

It is so healing to talk with other people who have the same challenges — strength together.

We need to know that we are not alone and that there is strength in this group.

It's calming to experience that you are not alone and that you want to do the right thing for yourself and your loved ones. You can open up your heart and expel all the fears and pain that you have.

Peer Support Group Influence on Intensive Care Unit Culture

Implementation of the peer support program at this VA hospital has changed the ICU culture to be more supportive of patient- and family-centered care. On a weekly basis, our team saw the value of human connection and empathy during critical illness. Too often, the humanity of the patient is missed, and providers forget that every patient has a story. Staff saw that the person in the corner of the ICU room was more than a body occupying space. This person was a wife, a mother, a child, or a friend full of emotions and fears, who are experiencing their own crisis. Before implementing our peer support program, this was not readily recognized. The peer support group provided our staff with insight into the perspectives and experiences of family members and friends and created a humanizing effect. We became better at connecting with families, recognizing their needs, and involving them in the daily care of the patients.

Implementation of the peer support program also helped to bring joy to the nursing staff. Nurses and other providers were rewarded by seeing how the peer support group was positively impacting family members. Staff also began to create special bonds with patients and family members. More so now than in the past, patients and family members return to the ICU after discharge to express their gratitude for the support they received during their critical illness admission.

DISCUSSION

The Nashville VAMC was able to successfully create a community for the promotion of health and well-being for those suffering from PICS and PICS-F via implementation of a peer support group program for critically ill Veterans and their family members. In conjunction with the Society of Critical Care Medicine THRIVE Peer Support Collaborative we have successfully sustained our peer support program for 3 years with a median of 3 participants per meeting. Our peer support program seems to be helpful in increasing patient and family member support for ICU recovery. Facilitation by a trained social worker and chaplain lent to the quality of peer support provided. Last, support from managing directors and ICU leadership for staff time lent to the stability and sustainment of our peer support program.

The implementation of the peer support program was the beginning of a new culture within the Nashville VAMC ICUs focused more intently on engaging with patients and family members more empathetically. Nurses and physicians described having a more real-life understanding of the suffering family members and patients experience during an ICU admission and while recovering from critical illness with ongoing physical, cognitive, and mental health impairments. Moreover, a number of VA staff and leadership began attending the meetings not as an observer, but as a participant in need of peer support for a personal ICU experience.

An Intensive Care Unit Survivor's Perspective

A key strength of our peer support program is the involvement of an ICU survivor as facilitator for peer support. Mr Gervasio's initial weekly attendance with the peer support group focused on his own cognitive issues, which allowed him to knit together things he could remember with those he could not. Ralph describes having issues during recovery, but they felt surmountable. Approximately 1 year after his first meeting, with his words coming out in the right order and with gratifying reassurances and support from the chaplain and social work facilitators, he attended not for himself, but for others. Per Ralph, so many patients have family members who need support and a break from the pressures of their loved one in a bad state. He offers himself as a survivor who can relate the effects of ICU delirium and other oddities the family members do not understand. He went through an ICU experience. Through his involvement in the peer support program, Ralph has become an incredible model of someone who has treated his recovery as an opportunity to give back. He inspires others in the ICU to help overcome barriers to patient- and family-centered care and clear misconceptions about ICU recovery. Ralph adds the following:

> When professional staff and clergy stopped short of asking deeply personal and poignant questions to support group participants, I had a more freedom, being an ICU ex-patient survivor and nonprofessional, to tap into the raw emotions of those who otherwise felt remiss to offer their true feelings. Often my comments/ questions spurred other PICS-F participants to speak more freely, having seen one member emote and thus wanting to support that person by sharing as well. I believe a veteran ICU survivor can sense through non-verbal cues when and

how to extract acute feelings from affected family members. I worked closely with my medical, social work, and pastoral partners for 2.5 years, to give back to those who gave me a second chance at life while helping others cope with the acute stress of having a loved one in the ICU.
—Ralph Gervasio, Vietnam Veteran and medical ICU survivor

Limitations

A limitation of this reported work is the single-center implementation of a peer support program at a VA hospital. Implementation in other contexts may require different processes, procedures, and approvals. However, we feel that providing details of our implementation decision-making process and final procedure will help others to develop a program that can work in their own context. Next, we did not evaluate whether symptoms of PICS and PICS-F are decreased by participation in our peer support program and this work needs to be done in future study. Finally, we have had the same multidisciplinary team overseeing and facilitating the peer support program since inception. Although we have sustained the program for 3 years, it is unclear how turnover in the implementation team will influence sustainment.

SUMMARY

We have developed a feasible and sustained process for peer support in the ICU and are now evaluating spread of the peer support program to the sister hospital in our middle Tennessee VA health care system. Our peer support group gave families a chance to tell a patient's story in a warm and supportive environment. ICU survivor peer presence helped family members hear from the perspective of a patient and gave great insight to what their loved one might be facing while being treated for critical illness. The multidisciplinary approach of having a chaplain, social worker, and nurse present to lead the peer support group provided a well-rounded and team-centered approach to care. Ultimately, the peer support group added significant value to the ICU experience by giving both family members of current patients and ICU survivors a chance to share stories while giving and receiving support.

Future research could focus on efficacy of peer support programs in reducing the mental health impairments associated with PICS and PICS-F and implementation strategies for sustained peer support group implementation. The post-ICU primarily nurse-led support group intervention was implemented with minimal financial resources and is offered as a replicable method of enhancing patient and family member recovery from critical illness.

ACKNOWLEDGEMENTS

Dr L.M. Boehm would like to acknowledge the leaders and membership of the Society of critical care medicine THRIVE peer support collaborative.

DISCLOSURE

L.M. Boehm is currently receiving grant funding from the NHLBI (#K12HL137943-01). The funding sources had no role in the design and conduct of the study; collection, management, analysis, and interpretation of the data; preparation, review, or approval of the article; and decision to submit the article for publication. The contents of this article are solely the responsibility of the authors and do not necessarily represent those of the National Institutes of Health, the Department of Veterans Affairs or Vanderbilt University.

SUPPLEMENTARY DATA

Supplementary data related to this article can be found online at https://doi.org/10.1016/j.cnc.2020.02.003.

REFERENCES

1. Prescott HC, Angus DC. Enhancing recovery from sepsis: a review. JAMA 2018; 319(1):62–75.
2. Harvey MA, Davidson JE. Postintensive care syndrome: right care, right now...and later. Crit Care Med 2016;44(2):381–5.
3. Needham DM, Davidson J, Cohen H, et al. Improving long-term outcomes after discharge from intensive care unit: report from a stakeholders' conference. Crit Care Med 2012;40(2):502–9.
4. Mikkelsen ME, Jackson JC, Hopkins RO, et al. Peer support as a novel strategy to mitigate post-intensive care syndrome. AACN Adv Crit Care 2016;27(2):221–9.
5. McPeake J, Hirshberg EL, Christie LM, et al. Models of peer support to remediate post-intensive care syndrome: a report developed by the society of critical care medicine thrive international peer support collaborative. Crit Care Med 2019; 47(1):e21–7.
6. Domestic violence evidence project. (n.d.). Available at: https://www.dvevidenceproject.org/. Accessed January 9, 2020.

Engaging Patients and Families to Help Research Inform and Advance Patient and Family–Centered Care in Critical Care Medicine

Peter Oxland, BASc[a], Nadine Foster, BN, RN[b],
Kirsten M. Fiest, PhD[c,d,e],*, Yoanna Skrobik, MD, FRCP(c), MSc, FCCM[f]

KEYWORDS

- Critical care medicine • Intensive care unit • Research • Engagement
- Patient-oriented research • Patients • Family members
- Patient centered and family centered

KEY POINTS

- Research engagement of intensive care unit (ICU) survivors and family members can mean involvement in generating project ideas; writing grants; leading and/or participating in qualitative research, committees, interviews, or focus groups; guideline production; result dissemination; and authorship.
- Family members and ICU survivors' lives are indelibly changed by their ICU experience. Making sense of this disruption can be achieved by purposeful narrative.
- Enabling and framing qualitative research initiatives provides credible feedback to critical care providers suggesting alternative and user-centered, rather than provider-driven, ways to offer ICU and post-ICU care.
- The qualitative projects highlighted herein suggest patient and family member–led qualitative research is feasible.

[a] Alberta Health Services, Critical Care, Patient & Community Engagement Researcher (PaCER), Department of Critical Care Medicine, University of Calgary, Ground Floor, McCaig Tower, 3134 Hospital Drive Northwest, Calgary T2N5A1, Canada; [b] Alberta Health Services, Critical Care, Department of Critical Care Medicine, Ground Floor, McCaig Tower, 3134 Hospital Drive Northwest, Calgary T2N5A1, Canada; [c] Department of Critical Care Medicine, Cumming School of Medicine, University of Calgary, Ground Floor, McCaig Tower, 3134 Hospital Drive Northwest, Calgary T2N5A1, Canada; [d] Department of Community Health Sciences, Cumming School of Medicine, University of Calgary, Ground Floor, McCaig Tower, 3134 Hospital Drive Northwest, Calgary T2N5A1, Canada; [e] Department of Psychiatry, Cumming School of Medicine, University of Calgary, Ground Floor, McCaig Tower, 3134 Hospital Drive Northwest, Calgary T2N5A1, Canada; [f] Department of Medicine, McGill University, 1650 Cedar Avenue, Room D6. 237, Montreal, Quebec H3G 1A4, Canada
* Corresponding author.
E-mail address: kmfiest@ucalgary.ca
Twitter: @nkwfoster (N.F.); @kmfiest (K.M.F.); @YoannaSkrobik (Y.S.)

Crit Care Nurs Clin N Am 32 (2020) 211–226
https://doi.org/10.1016/j.cnc.2020.02.004
0899-5885/20/© 2020 Elsevier Inc. All rights reserved.
ccnursing.theclinics.com

INTRODUCTION

Critical care units became integrated in hospitalized services in the 1970s. For the next three decades, caring for the critically ill focused almost exclusively on resuscitative medical care, both in clinical practice and in the literature. In the early 2000s, the first Society of Critical Care Medicine (SCCM)–sponsored family-centered guidelines,[1] updated in 2017,[2] described clinical observations from the bedside, bringing family experience and distress into the critical care literature. Subsequently, research corroborating the concept of post–intensive care syndrome, affecting both patients and families, further supported the importance of conceptually recognizing and researching family-centered care.[3] These first high-profile publications educated practitioners as to the collateral damage, and consequences, of the trauma experienced by families, highlighting the inextricable relationship between the quality of caring in the intensive care unit (ICU) and these sequelae.[4] In parallel, a Canadian led the first of many longitudinal studies[5] pointing out the physical and psychological sequelae experienced by patients[6] and families.[7,8] In 2005, ICUsteps, a United Kingdom–based intensive care patient support charity, reflected how ubiquitous and international post–intensive care caregiver challenges were, and highlighted the need for support on this difficult journey.

Integrating patients and family members in research was first instigated by individual researchers focusing on patient preferences for level of resuscitation,[9] and among critical care physicians asking about values and creating decision-making tools.[10] Patient preferences for which outcomes are studied became a collective effort in the partly critical care–based TechValueNet, in which patient involvement was framed not only in research participation but as an innovative model of knowledge translation. Collaborative research networks such as the Canadian Critical Care Trials Group formally created a family advisory board within its organization in February of 2015. Other researchers led Delphi-based inquiries to explore research priorities relevant to critical care survivors.[11]

In addition, inviting patients and families to take part in the writing process of professional guidelines, establishing recommendations determining their care, is a recent phenomenon. The Council of Medical Specialty Societies (CMSS) requirements mandate they be informed by families, caregivers, and other stakeholders; however, these recommendations do not define either process or level of involvement.[12] The American SCCM acquiesced in the requests of the chair of the Family-Centered Guidelines and the vice-chair of the Pain, Agitation, Delirium, Immobility and Sleep (PADIS)[13] to integrate patients and families as full partners. Including patients and family members on these work teams was an important recognition of the importance of acknowledging the input of "end users" of critical illness. Patients rank ordered proposed topic lists provided by each guidelines' expert panel, reordering priorities and in the process disrupting the traditional paternalistic self-attribution of the expert role long espoused by clinicians. In addition, the qualitative literature, including focus groups, surveys, and interviews of patients and families describing their experience, were considered in the family guideline evidence review and analysis.

The call for meaningful patient and family engagement in health care and research is increasingly mandated by clinical health care organizations, as well as becoming a prerequisite for research funding. Meaningful patient and family engagement requires health practitioners and researchers to actively partner with patients, families, and organizations to advance care and research. These partnerships and opportunities herald a departure from paternalism and the traditional disease-centered approach to health care and acknowledge, as has been proposed by the Canadian Critical Care Trials Group, that patients and families hold unique expertise and experiences that can improve clinical care and research.[14] Many factors motivate patient partnership, including influencing and improving health care.[15] Engagement in this context exceeds participation as an informant, and is instead a true partnership in the construct of advances or improvements in care.

As an example of this the authors describe our experiences with a collaborative patient engagement process. In 2014, University of Calgary and Alberta Health Services Department of Critical Care Medicine researchers initiated the "Reassessing Practices in the Daily Care of Critically Ill Patients: Building Capacity and Methodologies to Identify and Close Evidence Care Gaps" project. In conducting this study of the gaps in daily care of critically ill patients across the province of Alberta, Canada, the research team involved former ICU patients and family members as partners.

This article describes:

- Two qualitative research projects led by qualitative research–trained former patients and family members working with a local critical care research team
- How this exercise informed what is meaningful and important through ICU survivor and family member testimonials
- How this activity brought together the critical care community, including actionable items such as a prioritized list of critical care research topics

The following are highlighted in this article:

- A novel research model involving peer-to-peer qualitative researchers, to understand the ICU experiences of former ICU patients and family members (study A)
- Use of a second peer-to-peer qualitative research study to understand the experiences of patients and family members being transferred from ICU to a hospital ward (study B)
- Personal perspectives shared by the authors

STUDY A: UNDERSTANDING PATIENT AND FAMILY EXPERIENCES IN THE DAILY CARE OF CRITICALLY ILL PATIENTS
Background

Health care systems want to engage a broad spectrum of stakeholders to help identify and define patient care priorities for research and quality improvement.[16,17] Meaningful engagement of patients and families in this process can be challenging, and limited literature supports how this can best be implemented.[18] Barriers can be particularly salient in critical care, where contextual circumstances are often overwhelming.[19] Evidence suggests that patients and families may be more open to sharing their experiences with those who have had a similar experience.

Objective

This study was part of a larger initiative designed to identify and close evidence care gaps in ICUs in the province of Alberta, Canada. The objective was 2-fold:

- To understand the experiences of critically ill patients and their families
- To identify opportunities to improve the quality of ICU care for patients and families

Methods

Design
A novel program called Patient and Community Engagement Research[20] (PaCER)[21] was used to fully engage ICU patients and family members in this study. PaCER trains

patients, family, and community members to conduct peer-to-peer qualitative research. Overseen by university faculty and a PaCER lead, PaCER researchers apply a 3-phase framework: co-design/set, collect, reflect, to examine patient experiences from varied perspectives (**Fig. 1**). Participatory grounded theory, iterative data collection, and analysis cycles are used to test emerging data and cultivate a collective patient voice.

Participant recruitment

ICU patient care managers, social workers, and physicians provided information on the study to previous ICU patients. PaCER recruited 32 participants from 13 adult ICUs in 7 large and small urban centers in Alberta, Canada. Participants were former ICU patients and family members of ICU patients. Patients had a variety of admitting conditions, treatments, lengths of stay, and outcomes.

Data collection, analysis, and research method

Audio recordings of focus groups and interviews were transcribed verbatim. After coding by PaCER researchers, participants were invited to review, comment on, validate, and challenge emerging themes. All transcripts were also independently analyzed by 2 academic qualitative researchers blinded to the PaCER results.

Results

Thematic analysis produced 18 themes tied to 3 phases collectively describing the ICU "journey": (1) admission to ICU, (2) daily care in ICU, (3) after discharge from ICU. Themes within daily care (n = 14) were grouped into 5 higher-order themes that together highlighted a fragility of trust and comfort between patients and family members, and ICU providers (**Fig. 2**). Comfort and trust fluctuated with perceived appropriateness and quality of interactions (**Fig. 3**).

Key findings in each phase of the journey were:

- Admission to ICU: when first entering the ICU, family members usually experience extreme shock and disorientation. What is normal for staff feels alien for families. Families also outlined their need for support in getting clear, consistent, and complete information. Most patients had little memory of this experience.
- Daily care in ICU: family members need to be updated (day to day, in a timely manner when major changes in the patient's health occur and family is absent),

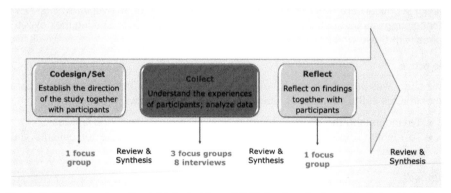

Fig. 1. PaCER research method. (*Adapted from* Gill M, Boulton D, Oswell D, Oxland P. Understanding patient and family experiences in the daily care of critically ill patients. Patient & Community Engagement Research (PaCER) report; 2014; with permission.)

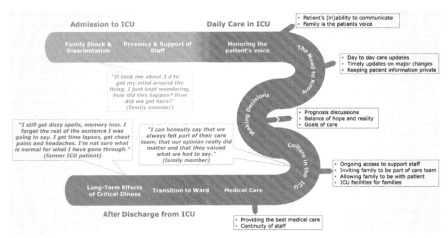

Fig. 2. The ICU journey. (*Adapted from* Gill M, Boulton D, Oswell D, Oxland P. Understanding patient and family experiences in the daily care of critically ill patients. Patient & Community Engagement Research (PaCER) report; 2014; with permission.)

heard, and involved in decisions to feel well cared for, respected, and valued. Interactions with the care team and efforts to establish comfort and trust in the ICU were integral to the notion of a community of caring. Families indicated the importance of honoring the patient's voice when patients were unable to speak for themselves. Readily sharing information regarding a loved one's health increased decision-making capacity and their sense of agency. Actions that left the family feeling less confident and in control included lack of visiting access and perceiving not being welcomed as an important part of the care team. These

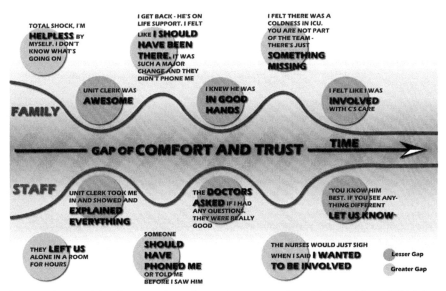

Fig. 3. Patient and family zone of comfort and trust over time. (*Adapted from* Gill M, Bagshaw S, McKenzie E, et al. Patient and family member-led research in the intensive care unit: a novel approach to patient-centered research. PLoS ONE 2016;11(8):e0160947.)

features, whether perceived or real, increased family member anxiety and reduced trust in the care team.

- Discharge from ICU was traumatic, expectations were not well understood, concerns were not always addressed, and symptoms sometimes went untreated. Specifically, inadequate preparation time for the move, perceived poor communication between ICU and ward providers, and limited knowledge on the part of ICU providers as to what would happen after ICU discharge were distressful. Discharge home triggered anxiety about physical, cognitive, and mental health symptoms suggestive of post-ICU syndrome. Patients and families were hesitant to rely on their primary care physicians, whom they perceived to have limited knowledge of the long-term sequelae of critical illness. A sense of abandonment and confusion as to where to turn for information was common.

Patients and families depended on ICU providers to invite them into a trusting and comforting relationship. These relationships are fragile, with trust being threatened with a single event or negatively perceived comment, regardless of the team's prior trust-building efforts. Patients and families perceive ICU providers as a team and need all team members working together for them to feel confident in their ongoing care.

Parallel Analysis

Academic researchers identified similar themes, but produced different interpretations and recommendations. This difference was most striking in interpretations of patient/family-provider communications. For example, PaCERs understood participants' need for improved communication skills such as improving providers' active listening skills, whereas academics interpreted this as improving the clarity of the content that providers deliver. The academic researchers also categorized the data into groupings of content, in contrast with the PaCER's organization of the data into a temporal journey.

Parallel levels of frustration in being heard are described in the very different context of primary care, where hurry/the need for throughput often leaves patients or families with unanswered questions and anxiety. Vulnerable individuals can perceive that their sense of agency is threatened, as has been described in European qualitative ICU patient experience studies.[22] Sites such as Discutons Santé (www.discutonssante.ca), a Web-based tool created to foster active patient engagement during medical consultations,[23] improves communication quality and chronic disease outcomes,[24] and promotes information recall. Patient focus groups confirm its value through stress reduction, empowerment, and improved partnering with the health care provider, with these empowerment initiatives significantly improving patient and family satisfaction. Physician interpretation, as in the PaCER example, differed from the patient and family perspective. One communication dimension related to the significant reduction in medication and diagnostic errors is a hereto unexplored aspect of communicating with patients and families in the critical care setting.

Recommendations for improvement made by patients and family members:

1. Provide a dedicated family navigator
2. Increase provider awareness of the fragility of family trust
3. Understand the importance of the mode, tone and content of provider communications
4. Improve ICU to hospital ward transitions
5. Inform patients about long-term effects of critical illness

Key Messages

Patients and families identified 9 themes, 14 subthemes, and 5 specific recommendations, based on their experiences in intensive care. Study results have since been used to inform and prioritize research and quality improvement initiatives in critical care across Alberta. Actionable guidance to enhance front-line ICU patient and family–centered care has included:

- ICU family presence guiding principles
- A 24-hour ICU supportive care bundle for patients and families
- A reconciliation process involving ICU clinicians and the results of this study (from ICU patients and families), which identified the 5 top priorities for critical care research going forward:
  1. Delirium screening
  2. Family presence and effective communication
  3. Transitions of care from ICU to hospital ward
  4. Transitions of care between ICU providers
  5. Early mobilization

Lessons Learned

Comfort and trust, and appropriate interactions with ICU providers, are important components in the common, collective ICU experience of patients and family members. Many opportunities exist for improvement in ICU care and research. Patients and family members are valuable partners for research and quality improvement. Engaging patients and family members as researchers is a viable strategy if institutional investments exist and patient and family–centered care prioritized. This approach could serve as a model for quality improvement across other settings. The PaCER method can identify opportunities for improving health care that academic researchers and front-line health care providers may not recognize or adequately elicit from research participants. Further, PaCER exemplifies the empower stage along the International Association for Public Participation (IAP2) spectrum and should be considered a viable model to foster public engagement in research and quality improvement across other settings.

STUDY B: PATIENT AND FAMILY EXPERIENCES WHEN MOVING FROM THE INTENSIVE CARE UNIT TO A HOSPITAL WARD
Background

ICU patients are among the sickest hospitalized patients. They receive constant, one-on-one, specialized care in an environment using life-support technologies and significant resources. When ICU patients' conditions improve and they no longer require this intensive care, they are usually transferred to a hospital ward. Here they become 1 patient among many,[25] and the nurse to patient ratio switches from 1 to 1 to 1 to many.[26] Moving vulnerable patients to an environment with limited resources is a high-risk medical transition and, because of the demand for ICU beds, patients may be given little advance notice of their move.[27]

In Canada, more than 250,000 patients will be transferred from ICUs this year. Many patients will experience adverse consequences during the transition, and 18,000 patients will be readmitted to the ICU,[28] an indication of both the risk associated with transfer and the challenges inherent to transitions within the health care system. Patients and their families often find the transition from ICU to a hospital ward challenging, given the fear of the unknown and the dependency fostered in the critical care setting[29] in contrast with hospital wards, which have fewer resources and lower nurse to patient ratios.

Objective

To understand the experiences of patients and family members when a patient is moved from the ICU to a hospital ward.

Methods

Patient engagement framework
Patients and family members led all aspects of the study. The project was led and conducted by PaCER interns, as part of their 1-year internship, supported by PaCER leadership.

Data collection
Two 5-hour focus groups were held with participants using the co-design/set (eg, establishing the direction of the study) and reflect (eg, to reflect on findings) method. Seventeen individual interviews were held with former ICU patients and family members.

Participant recruitment
Personal contacts, a PaCER lead, a research coordinator, and hospital recruitment posters helped recruit 22 participants from 5 adult ICUs in Alberta located in 2 cities (Calgary, Edmonton). ICU patients and family members of ICU patients participated. Patients had a variety of admitting conditions, treatments, lengths of stay, and outcomes.

Results: Experiences and Improvement Opportunities

Of the 17 themes, 6 described actions undertaken by families in response to a health emergency in the ICU, hospital ward, and/or elsewhere in the patient's health journey. These 6 themes were grouped in the What Families Do category (**Fig. 4**). Each of these actions can be viewed as an independent activity that families may have felt compelled to undertake to help care for the patients. Whether or not the families undertook these activities depended on whether they perceived they needed to, and whether they were able to intervene in the patients' care. Essentially, families do what they think needs to be done.

Four themes in the category What Families Do describe actions that families undertook to directly help with the patients' care and recovery: reduce vulnerability, provide care, figure it out and advocate, and keep the story. When these actions occur in isolation from ICU providers, their efficacy is perceived by family members as being limited. When these actions are combined with effective interactions with the staff, as depicted in **Fig. 5**, this capacity builds in a synergistic way, leading to a category called Positive Outcomes.

There are 4 main synergistic loops in **Fig. 5**, with each loop having enhanced interactions with providers at the center. Most patients and family members probably do not experience these loops in isolation from each other, which reinforces the importance of the common elements of all 3 loops: 2-way, caring, and informative interactions with the ICU providers.

We observed that patients and family members found it difficult to view the transfer experience from ICU to the hospital ward separately from their overall health journeys, because other experiences in their journeys influenced their perceptions of the transfer experience. **Fig. 6** shows how the hospital transfer experience is a subset of the challenging health journey.

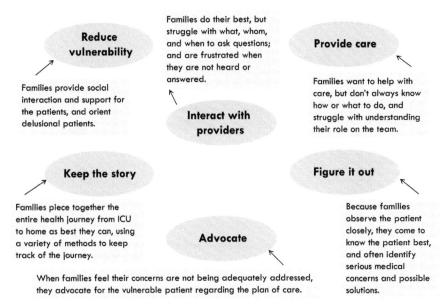

Fig. 4. What families do. (*Adapted from* Boulton D, Oswell D, Oxland, P. Patient and family experiences when moving from the intensive care unit (ICU) to a hospital ward. Patient & Community Engagement Research (PaCER) report; 2015; with permission.)

Recommendations

Six major recommendations were identified to help improve the transitions of care from ICU to a hospital ward:

1. Keep patients and family members informed about the move
2. Provide orientation to the ward
3. Facilitate family's attempt to keep the patient's story

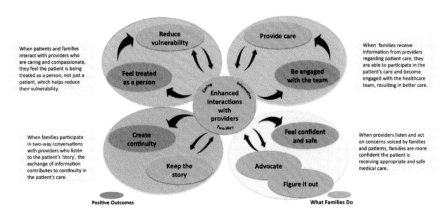

Fig. 5. Model for engaging families and patients. (*Adapted from* Boulton D, Oswell D, Oxland P. Patient and family experiences when moving from the intensive care unit (ICU) to a hospital ward. Patient & Community Engagement Research (PaCER) report; 2015; with permission.)

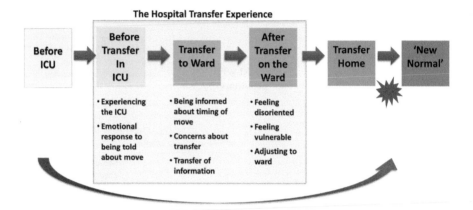

Medical care takes place in separate specialized units

Families create continuity between units by
Keeping the Story

Fig. 6. The hospital transfer experience. (*From* Oswell D, Oxland P. Patient and family experiences with critical care: Patient & Community Engagement Research (PaCER) project PowerPoint presentation; Critical Care Research Transitions in Care meeting. Sept 2018; with permission.)

4. Improve provider, patient, and family communications
5. Provide dedicated navigator/advocate
6. Engage families with the care team

Conclusion

The overarching message was to shift toward more meaningful engagement of families with the health care team, by valuing the benefits of family expertise and by giving them a role. Studies addressing the healing power of the narrative[30,31] and highlighting critical care caregivers as enablers for distressed families (sense-making theory[32]) are early descriptors of patient and family engagement benefits in research as in clinical care. Embracing diversity is universally beneficial,[33] but also requires hard work, genuine engagement rather than lip service, and trust. As with other models in which multidisciplinary partners engage in mutually respectful construction with a common goal, the benefits are likely to be numerous and multifaceted. How to best approach patient and family engagement, and an assessment of potential risks, should also be studied.

SUMMARY
Discussion

The Alberta critical care research team used a novel approach that involved patients and family members as qualitative researchers in 2 projects to better understand patient and family member ICU experiences and identify opportunities for improvement.

Former ICU patients and family members played different roles in different parts of the projects. Study participants described shared experiences in their ICU journeys and when moving from the ICU to a hospital ward. Ways to improve the experiences of ICU patients and family members were identified. Analyses by independent academic qualitative researchers in one project identified similar themes and suggestions for improvement,[34] but through a health system rather than patient and family lens. These projects have helped to better understand what is important to ICU patients and family members, and, together with the experiences of ICU providers, contributed to create a prioritized list of critical care research topics going forward, and had former ICU patients and family members meaningfully involved in the projects.

The role of patients and family members in research

Research studies have traditionally been conducted by health researchers. Members of the public with a health care experience usually serve as research subjects. Our experience shows that patients and families can play different, valuable roles when empowered to help with a research project.

Supporting members of the public in a qualitative research methodology training program is a major investment, which is intended to mirror a long-term commitment to patient and family–centered care. Our experience suggests this high level of qualitative research involvement is feasible and of interest to patients and family members, who value the opportunity to contribute to projects that can improve health care.

What former ICU patients and family members contribute should be shaped by their interests, abilities, and available energy and time. Locally, the critical care scientific research team embraced this involvement from grant writing, as project participants (committees, interviews, focus groups), in dissemination of results, and in publications (which informed the critical care community as a whole), and provided meaningful opportunity to the former ICU patients and family members involved.

Lessons for the Care of the Critically Ill

The two studies discussed in this article show the value of understanding the experiences of former ICU patients and family members, and the identified opportunities to improve their experiences. Patients and family members share common experiences, and initiatives to address identified opportunities for improvement can lead to improved care.

When a patient is in the ICU, an important covenant of trust is created between the family and ICU providers. In study A, families described how to foster that relationship, recognize the stress and disorientation when the patient is admitted, proactively orient the patient, invite the patient to be an active member of the care team (ie, by attending rounds, helping at the bedside as appropriate), and engaging the patient in bidirectional communication and decision making. In study B, it was found that, when a patient is transferred from ICU to a hospital ward, patients and family members experience distressing reactions to this transfer. They do not know what to expect, are hesitant with the transfer occurring, and family members wish to participate and have a role in the transfer process.

A recurring theme in both studies was that what is normal for health care providers is not normal for patients and families. Peer-to-peer qualitative researchers have the ability, through their lived ICU experiences, to gain the trust of ICU patient and family member study participants when facilitating interviews and focus groups. Our experience is that the creation of this safe, trusted, comfortable space for vulnerable former ICU patients is important and leads to an honest and rich sharing of their experiences.

Many opportunities for improving the experience of ICU patients and family members were identified in the two studies. When reconciled with the experiences of ICU providers, opportunities were created to identify and prioritize a dialogue that can lead to future research initiatives and eventually improved care.

AUTOBIOGRAPHICAL PERSONAL PERSPECTIVES
Peter Oxland

Our ICU experience was the most challenging time in our lives. My wife's deteriorating health over 12 months led to the late diagnosis of a rare malignant nasal-cavity tumor masquerading as chronic sinusitis,[35] expanding to involve her eyes and her brain. Over a 30-day period she was admitted to neurology, received cancer treatment, was discharged, was taken to emergency, and was admitted to the ICU, where she died 6 days later.

Soon after she died, I became a critical care family advisor with different committees focused on enhancing ICU care. Over time, I shared our story with audiences, a humbling, meaningful experience. Becoming a qualitative researcher with the University of Calgary's PaCER program involved a 1-year internship and helping conduct 2 qualitative research projects (studies A and B).

My experiences highlight considerations when engaging former ICU patients and family members in research:

- The often sacred stories of former ICU patients and family members should be acknowledged and honored. Balancing and leveraging these with the collective voice learned through qualitative research is also important.
- ICU stays have seriously affected the quality of life post-ICU for many patients and family members. Many interview and focus group participants, even after 2, 3, 4 years, had not shared their ICU experiences with others. Better post-ICU psychosocial and peer support could make a positive difference in the quality of their lives.
- ICU patient and family member experiences are often life changing. During interviews and focus groups, I was consistently aware of their interest in wanting to give back to the ICU, but ethics did not support their continued involvement. These passionate people are underused ICU resources whose continued involvement should be supported.
- Qualitative researchers with a lived experience similar to participants can provide safety and comfort in interviews and focus groups, especially with former, often vulnerable, ICU patients who struggle with their health and well-being. Our 5-hour focus groups involved participants sharing experiences, often the first time, resulting in meaningful, supportive, and intimate gatherings. In two individual scientific research team–led meetings, two patient-partners found (1) noisy environments, and (2) an overbearing presence of researchers. The researchers neither anticipated nor perceived these elements as threatening patient-partner sense of safety, highlighting how essential sensitizing is to ensure patient safety and comfort. Constant validation of a sense of safety is thus essential for this process so patients truly engage and choose to participate.
- The public becoming qualitative researchers is novel, as is the contrast with academic qualitative researchers, as shown in the different interpretations of next steps in this work. Performing data analysis from a patient/family (PaCER) versus from a health-system lens (academic researchers) is valuable.
- Public research capacities (interests, abilities, time, energy) vary and are often not well understood, resulting in the research team not knowing how each

member of the public can best contribute to research. Meaningful involvement deserves focus and good stakeholder communications.

- Creating published articles (important academically) does not seem balanced with regular/effective dissemination of research results. Proactively creating a visually appealing summary for each research project, and using this with front-line providers/clinicians and the public, would help ensure research results are used, plus help create awareness and generate enthusiasm.

Becoming a qualitative researcher and witnessing the increased involvement of former ICU patients and family members within the critical care community has been humbling, and a learning experience. I hope the collective voice of former ICU patients and family members is never forgotten, always considered, and, when combined with that of ICU providers/clinicians, leads to positive changes in care.

Nadine Foster

I have had the privilege to receive outstanding lifesaving ICU care. I have also been through unexpected end-of-life care with my mother in the ICU. As an interesting coincidence, my mother and I were both the only registered nurses (RNs) in the family. My mother was once a charge nurse in the ICU where she died. As a child, I remember my mother spoke about her patients always being asleep and her work uninterrupted by family visits. This happened in the 1970s. ICU care has come a long way from her nursing days. Patients are more alert now and families act as partners in care.

Although I am no longer a practicing RN, my previous career and my personal ICU experiences left me longing to contribute back to health care in a different way. I began simply by telling my own story. In my experience, telling my own story had an impact, particularly on front-line staff who often do not know what happens to patients when they leave the ICU. Sharing in this way can ideally express how grateful patients and families are for the difficult and important work they do every day. It also allows patients and families to discuss where things might have gone wrong, or what they would like to see change. Although I began by sharing my own story of being both a patient and a family member in the ICU, I came to the realization that there are common themes in the collective voice. This collective voice can be a powerful tool to help the critical care community understand ways in which to improve outcomes. These stories and voices were not heard when my mother was still working. Much to the credit of the critical care community, we are more welcome now.

In 2015, I joined my first patient and family–centered care group and have now sat on various similar committees in an effort to share patient and family views. I have been involved in the creation of tools for best practices for family presence, the MyHealth.Alberta ICU Delirium information page for patients and families, among many others.

Perhaps the most meaningful way to contribute is being involved in research. It is innovative to involve members of the public and embed them throughout the research process. This involvement can help to guide research in the direction of what patients and families think is important, while allowing patient and family partners to collaborate with multiple stakeholders to ensure all voices are heard and the best, most useful, ideas are put forth.

In both of the studies outlined in this article, the results and recommendations that emerged resonated strongly with me. I was able to relate to them personally, and they both helped me to see that my own story shares so many critical elements with the collective voice. Those results have been used to set priorities for projects and research provincially and have largely dictated the initiatives I have been a part of to date. It has been delightful to be a part of watching patient priorities become important research topics.

Kirsten Fiest

Collaborating with former ICU patients and family members in critical care research is a privilege. Instead of doing research for patients, research is now being done with patients; this shift has led to exciting research, including the studies described earlier. There is still much for researchers to learn, including how best to evaluate patient engagement initiatives. As clinicians focus on conducting research to ultimately improve patient care, they should continue to engage patients and family members in ways they find meaningful. This engagement can be achieved through an open and honest dialogue; expectation setting for all parties is essential to successful patient engagement in research. Although the research process is at times slow, I continue to be delighted by the progress that is being made in this area.

Yoanna Skrobik

Patients have been the primary source of what I learned about critical care over many years of practice. In this effort, as in other dimensions, welcoming their input in a safe, respectful environment is humbling; I echo the sense of privilege. I look forward to witnessing tangible change from an avuncular but paternalistic to deliverable patient-centered critical care.

SUMMARY

Many former ICU patients and family members are indelibly changed by their ICU experiences. Opportunities exist to meaningfully involve these individuals in many ways, including in research projects.

The recurring theme in both studies discussed in this article can be summarized as: what is normal for health care providers is not normal for patients and families, an insightful and important lesson to acknowledge, respect, and consider. ICU patient and family member experiences offered valuable perspectives of what is important to them through these two studies, and differed from insights brought forward by providers.

It is also important to acknowledge and respect the value of involving many different stakeholders (eg, ICU providers/clinicians, researchers, patients and families) in research projects. Involving the public in such projects requires focus and effort by the research team, with the opportunity over time to develop a trusted, valued working relationship, ultimately leading to improved ICU care.

ACKNOWLEDGMENTS

The authors wish to acknowledge Marlyn Gill and Donna Oswell for reviewing the current article.

DISCLOSURE

The authors have nothing to disclose.

REFERENCES

1. Davidson JE, Powers K, Hedayat KM, et al. Clinical practice guidelines for support of the family in the patient-centered intensive care unit: American College of Critical Care Medicine Task Force 2004-2005. Crit Care Med 2007;35(2):605–22.
2. Davidson JE, Aslakson RA, Long AC, et al. Guidelines for family-centred care in the neonatal, pediatric and adult ICU. Crit Care Med 2017;45:103–28.
3. Davidson JE, Jones C, Bienvenu OJ. Family response to critical illness: postintensive care syndrome-family. Crit Care Med 2012;40:618–24.
4. Griffiths J, Hatch RA, Bishop J, et al. An exploration of social and economic outcome and associated health-related quality of life after critical illness in general intensive care unit survivors: a 12-month follow-up study. Crit Care 2013; 17:R100.
5. Herridge MS, Cheung AM, Tansey CM, et al. One-year outcomes in survivors of the acute respiratory distress syndrome. N Engl J Med 2003;348(8):683–93.
6. Herridge MS, Chu LM, Matte A, et al, RECOVER Investigators and CCCTG. The RECOVER program: disability risk groups & one year outcome after ≥ 7 days of mechanical ventilation. Am J Respir Crit Care Med 2016;194(7):831–44.
7. Cameron JI, Herridge MS, Tansey CM, et al. Well-being in informal caregivers of survivors of acute respiratory distress syndrome. Crit Care Med 2006;34(1):81–6.
8. Cameron JI, Chu LM, Matte A, et al, RECOVER Program Investigators (Phase 1: towards RECOVER), Canadian Critical Care Trials Group. One-year outcomes in caregivers of critically ill patients. N Engl J Med 2016;374(19):1831–41.
9. Heyland DK, Lavery JV, Tranmer JE, et al. Dying in Canada: is it an institutionalized, technologically supported experience? J Palliat Care 2000;16(Suppl): S10–6.
10. Heyland DK, Barwich D, Pichora D, et al. Failure to engage seriously ill hospitalized patients and their families in advance care planning: results of a multicenter prospective study. JAMA Intern Med 2013;173:778–87.
11. Needham DM, Sepulveda KA, Dinglas VD, et al. Core outcome measures for clinical research in acute respiratory failure survivors. An international modified Delphi Consensus study. Am J Respir Crit Care Med 2017;196:1122–30.
12. Available at: https://cmss.org/wp-content/uploads/2017/11/Revised-CMSS-Principles-for-Clinical-Practice-Guideline-Development.pdf. Accessed October 1, 2019.
13. Devlin JW, Skrobik Y, Gélinas C, et al. Clinical practice guidelines for the prevention and management of Pain, agitation/sedation, delirium, immobility, and sleep disruption in adult patients in the intensive care unit. Crit Care Med 2018;46(9): e825–73.
14. Burns KEA, Misak C, Herridge M, et al, Patient and Family Partnership Committee of the Canadian Critical Care Trials Group. Patient and family engagement in the ICU: untapped opportunities and underrecognized challenges. Am J Respir Crit Care Med 2018;198(3):310–9.
15. McCarron TL, Noseworthy T, Moffat K, et al. Understanding the motivations of patients: a co-designed project to understand the factors behind patient engagement. Health Expect 2019;22(4):709–20.
16. Gill M, Boulton D, Oswell D, et al. Understanding patient and family experiences in the daily care of critically ill patients. Patient & Community Engagement Research (PaCER) Report 2014.

17. Concannon TW, Fuster M, Saunders T, et al. A systematic review of stakeholder engagement in comparative effectiveness and patient-centered outcomes research. J Gen Intern Med 2014;29(12):1692–701.
18. McCarron TL, Moffat K, Wilkinson G, et al. Understanding patient engagement in health system decision-making: a co-designed scoping review. Syst Rev 2019; 8(1):97.
19. Squires JE, Graham I, Bashir K, et al. Understanding context: a concept analysis. J Adv Nurs 2019;75(12):3448–70.
20. Available at: http://www.pacerinnovates.ca. Accessed October 1, 2019.
21. Marlet N, Emes C. Grey matters: a guide for collaborative research with seniors. University of Calgary Press; 2010. p. 344.
22. Laerkner E, Egerod I, Olesen F, et al. A sense of agency: an ethnographic exploration of being awake during mechanical ventilation in the intensive care unit. Int J Nurs Stud 2017;75:1–9.
23. Cegala DJ, Chisolm DJ, Nwomeh BC. Further examination of the impact of patient participation on physicians' communication style. Patient Educ Couns 2012; 89(1):25–30.
24. Richard C, Lussier MT. Measuring patient and physician participation in exchanges on medications: dialogue ratio, preponderance of initiative, and dialogical roles. Patient Educ Couns 2007;65(3):329–41.
25. Field K, Prinjha S, Rowan K. 'One patient amongst many': a qualitative analysis of intensive care unit patients' experiences of transferring to the general ward. Crit Care 2008;12(1):R21.
26. Boulton D, Oswell D, Oxland P. Patient and family experiences when moving from the intensive care unit (ICU) to a hospital ward. Patient & Community Engagement Research (PaCER) Report 2015.
27. Forsberg A, Lindgren E, Engstrom A. Being transferred from an intensive care unit to a ward: searching for the known in the unknown. Int J Nurs Pract 2011; 17(2):110–6.
28. Leeb K, Jokovic A, Sandhu M, et al. CIHI survey: intensive care in Canada. Healthc Q 2004;9(1):2.
29. Bench S, Day T. The user experience of critical care discharge: a meta-synthesis of qualitative research. Int J Nurs Stud 2010;47(4):487–99.
30. Waller N, Scheidt CE. Narration as a means of restoring self-coherency: thoughts on processing traumatic experiences. Z Psychosom Med Psychother 2010;56(1): 56–73 [in German].
31. Martino ML, Lemmo D, Gargiulo A, et al. Under fifty women and breast cancer: narrative markers of meaning-making in traumatic experience. Front Psychol 2019;10:618.
32. Davidson JE. Facilitated sensemaking: a strategy and new middle-range theory to support families of intensive care unit patients. Crit Care Nurse 2010;30(6): 28–39.
33. Available at: https://www.economist.com/business/2016/02/11/diversity-fatigue. Accessed October 1, 2019.
34. Gill M, Bagshaw S, McKenzie E, et al. Patient and family member-led research in the intensive care unit: a novel approach to patient-centered research. PLoS One 2016;11(8):e0160947.
35. McCulloch SG, Lau HY, Starreveld Y, et al. Esthesioneuroblastoma masquerading as chronic rhinosinusitis. Case Rep Clin Med 2015;4:303–8.

Impact of Patient and Family Involvement in Long-Term Outcomes

Christopher J. Grant, MD, FRCPC[a,b,c,*], Lauren F. Doig[c,d],
Joanna Everson, MN, NP[c,e], Nadine Foster, BN, RN[f],
Christopher James Doig, MD, MSc, FRCPC[a,c,g]

KEYWORDS

- Critical care • Critical illness recovery • Critical care outcomes
- Post–intensive care syndrome (PICS)
- Post–intensive care syndrome, family (PICS-F)

KEY POINTS

- Recovery from a critical illness includes addressing physical, cognitive, emotional, and functional effects that can persist for many months following discharge from an intensive care unit (ICU).
- Attending to patient and family care needs across the spectrum of care (in the ICU, on the ward, and in the community) is important to improve critical illness outcomes.
- Recovery resources following critical illness sometimes do not fully address the needs of patients and families; this represents an opportunity to improve care and outcomes.

Critical illness requiring care in an intensive care unit (ICU) is a harrowing event for patients and their families.[1] If aware, the patients face the risk of confronting their own mortality. Family members often overestimate the likelihood of ICU survival and/or a return to independent function at home, and underestimate the requirement of

[a] Department of Critical Care Medicine, Cumming School of Medicine, University of Calgary, Calgary, Alberta, Canada; [b] Department of Clinical Neurosciences, Cumming School of Medicine, University of Calgary, Calgary, Alberta, Canada; [c] Foothills Medical Centre, McCaig Tower, ICU Administration, 3134 Hospital Drive Northwest, Calgary, Alberta T2N 5A1, Canada; [d] Department of Occupational Therapy, Faculty of Rehabilitation Medicine, University of Alberta, Edmonton, Alberta, Canada; [e] Department of Critical Care Medicine, University of Calgary, Calgary, Alberta, Canada; [f] Department of Critical Care, Alberta Health Services, Foothills Medical Centre, McCaig Tower, ICU Administration, 3134 Hospital Drive Northwest, Calgary, Alberta T2N 5A1, Canada; [g] Department of Community Health Sciences, Cumming School of Medicine, University of Calgary, Calgary, Alberta, Canada
* Corresponding author. Foothills Medical Centre, McCaig Tower, ICU Administration, 3134 Hospital Drive Northwest, Calgary, Alberta T2N 5A1, Canada.
E-mail address: christopher.grant@ucalgary.ca

Crit Care Nurs Clin N Am 32 (2020) 227–242
https://doi.org/10.1016/j.cnc.2020.02.005
0899-5885/20/© 2020 Elsevier Inc. All rights reserved.
ccnursing.theclinics.com

physiologic intervention to sustain a patient's life.[2] As interventions are added that seem usual processes of care for staff, the family perception may be that they are seeing their loved one "slipping away."[3,4] Facing extreme uncertainty leads to a sense of chaos and loss of control, which is perpetuated by the physical transformation of the loved one.[5]

Survival and discharge from the ICU is often viewed as a moment for celebration.[6] This transition often occurs without the understanding that surviving critical care is often not as simple as being discharged from the ICU to the ward, then from the ward to home, and then life returning to what it was. ICU discharge is simply 1 transition in a complicated process of recovery that affects both the patient, the caregivers, and the family. Patients and families are hoping, expecting, and working toward full recovery, but changes in function and functional decline are a common experience after critical illness.[7–10]

Surviving a critical illness can have long-term effects for both patients and families. Former patients can be troubled by a myriad of symptoms that are often categorized under the umbrella of post–intensive care syndrome (PICS).[11] PICS is associated with myriad physical, psychological, emotional, and financial effects, which can result in important reductions in both quantity and quality of life. Recovery from a critical illness may take years, and is often incomplete. There may be a sense of ambiguous loss where individuals have difficulty coping, lacking an understanding of what has happened to them and why, and the conflict created in personal relationships identifying the dichotomy that, to family and others, survivors may seem physically better, but have significant psychological and neurocognitive residue.[12]

Academics and clinicians have recognized that the aftereffects of a critical illness also extend to families of critical illness survivors. PICS-family (PICS-F) is meant to help identify and stimulate examination and understanding of the effects and chronic burden, also physical, cognitive, psychological, and financial, on family members and caregivers of loved ones who were critically ill.[13] Both survivors and family members have to navigate a state of disruption as they attempt to regain their former selves or adapt to a new normal. The difficulties in recovery are hampered by a system that may not be aware or attentive to sequelae of critical illness and the struggles faced by ICU survivors and their families.[14] Despite interest, there remains a paucity of structured systems and follow-up for ICU survivors, ICU recovery care maps, and plans to guide patients and providers.[15,16] This situation is in contrast with other life-threatening diseases, such as cancer, for which the system of care is attentive to maintaining the physical and mental health of both patients and families as they receive specific cancer treatment.[11,17,18]

Family members play an essential role in the ICU survivors' recovery and potential adaptation to a new norm of health.[19] Using select anecdotes from patients and caregivers, this article describes some of the burden of recovery that starts in the ICU, and continues with patients and families long after they have left the ICU. It highlights some differences between the surviving patients and families, recognizing that both bear a potentially substantive burden. Addressing and influencing recovery trajectories for critically ill patients presents an immense challenge but also a tremendous opportunity. This article shares anecdotes and research about our experiences, with hopes the information will serve as a catalyst for changes in care.

PHYSICAL HEALTH EFFECTS OF SURVIVING CRITICAL ILLNESS

It was unbelievable how weak I was. I couldn't sit up by myself. My voice was a whisper. I felt like I didn't have the strength to breathe. I couldn't lift my arms and I couldn't walk. I felt like a child. The worst was when I went to the ward. I was so weak I needed help with everything, but the staff didn't seem to understand. The worst part was going to the bathroom. I'd ring the bell, somebody would answer, but nobody would come or at least not soon enough. It's embarrassing making a mess in the bed, and worse to then lie in it.

—Patient

I don't remember much … maybe the last day or so. I remember my chest tube being pulled, and my endotracheal tube being pulled. I remember how much it hurt.

—Patient

I was a triathlete … not professional, but able to compete. Nine months after ICU, I can barely work 4-hour shifts, and I can't run 5 km. If I do go for a run, that's it for the week because of how long it takes me to recover.

—Patient

I hated going into the ICU. My dad didn't look normal … swollen to almost unrecognizable proportions and covered with tubes from every hole. I didn't want to touch him for fear of harming him.

—Family member

It's a bit embarrassing to say, and selfish, but I was grossed out. I think everybody is physically attracted to their spouse … including the small physical flaws we each have. But when my wife came out, she had a big scar. She had a bag, and the rest of her body was totally different. She couldn't do anything we used to do together. It was as if a different person had come home with me.

—Family member

PICS includes substantial physical sequelae.[20,21] Some sequelae are unique to specific illnesses. For example, scars and stomas can be associated with complex abdominal surgery. Amputations can result from complicated soft tissue infections or trauma. Chronic renal failure can result from acute kidney injury in the ICU. However, it is now accepted that many physical effects that trouble patients after they leave the ICU are related more generally to the critical illness itself. In one of the seminal articles on the topic, Herridge and colleagues[22] followed acute respiratory distress syndrome (ARDS) survivors and showed substantial physical consequences that were not related to the respiratory system specifically. Herridge and colleagues[22] did show some organ-specific dysfunction, such as impaired pulmonary function, and this can be important. More generally though, these investigators showed profound and persisting weakness that was not obviously linked to lung function. For example, even 6 months after critical illness, survivors in this cohort averaged 64% of predicted for age-sex normative on the 6-minute walk tests. Other investigators have shown that survivors of ARDS are at higher risk of bone demineralization and fracture.[23] More research has shown the near-ubiquitous detrimental effect of critical illness on muscle volume and function. Estimates of loss of muscle volume are 3% to 4% per day in the early stages of the acute inflammatory stage of critical illness.[24] The complex pathobiology is not yet elucidated, but the biochemical and histologic changes described include impairment in mitochondrial function and contractility, collagen deposition, and apoptosis.[25] The practical reality is that patients may have significant decrements in muscle strength compared with age-sex normative values.[26]

Pain is common and can persist.[27] There may be pain specific to a medical procedure, such as postoperative pain, but neuropathic pain with dysesthesias and allodynia can also occur.[28] Chronic pain is associated with a myriad of physical and mental health consequences. Some chronic pain is debilitating and makes even simple daily tasks, such as dressing, extremely difficult. The personal recollections of Cheryl Misak, a survivor of sepsis, describe the severe pain experienced during her recovery at home.[29] A reader of her poignant story might wonder whether she had been a marathon runner, whether she could have "pushed through" her pain. Even if she did, how many cannot? Balanced against the pain is health care professionals' attention to excess opioid prescription and use, and a fear of habituating individuals to a state of dependency.[30] The physical effects of illness can be psychologically devastating. There is a potential effect on individuals' sense of personal worth and value with the loss of an inability to mobilize independently, to perform activities of daily living, and to swallow and speak. The change in physical appearance and self-image can be psychologically traumatizing. There is substantial evidence of the effect of body change and composition on a person's sense of self-worth, and the impact on personal relationships. The experience for the family member may be considerably different. Many health care providers do not understand the extent of the physical impact: the ambiguous loss, which may also be true for family.[24] Family members may not appreciate the physical changes at first. Loss of muscle mass in the ICU may be difficult to visualize because of edema fluid, or replacement by other subcutaneous tissue such as fat. The extent of the weakness and fatigue may not be appreciated. Radiographic abnormalities and their correlation to physiologic changes and functional limitations may not be known or understood by family: a normal appearance on the outside does not reflect profound anatomic changes internally. The impact on the ability to perform simple daily activities, such as walking, climbing stairs, and grocery shopping, may be significant. The slow trajectory of recovery may not be appreciated such that the ongoing consequences of recovery are difficult to comprehend. For example, a substantial proportion of ARDS survivors required ongoing informal care more than 1-year after hospital discharge.[31] At times, this can result in significant consequences to personal relationships. For example, a resentment that, if verbally expressed, might be equivalent to saying, "Why aren't you better yet," "How much longer until you're better," and resentment to a larger burden of work borne by the caregiver within the family/relationship. The physical changes may be difficult too. For spouses, the effect of change in body image can affect intimate relationships and worsen the perception of worth, value, or of being loved. Griffiths and colleagues[32] found that 45% of patients and 40% of their partners expressed dissatisfaction with their current sex lives. In addition, physical impacts of critical illness can have practical effects on patients and families. When can a person return to work? Who will be driving the ICU survivor to follow-up appointments? How will the mortgage be paid if the survivor is not yet back to work?

COGNITIVE AND EMOTIONAL CONSEQUENCES OF CRITICAL ILLNESS

I am not the same. I have difficulty in attention. I try to write an email, and it can take me an hour. Sometimes I can't remember the words. Sometimes I can't formulate the thought. Everything I do is exhausting, and it is far worse after I've been concentrating. My memory is terrible. I can get around some lapses by using lists. What's more distressing is forgetting individuals or losing the context of relationships. While I'm struggling, my husband looks at me and wonders what the hell is wrong with me: "it's been 6, 9, 12 months … are you just being lazy?" He may not say it straight out, but I can read between the lines. He doesn't get that I'm still not better.

—Patient

I hate not knowing what happened. I have blanks in my memory. There are weeks that are just gone … a black hole. I've read the diaries that my mum wrote. It sounds terrifying; mum was talking that I was dying. I can see her tears on the pages, yet I remember nothing. Not knowing what happened is reassuring — maybe I don't want to know. It's also difficult. I can't relate to what happened to my family because I can't remember.

—*Patient*

Sleeping is the worst part. We sleep in separate bedrooms now. I need a light on and sometimes I wake up in a panic or sweat. I can have vivid dreams. A few are peaceful but most are scary.

—*Patient*

I think the worst part was when he had delirium. The things he said (he's the politest man, but he was so rude). I couldn't comfort him, and he acted totally paranoid. It was tough, given how sick he had been, and everybody telling me he was getting better.

—*Family member*

It was just an emotional roller coaster. One doctor was very grim … I don't think he smiled. We seemed like an inconvenience in his busy day. When he did talk to us it was way above our heads. The next doctor was kinder, came (we think purposefully, but it seemed as if casually) and said "Hi" when we were at the bedside. He didn't take away our hope, while still being honest with how serious it was.

—*Family member*

My dad can't forgive himself. He really thought I was going to die. He planned my funeral during my stay. He now just can't or won't talk about it.

—*Family member*

How does anybody get better? The noise is unbelievable! Every machine beeps or alarms. We didn't understand how nurses ignored the alarms … aren't alarms important? What's on your phone that's more important than [an] alarm? The waiting was terrible too … you can wait for hours while the nurses "provide care," little do they know [you are] frustrated wondering if they're just on their phones.

—*Family member*

There are mental health and cognitive consequences associated with critical illness survival that can affect patients and their families in different ways. In circumstances in which patients are admitted to an ICU for a primary brain injury (eg, stroke or traumatic brain injury), families might be more prepared for cognitive changes. However, many family members are surprised by delirium and do not anticipate the long-term cognitive and psychological consequences that can follow. Most patients in ICU experience delirium, perhaps as part of or temporally associated with a systemic inflammatory response, with reports of prevalence between 50% and 80%.[33] The specific cause for delirium is unknown. Delirium might be a consequence of a multitude of risk factors, such as systemic inflammation, impairments in blood-brain function, the gut barrier function, the ICU environment, sleep disruption, pain, medication, or a combination of some or all. Further, it has been suggested that delirium should be considered as a primary brain injury with long-term cognitive consequences.[34]

Elderly survivors of critical care with delirium may experience significant intellectual impairment severe enough to prevent a return to independent living.[35] Impairment in intellectual dysfunction also affects younger individuals. As examples, there is evidence of impairments in spatial recognition, pattern recognition, and in tasks such as delayed matching to sample tests.[36] In the same report, animal models of sepsis showed that there are effects on pathways that include deficits in spatial memory. Electroencephalogram data from survivors also show abnormalities in frontal lobe function associated with disorders of habitual behavior.[37] Many individuals report abnormalities in executive function, such as concentration and integration of information. These abnormalities may have an effect on regaining employment in past occupations, and retraining and entering new careers. Research to date shows that approximately 50% of ICU survivors do not return to work after recovery, and in many despite no physical limitation.[38] Although commonly attributed to physical impairment, fatigue is also known as a common symptom of brain dysfunction.

Other mental health consequences may be just as significant as the cognitive consequences. It is well recognized that many patients experience effects to their memory. Many of these memories are false in that recalled events cannot be established as factual despite vivid, specific, and explicit recall by the patient.[39] Some of the memories are traumatic and associated with fear, anxiety, or panic; for example, the fear that somebody was trying to harm them. The phenomenon of Capgras delusion (a sense of a familiar replaced by an unknown or an alien) is common and frequently mentioned in reports of patient experiences.[40] Not all patients experience negative memories: some may be described as peaceful or calming (eg, a recollection of being rocked on a cruise ship, being in the north of Canada under the northern lights enveloped in a sleeping bag). Some can (with variable success) be explained (eg, the rocking cruise ship by the back-and-forth motion of a rocking mattress; description of a faceless staff member by a piece of vividly recalled clothing). These explanations may or may not provide relief for the patients. Some patients have virtually no recall of their ICU stays. Although at first glance this might seem potentially good (not having to remember being life-threateningly ill, or painful procedures being performed), the gap of not knowing what happened or why has been associated with contributing to residual psychological distress.

Apart from the effect on memories and cognition, many patients experience anxiety or depression that occurs during hospitalization and continues after hospital discharge. The use of standardized instruments such as the Hospital Anxiety and Depression Scale to screen for depression, the Generalized Anxiety Disorder 7-item (GAD-7) for anxiety, and the Impact of Events Score–Revised for traits associated with posttraumatic stress disorder is common in ICU follow-up clinics because of the frequency of these symptoms. Sleep disruption is common.[41,42] Initially these sleep changes are severe, and then they slowly improve over time. However, it is common for sleep pattern changes to persist to even a year after a critical illness. Pain and sleep disruption individually and together further impair physical and psychological recovery.

For families, the experience is different. Families often describe their stay as an emotional rollercoaster.[1] Although it is the rule for survivors of critical illness to have no or very little recall of the early hyperacute events in the ICU, family members often have intense and visceral recollections of events around the time when their loved ones were most ill. Invariably these are distressing memories. The environment for the family is often described by the foreign nature of the ICU. A physical environment with an overwhelming breadth of machines, and requisite supporting staff. A cacophony of light, odors, and noise from people, machines, and alarms. The physical appearance of the loved one may be difficult, and some have described a fear of touching the loved one for fear of causing damage or harm from misplacing a tube or device.[43] The complexity of illness and interventions can be intellectually and emotionally overwhelming. It may be hard to recognize improvement or recovery, and to emotionally navigate a balance between hope versus the fear of a fatal outcome.[44] The social and psychological environment is overwhelming too. Many

ICUs' processes of care are still seemingly steeped in paternalism in which the care provider knows best. Access may be explicitly restricted with limited visiting hours, locked doors, and interminable waiting; in other units, there is a functional restriction by staff providing care or busy with tasks. Individuals who are extremely important to patients but are not familial relatives may not therefore be recognized as family and may face particular barriers, including physical exclusion from visiting, and social exclusion from information.[45] Families notice loud, and therefore perceived as urgent, alarms that are often ignored without explanation. Staff answering phone calls seemed harried, but, in contradistinction, the use of personal devices may suggest inattentive or distracted staff. Communication can be difficult because of power imbalances, which can be contributed to by the multiplicity of teams and clinicians involved, none of whom may have had a prior relationship with the patient or family; the frequent change in staff; and the difficulty in finding an opportunity to speak to physicians or the person who is in charge. Families may perceive that care is more machines being manipulated rather than a patient being treated. Use of bed numbers not names and focusing on manipulating machines rather than providing care to a patient may be perceived as depersonalizing.[46] At the same time, patients and families can be extremely grateful for amazing recoveries, or compassionate end-of-life care; recognition of compassion and concerned care by an individual staff member of the team is common.

There is research on the effects on families, with significant reports of stress, anxiety, and mental health effects that are similar or greater in frequency and severity than for families supporting patients in many other health conditions, such as chronic dementia and cancer. Areas in which critically ill patients and family members share common experiences within the ICU are in the realms of mental health, quality of life, and fatigue. Like patients, many family members experience high levels of fatigue. Family member fatigue occurs early in the ICU admission, and persists for months after critical illness.[47] Anxiety and depression symptoms are prevalent in family members with loved ones in the ICU. Family members also show high levels of stress symptoms, even 6 months after ICU.[48] Three months after discharge from ICU, family members report changes in their quality of life. Unlike critical illness survivors, family members do not report changes in their physical health–related quality of life, but they do report substantial impairments in the mental components of quality of life.[49] Specifically, family members experience important reductions in social functioning, vitality, emotional role, and mental health functioning at 3 months after critical illness.

Significant research has been undertaken to understand the needs of families in an effort to improve care, communication, family support, and engagement while in the ICU. Attempts have been made to make family part of the care team.[50,51] Restricted visiting hours or access are being removed. National guidelines have been developed recommending ease of access and increased engagement by families.[52] The presence of family or individuals who are important to the patient may provide an important locus of reality for patients in the ICU because they are familiar or known. Attempts have been made to engage family in nontechnical care, and even in helping in the diagnosis of certain syndromes such as delirium. Diaries for families, including staff documenting information, help families explain and bring meaning to patients regarding the nature of their illnesses and what has happened.[53]

SOCIAL CONSEQUENCES OF CRITICAL ILLNESS: FINANCIAL AND RELATIONAL

I'm so tired I can't imagine having sex. I need help getting dressed. I need help with personal care. After dialysis I want to puke. After I eat, I want to puke. Sex is the last thing on my mind. I haven't even asked my wife. Do you think she wants to have sex with the person whose bum she has to wipe?

—Patient

I was the "hot wheels mama." I was an architect and good with spatial orientation. I lost that ability and couldn't work. That was hard but I guess okay. We were financially sound and I had long-term disability insurance. What wasn't okay was that one of my favorite relaxation time with my boys was to build complex hot wheels tracks. Losing my ability in spatial orientation meant I couldn't build these tracks. I think my kids thought I'd lost interest in them.

—Patient

I've struggled returning to work. I was a successful financial analyst. I used to rapidly evaluate a company's financial sheets. Now, I can do math, and read spreadsheets, but I can't integrate the information. I can't do my work anymore. I was the main bread winner for my family: the financial hardship is significant.

—Patient

It is irrational that after all of the work that dedicated physicians and nurses put into saving someone's life, when they do succeed, there is nothing after ICU except the resourcefulness of the family.[1]

—Family member

My husband had complex abdominal surgery, a stoma, fistulas. He had chronic renal failure. We had excellent follow-up appointments but so much was missing. I was overjoyed to have him home, but the regular daily care he needed was overwhelming. I stopped work to help him. I thought I was coping but I didn't realize the complexity. I still remember the day in the follow-up clinic, the worry on the doctor's face and his firmness with us that he needed readmission. I thought I had failed him.

—Family member

Many patients and their families experience not only emotional and physical consequences but also very practical financial impacts. Family members provide a substantial amount of informal (ie, nonprofessional) care, a role for which they are often untrained and unpaid.[54] The requirement for ongoing care for ICU survivors is substantial because major functional decline is the rule. Approximately 80% of ICU survivors with ARDS still required informal care 2 years after hospital discharge.[31] ICU survivors may need help with myriad physical, psychological, and cognitive problems, resulting in many hours of attention and care each day. In an Australian study of 71 families of ICU survivors surveyed 3 months after hospital discharge, family caregivers were providing 37 hours of care per week.[55] These family members only received 4 hours of caregiving support from friends and extended family, and paid daily caregiver support was the exception (8% of patients accessed daily paid caregiver support). Family and friends often coalesce around a patient to provide support during the ICU stay, but unfortunately, following discharge, often these supports return to their own lives, leaving families to cope using their own resources.

The role of caregiver is disproportionately borne by female spouses; male spouses often struggle in providing care and require more support.[55] The provision of care is often viewed as a consequence of filial obligation. At the same time, the strain of the responsibility is sometimes associated with stresses in personal relationships.[18,56] Although many studies have identified negative consequences, there are also studies that have suggested that not all effects are negative. For example, some families report that the sense of responsibility and physical, emotional, and financial costs are associated with a source of personal satisfaction. Caregiving has also been described as rewarding, with individuals providing gratification from providing complex care that in itself may help mitigate stress.

There may be specific detrimental effects on children of adult ICU patients. Children may have added difficulty contemplating the death of a parent and understanding the complexity of illness. Having a parent return home may require children to take over caregiving roles, jeopardizing educational, emotional, and social well-being.[57]

Financial stress is common for survivors and their families.[58] In 1 study, half of people who were fully employed before the critical illness had returned to work at the 1-year mark after the illness.[38] Research from US centers has shown that, in survivors of serious illness, a third of patients required caregiver assistance from family members, and, in 11% of cases, family members quit or take time off from work to provide this care.[59] Disturbingly, in this cohort, 31% reported losing most of their life savings as a result of their family member becoming ill.

Coupled with these increased financial stressors is the fact that rehabilitation can be expensive. Many health systems and health insurance providers do not cover the costs associated with rehabilitation following a critical illness. Coverage can seem arbitrary. For example, physiotherapy and targeted exercise programs provided to patients under the umbrella of cardiac rehabilitation after myocardial infarction; similarly ill patients with sepsis who have functional impairments analogous to heart failure may find that access to outpatient rehabilitation resources is not covered. The need for counseling for stress related to critical illness recovery months after hospital discharge may not be understood and therefore the counseling may be denied.

HOW SHOULD CRITICAL CARE AND HEALTH SYSTEMS RESPOND?

Six weeks in the ICU, 3 months in hospital, and then discharged home. The only thing I was told is "You might feel weaker when you go home, it might last for a few months." Nobody came to look at the house. I had a hospital bed in the living room because I was too weak to get up the stairs. I didn't have a shower on the same floor. I had appointments with specialists ... all on different days, all weeks to months after discharge, and I couldn't drive. The cost of my wife taking off work, of parking, was enormous. Physiotherapy and occupational therapy wasn't provided, and there was no way we could afford it.

—Patient

First, it is important that health care providers, particularly in a complex environment such as an ICU, recognize and embrace the essential role of the family in care provision.[60] Family members should not be viewed as passive bystanders. They should be viewed as partners in care, able to substantially contribute to the psychological and physical well-being of patients. Much work has already been done to identify family needs in the ICU, and ways to improve family satisfaction with care, but there needs to be broader and more systemic initiatives to maintain and build on improving the quality of care.[61] The first should be the environment. A family member advises us, "The environment of the ICU often serves the convenience of the ICU staff rather than the family unit, the objects of our care. Why is that ICU professionals believe their presence by the bedside to be more important than family members?"[62] One of the simplest measures is to improve access to patients,[63] not just improving physical access to the ICU bedside but improving how technology and care is perceived. Dehumanization and the physical barriers of technology are perhaps the greatest barriers to caring. ICUs should improve physical access to the ICU by minimizing time spent waiting. Limiting visitation hours is not respectful of the role of family, or the reality of coping with maintaining social structures, particularly when a stay in an ICU may be prolonged. It is possible to also have family engage in nontechnical aspects of care. This engagement may be as simple as passive range of motion, rubbing or massaging to relieve pain, or helping in the recognition of perturbations in a patient such as the recognition of delirium. In addition, clinicians have to be cognizant of the complexities in personal relationships that precede ICU admission, recognize that the traditional definition of family may not represent the reality for all individuals, and be inclusive in recognizing all of those close to a patient who may be emotionally invested and contribute to patient recovery and well-being.[45]

Second, clinicians need to improve the transitions in care and recognize the complexity of transfers/transitions and that care should not be compromised, or perceived to be compromised, at these transition points. One of the most negative aspects of transfer may be a perception that transfers are more associated with competing demands/interests for beds rather than based on patients' care needs.[64,65] There needs to be a recognition of relocation stress associated with transitions in care, and the necessity for enhanced support and communication.[65–67] There are considerable differences in the processes of care developed in the ICU and on wards: the change in these processes and the effect on interprofessional communication and communication with family may perpetuate psychological distress. The other transition in care is the transfer from hospital to home. In many health care systems, the primary contact for patients is a primary care practitioner, but individually these providers may only rarely have a patient who has been discharged from ICU, and an understanding of the complexities of PICS may be lacking. Professional education of providers, primary care, and other community health disciplines is important to help begin survivors in navigating resources and care available.[68]

Third, clinicians need to consider how to develop interdisciplinary interprofessional teams in a model of survivorship.[69–71] There are significant examples from other disease groups (eg, cancer) on how these models improve care and coping. The development of comprehensive follow-up clinics for ICU survivors is a needed first step.[72,73] These clinics should involve individuals that can address the physical or physiologic consequences of acute and chronic critical illness and the psychological and mental health effects in survivors and caregivers, be able to provide comprehensive rehabilitative and adaptive assessment, and be able to provide opportunities for care that are cognizant of the financial consequences of critical illness. The engagement of physiotherapists and kinesiologists focused on enhancing functional physical recovery; occupational therapists that can address cognitive capacity, evaluate potential for employment, and help individuals adapt in complex environments; mental health counselors who can address psychological sequelae; and rehabilitation physicians with expertise in coordinating complex care requirements among multidisciplinary teams is needed. Part of this work needs to focus on agreed outcome measures that focus on functional recovery and measure adaptation or return to normal function, or function related to activities of daily living rather than organ-specific measures, or measures of physiologic function.[21] Part of care should include engagement of survivors and caregivers with other survivors and their families in a mechanism of peer support.[74] Although evidence has been limited, there is increasing attention to peer support as a mechanism to decrease social isolation, improve psychological morbidity, and improve the understanding of the journey of recovery.[75] The Intensive Care Foundation and ICUSteps in the United Kingdom has published a guide to facilitate setting up peer support groups. Twenty four cities in England and Scotland have these groups running.[76] To supplement this, criticalcarerecovery.com has developed online forums that are localized to specific centers where patients and families can share their experiences. The evidence on the effectiveness of these interventions is

> **Box 1**
> **Potential strategies to improve caregiver outcomes**
>
> The ICU environment
> - Increase communication
> - Decrease the strain of the environment
> - Include and engage families in care
> - Provide information
> - Screen for stress and develop multidisciplinary support
> - Show through words and action the principle of patient and family–centered care
> - Thoughtful and compassionate decision making
> - Prepare for ICU postcare
>
> Following discharge
> - Facilitate patient adaptation
> - Develop support networks
> - Manage psychological consequences
> - Provided access to respite care
> - Screen for stress
> - Increase social support; decrease social isolation

still to be determined, but they represent innovative approaches to address patient and family needs after ICU.

In addition to the strategies shown in **Box 1**, ongoing research is needed to improve the quality of survivorship. Although ICU research dedicated to understanding the complex pathobiology of critical illness and addressing translational therapies for the bedside is essential to improve ICU survivorship, concurrently there is a need to increase the understanding of the quality of survivorship and develop mechanisms to improve survivorship for patients and caregivers. Survivorship research should include the development of multidisciplinary research networks.[77,78] Further, research on survivors should engage multidisciplinary partners outside of critical care.

SUMMARY

Recovery following a critical illness is a complex process. There are many aspects associated with critical illness recovery. These aspects include physical, emotional, cognitive, relational, and financial changes. These changes affect patients as well as their families long after they leave the ICU.

It is important for care providers not to be nihilist about the work they do. What happens in an ICU is foundational. But for the care provided in the ICU, many patients and families would not have the opportunity to even attempt healing and recovery. However, much of the work associated with critical illness recovery happens beyond the walls of an ICU.

To improve ICU outcomes, clinicians must continue to provide excellence in care within the unit. They also must be practical about the challenges that patients and their families face after they leave. Supporting and empowering patients and their families across the continuum of care is key to improving critical illness outcomes.

DISCLOSURE

The authors have nothing to disclose.

REFERENCES

1. Dyzenhaus D. One family's perspective on the legacy of critical illness. In: Stevens RD, Hart N, Herridge M, editors. Textbook of post-ICU medicine: the legacy of critical care. Oxford (England): Oxford University Press; 2014. p. 130–3.
2. Azoulay E, Chevret S, Leleu G, et al. Half the families of intensive care unit patients experience inadequate communication with physicians. Crit Care Med 2000;28(8):3044–9.
3. Unroe M, Kahn JM, Carson SS, et al. One-year trajectories of care and resource utilization for recipients of prolonged mechanical ventilation: a cohort study. Ann Intern Med 2010;153(3):167–75.
4. Cox CE, Martinu T, Sathy SJ, et al. Expectations and outcomes of prolonged mechanical ventilation. Crit Care Med 2009;37(11):2888–94 [quiz: 2904].
5. Agard AS, Harder I. Relatives' experiences in intensive care–finding a place in a world of uncertainty. Intensive Crit Care Nurs 2007;23(3):170–7.
6. Chaboyer W, Kendall E, Kendall M, et al. Transfer out of intensive care: a qualitative exploration of patient and family perceptions. Aust Crit Care 2005;18(4):138–41, 143–5.
7. McPeake J, Mikkelsen ME. The evolution of post intensive care syndrome. Crit Care Med 2018;46(9):1551–2.
8. de Grood C, Leigh JP, Bagshaw SM, et al. Patient, family and provider experiences with transfers from intensive care unit to hospital ward: a multicentre qualitative study. CMAJ 2018;190(22):E669–76.
9. Gill M, Bagshaw SM, McKenzie E, et al. Patient and family member-led research in the intensive care unit: a novel approach to patient-centered research. PLoS One 2016;11(8):e0160947.
10. Li P, Boyd JM, Ghali WA, et al. Stakeholder views regarding patient discharge from intensive care: suboptimal quality and opportunities for improvement. Can Respir J 2015;22(2):109–18.
11. Needham DM, Davidson J, Cohen H, et al. Improving long-term outcomes after discharge from intensive care unit: report from a stakeholders' conference. Crit Care Med 2012;40(2):502–9.
12. Johnston LB. Surviving critical illness: a case study in ambiguity. J Soc Work End Life Palliat Care 2011;7(4):363–82.
13. Davidson JE, Jones C, Bienvenu OJ. Family response to critical illness: postintensive care syndrome-family. Crit Care Med 2012;40(2):618–24.
14. van der Schaaf M, Beelen A, Dongelmans DA, et al. Functional status after intensive care: a challenge for rehabilitation professionals to improve outcome. J Rehabil Med 2009;41(5):360–6.
15. Lasiter S, Oles SK, Mundell J, et al. Critical care follow-up clinics: a scoping review of interventions and outcomes. Clin Nurse Spec 2016;30(4):227–37.
16. Kahn JM, Angus DC. Health policy and future planning for survivors of critical illness. Curr Opin Crit Care 2007;13(5):514–8.
17. Mewes JC, Steuten LM, Ijzerman MJ, et al. Effectiveness of multidimensional cancer survivor rehabilitation and cost-effectiveness of cancer rehabilitation in general: a systematic review. Oncologist 2012;17(12):1581–93.
18. Bevans M, Sternberg EM. Caregiving burden, stress, and health effects among family caregivers of adult cancer patients. JAMA 2012;307(4):398–403.

19. Erb C, Siegel M. Caring for the ICU survivor: the family caregiver burden. In: Stevens R, Hart N, Herridge M, editors. Textbook of post-ICU medicine: the legacy of critical care. Oxford (England): Oxford University Press; 2014. p. 108–22.

20. Desai SV, Law TJ, Needham DM. Long-term complications of critical care. Crit Care Med 2011;39(2):371–9.

21. Aitken LM, Marshall AP. Monitoring and optimising outcomes of survivors of critical illness. Intensive Crit Care Nurs 2015;31(1):1–9.

22. Herridge MS, Cheung AM, Tansey CM, et al. One-year outcomes in survivors of the acute respiratory distress syndrome. N Engl J Med 2003;348(8):683–93.

23. Rawal J, McPhail MJ, Ratnayake G, et al. A pilot study of change in fracture risk in patients with acute respiratory distress syndrome. Crit Care 2015;19:165.

24. Field K, Prinjha S, Rowan K. One patient amongst many': a qualitative analysis of intensive care unit patients' experiences of transferring to the general ward. Crit Care 2008;12(1):R21.

25. Kress JP, Hall JB. ICU-acquired weakness and recovery from critical illness. N Engl J Med 2014;370(17):1626–35.

26. Solverson KJ, Grant C, Doig CJ. Assessment and predictors of physical functioning post-hospital discharge in survivors of critical illness. Ann Intensive Care 2016;6(1):92.

27. Battle CE, Lovett S, Hutchings H. Chronic pain in survivors of critical illness: a retrospective analysis of incidence and risk factors. Crit Care 2013;17(3):R101.

28. Choi J, Hoffman LA, Schulz R, et al. Self-reported physical symptoms in intensive care unit (ICU) survivors: pilot exploration over four months post-ICU discharge. J Pain Symptom Manage 2014;47(2):257–70.

29. Misak C. Survival and recovery: a patient's perspective. In: Stevens RD, Hart N, Herridge M, editors. Textbook of post-ICU medicine: the legacy of critical care. Oxford (England): Oxford University Press; 2014. p. 125–9.

30. Puntillo KA, Naidu R. Chronic pain disorders after critical illness and ICU-acquired opioid dependence: two clinical conundra. Curr Opin Crit Care 2016; 22(5):506–12.

31. Cameron JI, Herridge MS, Tansey CM, et al. Well-being in informal caregivers of survivors of acute respiratory distress syndrome. Crit Care Med 2006;34(1):81–6.

32. Griffiths J, Gager M, Alder N, et al. A self-report-based study of the incidence and associations of sexual dysfunction in survivors of intensive care treatment. Intensive Care Med 2006;32(3):445–51.

33. Svenningsen H, Tonnesen EK, Videbech P, et al. Intensive care delirium - effect on memories and health-related quality of life - a follow-up study. J Clin Nurs 2014;23(5–6):634–44.

34. Girard TD, Jackson JC, Pandharipande PP, et al. Delirium as a predictor of long-term cognitive impairment in survivors of critical illness. Crit Care Med 2010; 38(7):1513–20.

35. Balas MC, Happ MB, Yang W, et al. Outcomes associated with delirium in older patients in surgical ICUs. Chest 2009;135(1):18–25.

36. Andonegui G, Zelinski EL, Schubert CL, et al. Targeting inflammatory monocytes in sepsis-associated encephalopathy and long-term cognitive impairment. JCI Insight 2018;3(9) [pii:99364].

37. Hosokawa K, Gaspard N, Su F, et al. Clinical neurophysiological assessment of sepsis-associated brain dysfunction: a systematic review. Crit Care 2014; 18(6):674.

38. Norman BC, Jackson JC, Graves JA, et al. Employment outcomes after critical illness: an analysis of the bringing to light the risk factors and incidence of

neuropsychological dysfunction in ICU survivors cohort. Crit Care Med 2016; 44(11):2003–9.

39. Storli SL, Lindseth A, Asplund K. A journey in quest of meaning: a hermeneutic-phenomenological study on living with memories from intensive care. Nurs Crit Care 2008;13(2):86–96.

40. Jones C. Narratives of illness and healing after the ICU. In: Stevens RD, Hart N, Herridge M, editors. Textbook of post-ICU medicine: the legacy of critical care. Oxford (England): Oxford University Press; 2014. p. 597–620.

41. Altman MT, Knauert MP, Pisani MA. Sleep disturbance after hospitalization and critical illness: a systematic review. Ann Am Thorac Soc 2017;14(9):1457–68.

42. Solverson KJ, Easton PA, Doig CJ. Assessment of sleep quality post-hospital discharge in survivors of critical illness. Respir Med 2016;114:97–102.

43. Eriksson T, Lindahl B, Bergbom I. Visits in an intensive care unit–an observational hermeneutic study. Intensive Crit Care Nurs 2010;26(1):51–7.

44. Engstrom A, Soderberg S. The experiences of partners of critically ill persons in an intensive care unit. Intensive Crit Care Nurs 2004;20(5):299–308 [quiz: 309–10].

45. Brown SM, Rozenblum R, Aboumatar H, et al. Defining patient and family engagement in the intensive care unit. Am J Respir Crit Care Med 2015;191(3): 358–60.

46. Cypress BS. The intensive care unit: experiences of patients, families, and their nurses. Dimens Crit Care Nurs 2010;29(2):94–101.

47. Choi J, Tate JA, Hoffman LA, et al. Fatigue in family caregivers of adult intensive care unit survivors. J Pain Symptom Manage 2014;48(3):353–63.

48. Anderson WG, Arnold RM, Angus DC, et al. Posttraumatic stress and complicated grief in family members of patients in the intensive care unit. J Gen Intern Med 2008;23(11):1871–6.

49. Lemiale V, Kentish-Barnes N, Chaize M, et al. Health-related quality of life in family members of intensive care unit patients. J Palliat Med 2010;13(9):1131–7.

50. Bain S, Littlepage M. A promising new therapy may assist efforts to combat ICU-acquired weakness. Crit Care 2014;18(5):573.

51. Page P. Critical illness survivorship and implications for care provision; a constructivist grounded theory., in School of Health Sciences. London: University of London; 2016.

52. Davidson JE, Aslakson RA, Long AC, et al. Guidelines for family-centered care in the neonatal, pediatric, and adult ICU. Crit Care Med 2017;45(1):103–28.

53. Garrouste-Orgeas M, Perier A, Mouricou P, et al. Writing in and reading ICU diaries: qualitative study of families' experience in the ICU. PLoS One 2014; 9(10):e110146.

54. Van Pelt DC, Schulz R, Chelluri L, et al. Patient-specific, time-varying predictors of post-ICU informal caregiver burden: the caregiver outcomes after ICU discharge project. Chest 2010;137(1):88–94.

55. Foster M, Chaboyer W. Family carers of ICU survivors: a survey of the burden they experience. Scand J Caring Sci 2003;17(3):205–14.

56. Van Pelt DC, Milbrandt EB, Qin L, et al. Informal caregiver burden among survivors of prolonged mechanical ventilation. Am J Respir Crit Care Med 2007; 175(2):167–73.

57. Aldridge J, Becker S. Children as carers: the impact of parental illness and disability on children's caring roles. J Fam Ther 1999;21(3):303–20.

58. Kamdar BB, Huang M, Dinglas VD, et al. Joblessness and lost earnings after acute respiratory distress syndrome in a 1-year national multicenter study. Am J Respir Crit Care Med 2017;196(8):1012–20.

59. Covinsky KE, Goldman L, Cook EF, et al. The impact of serious illness on patients' families. SUPPORT Investigators. Study to understand prognoses and preferences for outcomes and risks of treatment. JAMA 1994;272(23):1839–44.

60. Carman KL, Dardess P, Maurer M, et al. Patient and family engagement: a framework for understanding the elements and developing interventions and policies. Health Aff (Millwood) 2013;32(2):223–31.

61. Kynoch K, Chang A, Coyer F, et al. The effectiveness of interventions to meet family needs of critically ill patients in an adult intensive care unit: a systematic review update. JBI Database System Rev Implement Rep 2016;14(3):181–234.

62. Levy MM, De Backer D. Re-visiting visiting hours. Intensive Care Med 2013;39(12):2223–5.

63. Cappellini E, Bambi S, Lucchini A, et al. Open intensive care units: a global challenge for patients, relatives, and critical care teams. Dimens Crit Care Nurs 2014;33(4):181–93.

64. Lin F, Chaboyer W, Wallis M, et al. Factors contributing to the process of intensive care patient discharge: an ethnographic study informed by activity theory. Int J Nurs Stud 2013;50(8):1054–66.

65. McKinney AA, Deeny P. Leaving the intensive care unit: a phenomenological study of the patients' experience. Intensive Crit Care Nurs 2002;18(6):320–31.

66. Mitchell ML, Courtney M, Coyer F. Understanding uncertainty and minimizing families' anxiety at the time of transfer from intensive care. Nurs Health Sci 2003;5:207–17.

67. Mitchell ML. Family-centred care – are we ready for it? An Australian Perspective. Nurs Crit Care 2005;10:54–5.

68. Kiernan F. Care of ICU survivors in the community: a guide for GPs. Br J Gen Pract 2017;67(663):477–8.

69. Hart N. Therapeutic and rehabilitation strategies in the ICU. In: Stevens RD, Hart N, Herridge M, editors. Textbook of post-ICU medicine: the legacy of critical care. Oxford (England): Oxford University Press; 2014. p. 419–20.

70. Elliott D, Davidson JE, Harvey MA, et al. Exploring the scope of post-intensive care syndrome therapy and care: engagement of non-critical care providers and survivors in a second stakeholders meeting. Crit Care Med 2014;42(12):2518–26.

71. Allen D, Gillen E, Rixson L. The effectiveness of integrated care pathways for adults and children in health care settings: a systematic review. JBI Libr Syst Rev 2009;7(3):80–129.

72. Connolly B, Douiri A, Steier J, et al. A UK survey of rehabilitation following critical illness: implementation of NICE Clinical Guidance 83 (CG83) following hospital discharge. BMJ Open 2014;4(5):e004963.

73. Cotton K. NICE CG83 - rehabilitation after critical illness: implementation across a network. Nurs Crit Care 2013;18(1):32–42.

74. McPeake J, Hirshberg EL, Christie LM, et al. Models of peer support to remediate post-intensive care syndrome: a report developed by the society of critical care medicine thrive international peer support collaborative. Crit Care Med 2019;47(1):e21–7.

75. Haines KJ, Beesley SJ, Hopkins RO, et al. Peer support in critical care: a systematic review. Crit Care Med 2018;46(9):1522–31.

76. ICUSteps. Guide to setting up a patients and relatives intensive care support group. In: Intensive Care Foundation, ICUSteps. London: Intensive Care Foundation, ICUSteps. 2010. p. 8.

77. RECOVER program. Canadian critical care trials group. Available at: https://www.ccctg.ca/Programs/RECOVER.aspx. Accessed December 5, 2019.

78. Outcomes after critical illness and surgery. Johns Hopkins Medicine. Available at: https://www.hopkinsmedicine.org/pulmonary/research/outcomes_after_critical_illness_surgery/. Accessed December 5, 2019.

Implementation of a Standardized Patient/Family Communication Bundle

Carrie Sona, RN, MSN, CCRN, CCNS, ACNS-BC, FCCM[a],*,
Kathryn A. Pollard, MD[b], Marilyn Schallom, RN, PhD, CCNS, FCCM[c],
Anne Schrupp, RN, BSN, CCRN[a], Brian T. Wessman, MD, FCCM[d,e]

KEYWORDS

- Communication • Family • Engagement • Satisfaction • Surrogate • Decision
- Goals • End-of-life

KEY POINTS

- Implementation of a patient and family communication bundle helps align the care provided with the patient goals and wishes.
- Align goals of care with patient wishes.
- Documentation of family discussions in the electronic health record improves communication among the healthcare team and patient and healthcare team satisfaction.

INTRODUCTION

Critical illness is a stressful time for patients and families; thus, providing patient-centered care is the accepted standard. Starting in 2002, the Centers for Medicare and Medicaid Services partnered with the Agency for Healthcare Research and Quality to develop a discharge survey to measure patient experiences. This survey, known as the Hospital Consumer Assessment of Healthcare Providers and Systems (HCAHPS), has further driven practice changes in hospitals to improve patient experience. In 2017, the Society of Critical Care Medicine (SCCM) published new Guidelines for Family-Centered Care in the Neonatal, Pediatric, and Adult ICU.[1] These guidelines summarize the current literature for patient-centered care practices and highlight areas that are valued by patients and family. These guidelines varied from the 2007 guidelines in that they reviewed all published literature since 1984, and

[a] Surgical/Burn/Trauma ICU, Barnes Jewish Hospital, St Louis, MO, USA; [b] Critical Care and Emergency Medicine, Indiana University Health Methodist Hospital, Indianapolis, IN, USA; [c] Department of Research for Patient Care Services, Barnes Jewish Hospital, St Louis, MO, USA; [d] EM/CCM, Department of Anesthesiology, Washington University in Saint Louis, School of Medicine, St Louis, MO, USA; [e] EM/CCM, Department of Emergency Medicine, Washington University in Saint Louis, School of Medicine, St Louis, MO, USA
* Corresponding author. 1 BJH Plaza, Mailstop 90-59-346, St Louis, MO 63110.
E-mail address: carrie.sona@bjc.org

Crit Care Nurs Clin N Am 32 (2020) 243–251
https://doi.org/10.1016/j.cnc.2020.02.006
0899-5885/20/© 2020 Elsevier Inc. All rights reserved.
ccnursing.theclinics.com

patients and families were involved in the development of the guideline. The amount of literature available in this area has exponentially increased since the 2007 SCCM Guidelines and the HCAHPS survey initiation. The comprehensive multiprofessional authorship group independently and anonymously rated the existing evidence. Despite the increase in literature, no evidence was rated as "strong" in the 2017 guidelines, which highlights the need for more work to be done. Areas identified as meaningful to critically ill patients and their support systems were separated into 5 categories that included family presence, family support, family communication, consultations and team, and organizational/environmental.

As part of a collaborative with the SCCM and the Patient-Centered Outcomes Research Institute (PCORI) to improve family engagement in the intensive care unit (ICU), our unit participated in a multicenter quality improvement project.[2] As a first step in the project, a unit self-assessment was completed using the Patient and Family-Centered Care Self-Assessment inventory contained within the SCCM Guidelines described previously.[1] Based on the gap analysis, our team identified the need to improve family communication as our priority to improve patient-centered care. This project was conducted in a 36-bed Surgical, Burn, Trauma ICU in a quaternary care academic, magnet-certified hospital with a closed ICU model; all patients having an intensivist-led care team coordinating care. Other specialties round separately when involved in the patient's care. In the academic setting, each hospital team may have multiple layers of team members (interns, residents, advanced practice providers [APPs], fellows, attending). This type of academic model can lead to poor patient/family communication with informal communication and fragmented messages. Fragmentation also can be stressful for ICU providers who witness this fragmented family communication model. Previous unit initiatives to improve end-of-life (EOL) care were implemented to address family support and team involvement.[3]

These prior published initiatives involved the creation of a multidisciplinary goals-of-care/EOL (GOC/EOL) team, the development of educational and communication tools for providers, patient/family and standardized EOL order sets, educational pamphlets regarding introduction to the ICU, and end-of-life educational materials for families and staff on EOL care. This current project sought to address the gap analysis of improving family communication and involvement throughout the ICU stay; not just at the EOL. We formulated a communication bundle with 3 components: (1) provider education and resources, (2) clearly identifying surrogate decision makers and existing advanced directives within 48 hours of ICU admission, and (3) thoroughly document these discussions in the medical record.[3] Our goal for the communication bundle was to improve patient/family satisfaction as well as medical provider satisfaction.

PROJECT

The multidisciplinary GOC/EOL team performed a review of the literature using the search terms *family, decision making, intensive care unit, communication,* and *goals of care*. Huffines and colleagues[4] implemented a family communication algorithm with a communication bundle of interventions provided at 24, 72, and 96 hours after admission to the ICU. The 24-hour meeting focused on ICU introductions, spokesperson identification and documentation, and health care legal document review. Patients were identified for a family meeting at 72 to 96 hours that was most frequently triggered by an Acute Physiology and Chronic Health Evaluation score predicting mortality greater than 40%. Most meetings did not prompt a change in level of care; however, 42% of meetings resulted in decisions about treatment limitations. Using the Critical Care Family Satisfaction Survey, the researchers found that family satisfaction scores increased, particularly for participation in decision making and perception of ICU staff teamwork. The primary barrier for family meeting completion was arranging the meeting to accommodate family members' and ICU team members' schedules. This same barrier was identified by Daly and colleagues.[5] They held scheduled family meetings within 5 days of ICU admission and weekly thereafter and found no improvement in mortality, length of stay, treatment limitation orders, or tracheostomy. Investigators did note that their structured family meetings may improve family information and support needs. In addition, Hurd and Curtis[6] identified education on family conferences as an important aspect of critical care physician training. Black and colleagues[7] treated patient/family communication like other clinical guidelines, such as surviving sepsis and eliminating hospital-acquired infections, and found that compliance was significantly better on day 1 than day 3. This contributed to our decision to achieve bundle compliance by 48 hours of ICU admission.

Based on the review of the literature and information obtained from the educational materials on conducting family care conferences on the VitalTalk.org Web site, we developed an initial discussion meeting outline and adopted the VitalTalk content for use as a standard communication pocket card (**Fig. 1**).[8] The initial discussion elements included team members who would be present at the family meeting, introductions with identification of surrogates with or without legal documents, allowing the family to speak, a brief overview of the ICU, medical update in simple language, time for questions, plan of care, and scheduling future meetings as needed. After the meeting, the conversation was to be documented in the electronic medical record (EMR) using our previously developed template (**Fig. 2**). Our goal was to conduct conversations with all families of patients with an ICU length of stay greater than 48 hours who were not being transferred or discharged on that day. Conversations were to be led by the ICU fellow, the ICU APP (nurse practitioner or physician assistant), or the ICU attending. To inform all providers on the team that the conversation had occurred, a communication method was developed using a visual cue on the patient's glass door, a standardized communication method used by the health care team.[9] A chat

PCORI Patient and Family Communication ALL patients admitted to SICU >48h	SUGGESTIONS FOR WHAT TO SAY
❶ PRE-MEET WITH TEAM—Include the bedside RN • Agree on key points, share what you know about family • Who will speak about what?	
❷ INTRODUCE • Hold conference in private area, hand over phone/pager or on vibrate • Identify roles and names of family and the medical team • State purpose, anything family would like covered?	"Tell me about your _____." "Do you have any specific concerns we should address?"
❸ ASSESS/EXPLAIN/UPDATE • Assess understanding of current medical condition • Give information in parts, avoid one long lecture, use plain language • Pause for questions, end with big picture	"So I know where to begin, what have you heard already?" "Increased support from the ventilator" instead of increasing PEEP "The most important piece of news is [...]"
❹ EMPATHIZE • Acknowledge emotions • Pause and give time to process	"I can see you are really concerned" "I am impressed you've been here to support [patients name]" "I wish we could_____, but_____."
❺ PRIORITIZE/HIGHLIGHT • Elicit patient and family values and preferences • Identify POA/surrogate decision maker • Any advance directive? Current patient goals	"Could you tell me about [patient's name] as a person?" "Does [patient name] have an advance directive or living will?" "If [patient name] could talk to us now, what do you think he/she would say"
❻ PLAN/ALIGN • Align medical care plan with patient's values • SHARED DECISION MAKING • Allow all parties to express viewpoint—try not to take sides • Offer recommendations if family unsure or uncertain	"What is your understanding of what we discussed today?" "Knowing what I know about [patient name]'s values and the medical situation, can I make a recommendation?" "Is there anything else you'd like to share, any questions?"
❼ DOCUMENT/UPDATE • Enter "Family Discussion Note" in Compass • Update Code Status if necessary • Update surgical/consulting services re: changes	

Fig. 1. Communication pocket card.

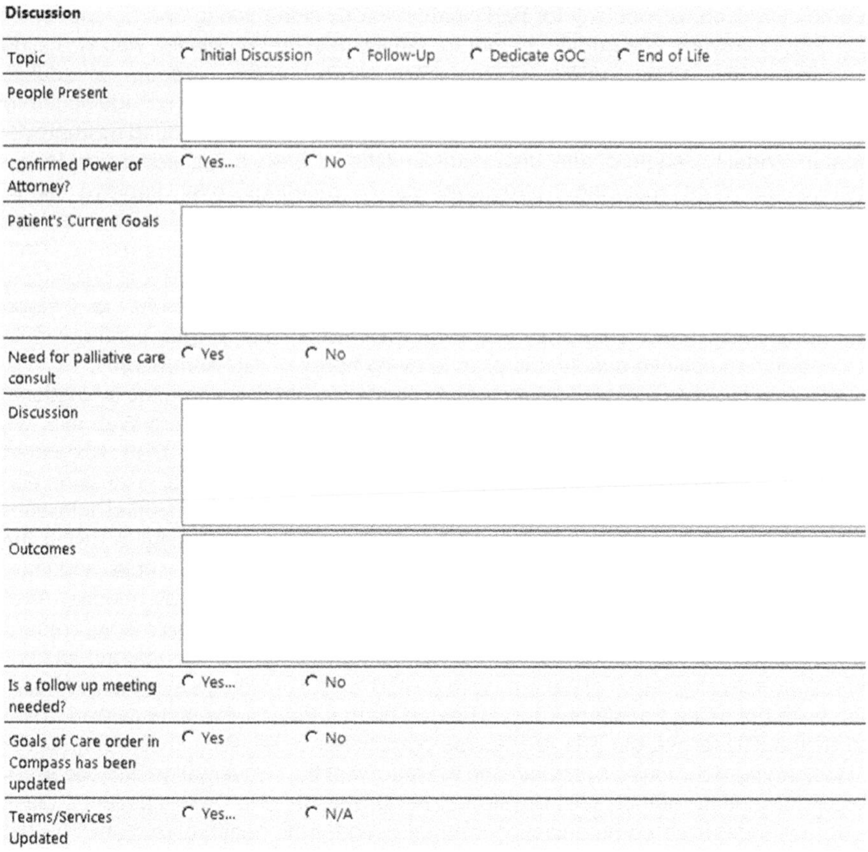

Discussion

Topic	⊙ Initial Discussion	⊙ Follow-Up	⊙ Dedicate GOC	⊙ End of Life
People Present				
Confirmed Power of Attorney?	⊙ Yes...	⊙ No		
Patient's Current Goals				
Need for palliative care consult	⊙ Yes	⊙ No		
Discussion				
Outcomes				
Is a follow up meeting needed?	⊙ Yes...	⊙ No		
Goals of Care order in Compass has been updated	⊙ Yes	⊙ No		
Teams/Services Updated	⊙ Yes...	⊙ N/A		

Fig. 2. Family discussion note template.

emoji bubble was checked when the family meeting had occurred and was documented in the EMR.[9]

After development of the communication bundle and improved process, baseline metrics of both the ICU team and the family were obtained before initiation. These metrics were universal for all sites participating in the multicenter PCORI collaborative using validated tools. The patient and family survey used the Family Satisfaction in the ICU 24 (FS-ICU).[9] This tool uses a Likert scale focused on questions related to the decision-making process, level of inclusion, frequency of communication, and the medical team participants. The clinician survey was assessed using the Patient- and Family- Centered Care Self-Assessment Inventory.[1] This survey assessed provider role, years of experience, perceptions about patient-centered care, participation in family meetings, and identification of surrogates. An ICU staff registered nurse (RN) participating in a hospital-based evidence-based practice (EBP) fellowship performed the family interviews and data collection.

Following the baseline assessment of families and staff, all team members were educated on the communication bundle. Bundle education included didactic sessions, electronic distribution of materials, and role play scenarios. Education of all bundle elements was performed by the multiprofessional EOL/GOC team, including the attending physician champion, an ICU fellow champion, the unit clinical nurse specialist, and the ICU RN in the EBP fellowship. All members of the ICU nursing staff, critical care fellows, APPs, and attending physicians were educated on the bundle. Bundle elements included staff education, communication, and documentation (**Fig. 3**). Based on findings in the pre-clinician survey, staff were also educated on several existing resources that scored very low and identified lack of knowledge, such as family resources in the unit and hospital. The educational materials were added to the orientation process for all ICU providers to assist with sustainment of the initiatives. On completion of staff education, family meetings for all patients who had been in the ICU for longer than 48 hours were expected to occur by the ICU medical provider (the ICU fellow, attending, or APP). The purpose of the initial family meeting was to designate a spokesperson, clarify the Durable Power of Attorney (DPOA) and advance directive (AD) status if legal documents existed, address code status, and discuss the patient/family goals with potential for revision of medical goals of care. Residents and medical students were encouraged to attend and participate in family meetings but not lead the discussions. After completion of the family meeting, the conversation and any changes to the patient's code status were documented in the EMR using the designated template. Patients were considered to have all elements of the bundle addressed when a family meeting occurred, a family discussion note was present, the AD/DPOA was documented, the patient's goals of care were updated after the family discussion, and the glass door chat emoji was checked. Nursing documentation of the AD status was also audited for matching documentation present in the medical record.

Weekly audits for bundle compliance were conducted for 22 weeks and reviewed as part of weekly discharge rounds in the ICU. The multiprofessional team members present during weekly discharge rounds included the unit social worker, clinical nurse specialist, ICU attending, and based on unit staffing, the ICU fellow. A weekly reminder e-mail was sent to ICU providers with bundle compliance data and a list of patients/families who were eligible but did not receive the bundle by the EBP ICU RN. On

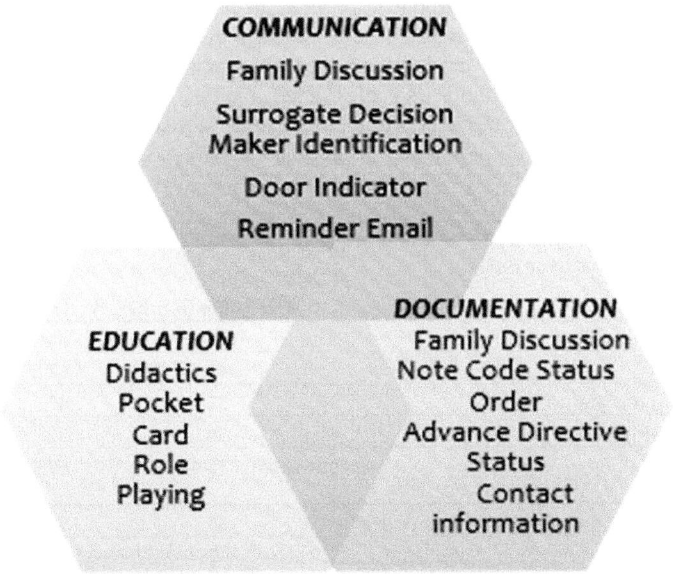

COMMUNICATION

Family Discussion

Surrogate Decision
Maker Identification

Door Indicator

Reminder Email

EDUCATION
Didactics
Pocket
Card
Role
Playing

DOCUMENTATION
Family Discussion
Note Code Status
Order
Advance Directive
Status
Contact
information

Fig. 3. Bundle elements.

completion of the 22-week process improvement, families and clinicians were reassessed using the FS-ICU 24 and PCORI clinician survey. For the post FS-ICU 24, additional questions related to the process improvement also were asked. For our project, families were asked to rate several statements regarding family care conferences.

RESULTS

FS-ICU surveys were completed by 27 family members before the communication bundle implementation and 33 family member after implementation. Female respondents were higher in both pre and post time intervals, with an older mean age in the post-survey respondent group. The percentage of respondents who lived more than 1 hour away from our facility was 52% on the pre-implementation period and 42%, post-implementation. Both inclusion in decision making rated as "very included" and completeness of information rated as "excellent" decreased by 10% after the implementation of the bundle. The frequency of RN communication was rated as excellent 79% of the time before and 69% after, whereas the frequency of physician communication rated as excellent increased from 44% to 54%. Changes to the key elements were seen in the percentage of families that felt "very included" and "very supported" in decision making after implementation of the bundle (**Table 1**). The survey identified a need to improve orientation to the ICU. Questions asked only post-implementation to address if families liked the family care conferences, thought the family care conferences were helpful, gave confidence in the health care team, impacted care of the patients, and reduced worry about family members had mean scores that ranged from 3.9 to 4.5, with an overall mean of 4.5 (possible scores 1–5). The percentage of respondents who strongly agreed with liking family care conferences, thought the family care conferences were helpful, gave confidence in the health care team, impacted care of the patients, and reduced worry about family members were 43.5%, 52.2%, 62.5%, 62.5%, and 62.5%, respectively.

Clinician survey respondents were most often completed by RN and MD providers with an average mean ICU year experience of 7.6 years pre and 7.1 years post. Staff reported a decrease in the opportunity to participate in multidisciplinary meetings after bundle implementation. There was a 10.5% increase in identification of surrogates to participate in care; however, the increase was not significant. Other significant staff survey results included rating use of diaries higher, 7% pre and 26% post ($P = .002$) and availability of pet therapy significantly higher, 7% pre and 41% post ($P<.001$) (**Table 2**).

Table 1 Family satisfaction survey results		
Survey response	Pre (n = 27), %	Post (n = 33), %
Gender, female/male	84/16	64/36
Age, y, mean[a]	49.6 ± 13.5	62.5 ± 14.2
Proximity to hospital >1 h away	52	42
Previous intensive care unit exposure	64	67
Frequency of communication, registered nurse/physician "Excellent"	75/44	69/54
Inclusion in decision making: "Very Included"	56	65.4
Completeness of information: "Excellent"	72	62

[a] $P\leq.05$.

Table 2
Clinician survey results

Survey response	Pre (n = 106), %	Post (n = 46), %
Registered nurse	41.5	36.4
Physician	32	40
Advanced practice provider	8.5	11.4
PharmD	2	0
Therapist	10.4	5.3
Other	5.6	6.8
Intensive care unit experience, y, mean	7.6	7.1
Opportunity to participate in multidisciplinary family meetings	26.2	15.2
Identify family members to participate in care (surrogates)	24.3	34.8 (P = .48)
Use of diaries higher post, 7% pre and 26% post (P = .002) and	7	26 (P = .002)
Availability of pet therapy	7	41 (P<.001)

A total of 680 total patients were screened for bundle eligibility, of whom 393 (57.9%) were in the ICU for more than 48 hours without planned transfer or discharge. Compliance was measured as family meeting occurred, family discussion note present, the AD/DPOA documented, the patient's goals of care updated after the family discussion occurred, and the glass door chat emoji checked. Of the 393 patients who met criteria for the family meeting, total compliance was observed in 27 patients (7%) (**Fig. 4**). Over the 22-week intervention period, 204 (51.8%) had an family discussion note (FDN) documented (**Fig. 5**). Sixty-six (16.8%) patients had an updated GOC after a family discussion. No newly admitted patients had their code status documented before admission to the ICU. GOCs were documented in 307 (78%) of patients with matching medical record documentation in 250 patients (63%).

SUMMARY

The 2017 SCCM Guidelines for Family-Centered Care in the Neonatal, Pediatric, and Adult ICU highlight focus areas for critical care providers to improve care. Our team improvements focused on improving family communication. Provider education on the importance of early identification of surrogates and the process for communicating with patients and families has been built into the onboarding educational curriculum for critical care nurses and fellows. Identification of surrogates and documentation of patient wishes has been adopted into the standard work of many of our staff and sustained over time but is variable among providers. The ease of use of the designated documentation template in the EMR improved documentation compliance and communication of the family discussion to all team members and was adopted by other ICUs and care teams. Numerous consult providers, such as wound care and palliative care, provided positive feedback regarding the family discussion note documentation in the EMR. Unfortunately, the family discussion note documentation compliance has not been sustained over time due to our recent system-wide conversion to a new EMR and decreased the momentum of our project. We are currently requesting documentation enhancements to allow for ease of documentation and

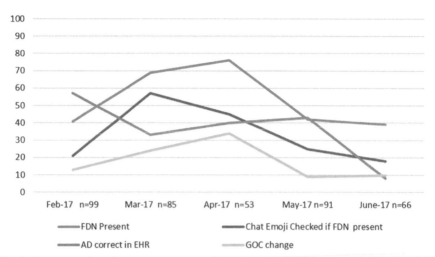

Fig. 4. Percentage bundle component compliance by month. AD, advanced directive; EHR, electronic health record; FDN, family discussion note; GOC, goals of care.

chart review that was lost in the transition. A direct mechanism to provide feedback to providers on documentation compliance, such as an inbox message or best practice advisory, may be a helpful next step to improve documentation and increase the number of conversations that occur. The practice of having family discussions is more common among our sickest patients, but expanding the practice to all patients remains an opportunity for improvement in our unit. A change to the culture in which family discussions are held as a standard of care may allow patients to participate in the conversation and designate their own decision makers or open conversations with family members for future hospitalizations. Increasing staff comfort with engaging patients and families in these conversations may improve our clinical care to align with the patient wishes.

Although the FS-ICU post-survey results showed a positive impact of family meetings on care perceptions by families, it is interesting to note that clinicians reported less opportunity to participate in family meetings after the implementation of the bundle. This could be an effect of increased awareness of the importance of family meetings by team members and inconsistent clinical practice among rotating providers, or the increased volume of meetings given the expansion of the practice.

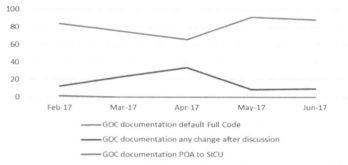

Fig. 5. Goals of care documentation. GOC, goals of care; POA, present on admission; SICU, surgical ICU.

Standardizing family meetings for all comers could decrease variability among team members. The disappointing overall bundle compliance may be responsible for the negligible impact in other areas. As described earlier, Huffines and colleagues[4] and Daly and colleagues[5] also reported difficulties in coordinating care conferences with necessary stakeholders in a timely fashion and in changing patient outcomes as a result of care conferences. This work highlights the importance of identifying improved methods of communication with families in an effort to provide timely, relevant, and meaningful support to families and minimize the impact of posttraumatic stress after critical illness.

The next steps for our team are to continue to improve our new EMR to allow for documentation of family meetings and goals of care conversations so the information is easily communicated among the care team. The FS-ICU results identified a need to provide a better orientation to the ICU and we are developing introductory videos to explain the ICU personnel, daily rounds, equipment, and resources. We will continue to strive to provide care that is consistent with the patient and family wishes and support improved patient and family communication.

DISCLOSURE

The authors have nothing to disclose.

REFERENCES

1. Davidson JE, Aslakson RA, Long AC, et al. Guidelines for family-centered care in the neonatal, pediatric, and adult ICU. Crit Care Med 2017;45(1):103–28.
2. Kleinpell R, Zimmerman J, Vermoch K, et al. Promoting family engagement in the ICU: experience from a national collaborative of 63 ICUs. Crit Care Med 2019; 47(12):1692–8.
3. Wessman B, Sona C, Schallom M. Improving caregivers' perceptions regarding patient goals of care/end-of-life issues for the multidisciplinary critical care team. J Intensive Care Med 2017;32(1):68–76.
4. Huffines M, Johnson KL, Smitz Naranjo LL, et al. Improving family satisfaction and participation in decision making in an intensive care unit. Crit Care Nurse 2013; 33(5):56–69.
5. Daly BJ, Douglas SL, O'Toole E, et al. Effectiveness trial of an intensive communication strategy for families of long-stay ICU patients. Chest 2010;138(6):1340–8.
6. Hurd CJ, Curtis JR. The intensive care unit family conference: teaching a critical intensive care unit procedure. Ann Am Thorac Soc 2015;12(4):469–71.
7. Black MD, Vigorito MC, Curtis JR, et al. A multifaceted intervention to improve compliance with process measures for ICU clinician communication with ICU patients and families. Crit Care Med 2013;41(10):2275–83.
8. Conduct a family conference. Available at: http://www.vitaltalk.org/clinicians/family. Accessed February 13, 2017.
9. Wessman B, Sona C, Schallom M. A novel ICU hand-over tool: the glass door of the patient room. J Intensive Care Med 2016;32(8):514–9, 1-6.

One Team's Experience with Integrating Flexible Visitation in the Medical Intensive Care Unit

Chris Winkelman, PhD, ACNP, CCRN, FCCM[a],*,
Kathleen Kerber, MSN, APRN- CNS, CCRN, CNRN[b],
Jessica Zangmeister, BSN, RN[c], Molly McNett, PhD, RN, CNRN, FNCS[d]

KEYWORDS

• ICU • Patient visitors • Family presence • Simulation • Quality improvement

KEY POINTS

• This article discusses a unit-specific journey and outcomes over the course of 18 months to implement flexible visitation in a medical intensive care unit.

• To reinforce the value of family at the bedside and boost uptake related to flexible visitation, particularly as staff transitioned into a new physical space, simulation was used to prepare nursing staff for family presence during all aspects of care. Actors portrayed family visitors during a simulated cardiopulmonary arrest exercise.

• In addition to staff and family satisfaction, patient safety events were examined, and a trend was identified toward reduce adverse events following implementation of flexible visitation.

Several professional organizations advocate flexible visitation hours for family members of patients hospitalized in the intensive care unit (ICU).[1,2] Federal and accrediting agency policies support visitation practices that reflect patient preferences.[3,4] Terms used to describe flexible visitation in the ICU are open, liberal, enhanced, extended, or unrestricted. Flexible visiting includes daily visiting times that range from 4 to 6 hours[5,6] to 24 hours daily.[2,7] Flexible visitation in the ICU can also refer to the removal of

[a] Frances Payne Bolton School of Nursing, Case Western Reserve University, 10900 Euclid Avenue, Cleveland, OH 44106, USA; [b] The MetroHealth System, 2500 MetroHealth Drive, Cleveland, OH 44109, USA; [c] Medical Intensive Care Unit, The MetroHealth System, 2500 MetroHealth Drive, Cleveland, OH 44109, USA; [d] Clinical Nursing, Implementation Science Core, The Helene Fuld Health Trust National Institute for Evidence-Based Practice in Nursing & Healthcare, College of Nursing, The Ohio State University, 760 Kinnear Road, Columbus, OH 43212, USA
* Corresponding author.
E-mail address: cxw26@case.edu

Crit Care Nurs Clin N Am 32 (2020) 253–264
https://doi.org/10.1016/j.cnc.2020.02.007
0899-5885/20/© 2020 Elsevier Inc. All rights reserved.
ccnursing.theclinics.com

restrictions around age or family membership as a requirement to spend time with a critically ill patient.[5] Flexible visitation might also include removing constraints around special circumstances, such as allowing family presence during procedures and cardiac or respiratory arrest.

Despite more than a decade of published support for flexible visitation in the ICU, restrictive policies remain common.[8,9] The purpose of this quality improvement project was to implement flexible visitation in the medical ICU (MICU) by increasing the hours for visitors, removing restrictions around family membership, and increasing nurse discretion around timing and duration of visitation.

The process of integrating flexible visitation in the MICU began as an internal, site-specific effort in 2015. In May 2016, we joined with other ICU teams the Society of Critical Care Medicine (SCCM) in a Patient-Centered Outcomes Research Institute (PCORI)–funded collaborative designed to help hospitals implement patient and family engagement programs. This article describes the processes and outcomes during planning, initial implementation, and transition to a new building. It describes a unit-specific journey and outcomes over the course of 18 months, and includes data about staff attitudes collected only during the SCCM collaborative.

PROBLEM DESCRIPTION AT THE MEDICAL INTENSIVE CARE UNIT: WHERE DID WE START?

Before 2015, the MICU endorsed a restricted visiting policy that included a maximum of 2 family members at the bedside during the hours of 10 AM and 2 PM, and again at 4 to 8 PM. Typically, the patient named the family members allowed to visit, or, if the patient was not able to communicate, the visitor self-identified as a family member. When possible, the patient or 1 family member (or designated individual) overseeing care and providing consent for the patient identified a password, and visitors were required to say the password to enter the unit.

Multiple staff members in the MICU recognized that restricted visiting times did not meet the needs of patients and their significant others. The MICU Nursing Practice Council members reported that some families reported challenges attending during posted visiting hours caused by work schedules, transportation issues, and childcare arrangements. Paid time off work or flexible work schedules were not available for many visitors. Based on the values of our institution, a review of the literature, and trending practice reported at professional meetings, the MICU Nursing Practice Council, nurse manager, and clinical nurse specialist (CNS) decided to develop a flexible visitation policy.

Context

As a public safety-net hospital, an important mission of the institution continues to be to treat patients regardless of their ability to pay, and many patients and visitors have limited resources. Flexible visitation would permit visitors the means to match their resources of time and transportation to support care and communication at the bedside. The MICU is a closed unit: physician intensivists are scheduled and accessible during daytime hours and provide all admissions and orders by phone to the physician residents providing overnight care during an ICU rotation of 4 weeks. In addition, an MICU fellow on service is available to both residents and nursing staff for care-related issues most days of the week. Registered nurses typically provide direct care for no more than 2 patients with a critical care designation and 3 patients when designated as intermediate or step-down care. The unit admits approximately 1700 patients annually, with a mean patient acuity–nurse workload score of 2.9 ($\pm$ 0.15) during the project period.[10,11] The mortality of this very ill population was approximately 40% between 2015 and 2017. Support was received from nursing and medical administrators in endorsement of this effort. However, no administrator directly participated in the planning, implementation, or evaluation of the transition and maintenance of flexible visitation in the MICU. The MICU medical director was involved in decisions such as the restriction at change of shift and final editing of the visitor brochure and assisted with educating medical staff about visitation policy and practices during orientation to the MICU.

INTERVENTION

A flexible visitation policy affects not only patients and their visitors but also clinicians who provide direct care, such as nurses, physicians, respiratory therapists, clerical support, housekeepers, and admissions staff. It was recognized that nurses were critical to the success of visitation in an ICU. For example, the nurse often asks questions that may clarify relationships that reflect familial affiliations, such as, "We are not married, but we have been together for many years," or "I am not legally an adopted son, but I grew up in her home." The first step was to define flexible visitation for everyone.

Phase 1: Team Building and Initial Implementation

The leadership of the MICU nurse manager and the MICU-based CNS identified a team of nurses willing to work on the transition to flexible visitation. This team ultimately defined flexible visitation as unrestricted by hours and bounded by patient and family requests. One hour, twice daily at change of shift (7–8 AM and 7–8 PM) was designated as closed to visitors to reduce the risk to confidentiality. This unit used walking rounds; private patient information could be overheard between rooms with this format in certain visitation areas. The team acknowledged that the nurse could modify visitation, such as asking visitors to stay within a patient's room during walking rounds. Alternatively, verbally abusive or inappropriate behavior by visitors could create or escalate restrictions to visitation.[2,12]

Education was the primary intervention to support implementation. Following endorsement by the MICU nurse manager and Practice Council, the CNS disseminated the changes planned by the team to MICU interdisciplinary and ancillary staff and collected feedback. Additional individual face-to-face discussions with attending physicians and unit secretaries who greet visitors to the MICU occurred. Publications about the evidence for benefits to flexible visitation were made available to staff on bulletin boards and during regular meetings. To address concerns about privacy and safety, the CNS and MICU team developed a brochure to guide visitors and clinicians in making visitation decisions that centered on patient and care goals. This brochure underwent several revisions and provided an opening for dialogue with unit-based champions for open visitation. Once the team finalized the brochure, a date for change was announced at staff meetings and during rounds the week before adoption. In mid-2015, the MICU went from restricted visitation to flexible visitation.

During the course of this initial implementation, the health system began construction on a new critical care pavilion that included moving the MICU into a new physical space, planned to occur in late 2016. Specific and deliberate planning centered on creation of a welcoming environment for patients and families. Family members, ICU patients, and MICU interdisciplinary staff participated in focus groups and planning committees to create a new space that accommodated visitors and remained respectful of multiple needs for privacy during care and communication. The newly designed critical care pavilion included 18 MICU beds, an increase from the prior unit capacity of 15 beds. Individual rooms went from 19.9 m² (214 square feet) to an average of 29.9 m² (322 square feet). Built-in window benches for visitors to sit and sleep on at night were a welcome improvement in the new rooms. In addition, the designers used floor patterns to create a zone of workflow that allowed visitors to stay in the room while maintaining working space for clinicians. **Fig. 1** shows the darker/green swirl, which is the safe zone where presence at the immediate bedside needs to be limited for care (eg, privacy or dignity concerns) or a procedure (eg, safety or sterility concerns). **Fig. 2** shows the flow of work for implementing MICU flexible visitation.

Phase 2: Sustaining Flexible Visitation After the Move to the Critical Care Pavilion

To reinforce the value of family at the bedside and boost uptake related to flexible visitation, particularly as staff transitioned into a new physical space, a second intervention was implemented to prepare nursing staff for family presence during all aspects of care, using the enhanced design features. Simulation scenarios were created for interdisciplinary staff to practice incorporating family presence in the new location. One specific simulation included an interactive manikin that simulated a cardiac or respiratory arrest while visitors were present in the newly constructed MICU. Professional actors portrayed visitors who witnessed the cardiac or respiratory arrest in the new MICU. Similar to standardized patients used for simulation or objective structured clinical examination,[13] these actors were standardized family members present during this stressful situation. Nursing staff could use the resources available to them in the new MICU environment, such as the zones of workflow or pastoral care and security. Staff practiced using the MICU rooms by having visitors remain in the safe zone designated by floor markings or requesting that visitors move to a communication or waiting room. This simulated experience was designed to be congruent with the hospital's value of respect for individuals. The simulation allowed the code team to select among options for visitor location in or out of the room when patient safety was a concern. The actors portrayed spouses, adult siblings, and estranged family members in various scenarios. They were helpful or uncooperative based on the simulation script. The script provided opportunities for the code team to make decisions. Debriefing allowed team members to acknowledge successes, failures, and alternate strategies with visitor interactions and to process the challenges of engaging visitors during high-stress situations. Seventeen sessions were delivered and 276 people were trained, including nurses, doctors, respiratory therapists, and service representatives (front desk personnel).

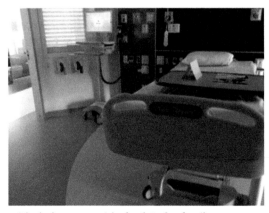

Fig. 1. Floor zones with dark green swirl of safety for family.

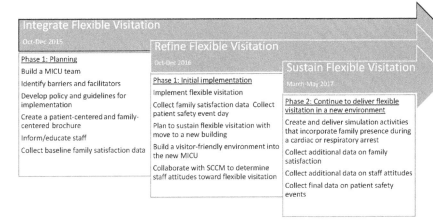

Fig. 2. MICU timeline.

Shortly after the MICU transitioned to the new physical space, SCCM PCORI investigators selected the MICU to participate in a national effort to improve family-centered care in ICUs. Participation in this project allowed staff to explore attitudes toward flexible visitation in the new space, along with evaluating the impact of the new visitation and physical location on patient/family satisfaction. Additional data were gathered on patient acuity, length of stay, and number of adverse events before and after the transition periods. Engagement in the SCCM PCORI project provided an opportunity for trending of data over time, from early onset of the project in the old unit, and throughout the transition to a new policy and practice and follow-up periods in the new unit.

MEASURES

The team considered how to measure outcomes for this change in practice and policy. They decided to focus on the effect on family and visitors, developing a 6-item satisfaction survey. **Table 1** details the 6 items. The team recruited volunteer respondents immediately before (time 1), 6 months after the visitation practice change (time 2) in the old MICU, and after the move into the new MICU (time 3). The survey used a paper-pencil format and a 5-point Likert response scale. The team evaluated the questions for face and content validity; no reliability evaluation occurred because no gold standard for comparison was identified. There was discussion to use the survey to compare between 2 groups of visitors. However, the team thought that dividing visitors into groups of restricted or flexible visitation would be challenging, because visitors clearly expected flexible visitation. Questions from the SCCM PCORI-funded project were used to examine staff attitudes toward flexible visitation in the MICU at time 3 only. The SCCM PCORI research team developed and deployed the measures via a shared REDCap database.[14]

Visitor satisfaction data were collected for 30 days at each period (ie, times 1, 2, and 3). The CNS and team members involved in developing the flexible visitation policy distributed the survey. The hospital institutional review board (IRB) approved this project as exempt. Visitors could decline to complete the survey. Surveys were anonymous and contained no personal or health-protected data. In addition, the PCORI collaborative effort received IRB approval through Rush University.

Table 1
Mean scores by item and total

Visitor Satisfaction 6-Item Tool	Preintervention Mean Score (Standard Deviation) n = 28	Postintervention Mean Score (Standard Deviation) n = 20	t-test Value (P) Comparing Preintervention with Postintervention Scores	90% Confidence Intervals	After the Move: Mean Scores (Standard Deviation) n = 16	t-test Value (P) Comparing Preintervention with Postmove Scores	90% Confidence Intervals
I felt comfortable with the care provided by the nurses in the MICU	4.86 (0.356)	4.70 (0.470)	1.282 (.209)	−0.085–0.405	3.63 (0.500)	8.698 (.000)[a]	0.952–1.507
Nurses were attentive and addressed concerns in a timely manner	4.72 (0.455)	4.75 (0.550)	−0.201 (.842)	−0.313–0.253	3.56 (0.629)	6.472 (.000)[a]	0.809–1.511
I felt welcome in the MICU	4.79 (0.418)	4.90 (0.308)	−1.050 (.299)	−0.315–0.095	3.56 (0.814)	5.635 (.000)[a]	0.802–1.658
Nurses were available to answer questions during my stay/visits	4.75 (0.518)	4.76 (0.539)	−.064 (.949)	−0.314–0.294	3.69 (0.602)	5.904 (.000)[a]	0.708–1.412
Visitation times met my need	4.62 (0.518)	4.65 (0.587)	−0.179 (.859)	−0.358–0.298	3.69 (0.479)	5.815 (.000)[a]	0.617–1.243
The nurse helped me (family member) manage pain/discomfort	4.60 (0.549)	4.43 (1.121)	0.973 (.339)	−0.264–0.784	3.69 (0.479)	6.311(.000)[a]	0.689–1.311
TOTAL score (potential range 6–30)	28.85 (2.167)	28.45 (2.86)	.527 (.602)	−1.107–1.900	21.813(2.903)	11.280 (.000)[a]	5.400–8.586

Comparison of scores at preintervention/time 1, postintervention/time 2, and after the move/time 3.
[a] Significant differences.

RESULTS

Phase 1

There were 28 visitors who completed the survey before the implementation of unrestricted visitation, and 20 who completed the survey at 3 months after implementing flexible visitation. **Table 1** shows the scores at preintervention and postintervention. There were no differences between the average scores or for any single item.

Phase 2

Sixteen visitors completed the family satisfaction survey after the move into the new ICU pavilion and new MICU. There were significant differences ($P<.01$) in all items and the total score, with decrements universal after the move. **Table 1** details these results.

The staff attitude toward flexible visitation consisted of 23 respondents. Respondents used a 1 to 5 Likert scale of agreement (1 = strongly disagree; 5 = strongly agree). The PCORI research team developed these items, detailed in **Table 2**. Two positive responses were more than 4 (ie, "During rounds, in accordance with patient preferences, families can remain with the patient" and "Policies and practices encourage patient and family involvement in decision making regarding their health care"). The highest degree of agreement (4.5) was associated with a negative item: "Having nonrestricted/open visitation results in more work for the staff." The lowest agreement score was 2.5 for "Patient care has improved since having nonrestricted/open visitation."

Additional Data

Data were collected on 3 other variables as a mean average over the 3 months surrounding each data collection period: safety events (PSEs), patient length of stay, and patient acuity. A 3-month average was used to provide more nuanced trend data than a single monthly report (**Fig. 3**). PSEs were defined as reports filed in an electronic safety event recording system. Reports were filed according to institutional policy, recording an event that may or did cause harm to a patient. The team elected to consider this variable because they wondered whether more visitors, or visitors staying for longer periods, would distract staff, creating or increasing PSEs. Trend data in **Fig. 3** suggested a decrease in reported PSEs at times 2 and 3 compared with time 1, although there were too few data to analyze statistically.

Length of stay varied from a mean average of 4 days to a mean average of 6 days at the 3 time points. The greatest duration of stay occurred after the move. Patient acuity, measured with the QuadraMed Acuity Plus system tool,[11] ranged from 2.82 to 3.01 with the peak after the move. Trend data seemed to suggest that acuity and length of stay were related, and both increased over time as the unit expanded into the new space. QuadraMed Acuity uses a range of 1 to 4 to describe patient status; the higher score indicates a greater nurse workload. There is no published information about whether an increase of 0.2 in the 1 to 4 scale is clinically important.

Anecdotally, no barriers were noted in the uptake of flexible visitation during either phase 1 or 2. Signage reflecting restricted hours was removed from the waiting rooms immediately before adoption of the new practice and policy. Signage in the new building in patient waiting areas reflected flexible times, rather than the restricted hours. Brochures were readily available at the entrance desk to the ICUs and at central desks in the MICU.

DISCUSSION

Despite more than 10 years of recommendations for flexible visitation, it is difficult for units to change from restrictive visitation policies and practices.[8,15] Further, recent publications suggest that it is not simply visitation but participation in care that drives family satisfaction.[15,16] Family participation in care was not measured.

Visitors initially reported a high satisfaction with (restricted) visitation practices in the ICU, averaging more than 28 on a 30-point measure. Implementing flexible visitation in the old building did not change visitor satisfaction scores from time 1 (scheduled visitation) to time 2 (flexible visitation in the old building) but decreased at time 3 (after a move to a new space). We recognize that newly built space. We speculate that the reduced intimacy in space and visibility caused by single-room built space in the new building affected both staff and family visitor responses. This finding is supported by a 2015 report of patient and staff experiences after a move into all-single-room hospital accommodation that indicated an increased feeling of isolation and reduced opportunity to discuss care with colleagues.[17]

The decrease of visitor satisfaction at time 3 (after the move) was unexpected. Scores decreased in all items by about 1.2 out of 6 points and overall by 7 out of 30 points. Although visitation times did not change from after implementation to after the move, participants were less satisfied with visitation-related issues after the

Table 2
Staff responses to flexible visitation[a]

Item	Average Score Range 1–5
Family members are not viewed as visitors; they are always welcome to be with the patient in accordance with patient preference	3.3
Families can remain with the patients during nurse change of shift, in accordance with patient preference	4.2
During rounds, in accordance with patient preferences, families can remain with the patients	4.4
During rounds, in accordance with patient preferences, families can participate with rounds	3.5
Patients and families are viewed as integral members of the health care team	3.5
Policies and practices encourage patient and family involvement in decision making regarding their health care	4.2
I prefer when there is nonrestricted/open visitation for the ICU	2.8
Communication with family members has improved since having nonrestricted/open visitation for the ICU	3.4
Patient care has improved since having nonrestricted/open visitation	2.5
Having nonrestricted/open visitation has been beneficial for the ICU	3.0
Having nonrestricted/open visitation has been beneficial for patients	2.8
Having nonrestricted/open visitation has been beneficial for families	3.6
Having nonrestricted/open visitation results in more work for the staff	4.5

[a] Collected 18 months after implementation and after the move to new MICU.

move. Adjustment to a newly built space may account for the decrement.[17,18] Importantly, the move did not cause a change in behavior: flexible visitation remained operational in the newly built space. Because trend data indicated increased length of stay and acuity at time 3 (after the move), compared with times 1 and 2 (before and after implementation in the old building), visitors and staff may have had a general negativity associated with the stress of more severe illness, rather than a specific reflection on satisfaction with visitation. It may be that there was a decrease in visitor awareness of flexible visitation in the MICU in the new building. It may be that the smaller sample size captured after the move was less representative of all visitors or captured a greater proportion of dissatisfied visitors. We also speculate that the more spacious environment after the move decreased the visibility of staff, and this reduced visibility influenced communication and satisfaction with each visit. The changes in visibility and need to alter teamwork and communication workflow has previously been reported in hospitals designed with both single-room accommodation and more centralized support staff.[17]

The increased floor space and long hallways in the new unit changed the workflow patterns for nurses and the accessible path to connect with hospital personnel for visitors. In the old MICU, a secretary sat at the entrance desk and greeted visitors as they entered. Now there is a single desk and secretary at the entrance to 5 ICUs. Now, visitors must leave the bedside and the MICU to locate this secretary if questions or concerns arise and staff are not immediately visible. Increased distance in rooms and between rooms may reduce the feeling of shared experiences and intimacy with visitors. Perceived reduced staff visibility may be stressful, reducing satisfaction. It is possible that decreased time in waiting areas (and more time in the patient room) means less peer family support and information, leading to decreased visitor satisfaction. The authors also considered the explanation that the culture of the MICU changed in the new building with the addition of new staff, new patterns of workflow, and the stress of relocation. Although we do not have new data to report, clearly a follow-up survey would help us to understand whether this decrement was permanent or simply a transient decrease from the burdens of any move that ease over time. Despite the challenges of accommodating a new environment, staff did not challenge or change the flexible visitation policy after the move and it remains an active priority in patient care and is reinforced with simulation, using actors to portray visitors during training in the new building.

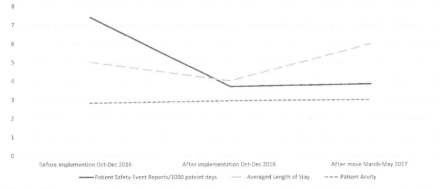

Fig. 3. Three-month data for patient safety event reports, length of ICU stay, and patient acuity at each period.

Overall, there was a downward trend in reported number of adverse events during the transition to both flexible visitation and to the new unit. Although there were not sufficient data to definitively infer causation or reach statistical significance, the trend was encouraging. Few studies have investigated effects of flexible or open visitation on adverse events within critical care units. Our decreased trend suggests that increasing visitor access to patients may not have a negative effect on nursing time that would result in harm to other patients, nor would flexible visitation increase risk for patient harm. One interpretation is that the presence of visitors prevented patient safety events, perhaps because of communication or a sense of increased vigilance from visitors. However, additional research is warranted to better elucidate this relationship. The trend in decreasing reported patient safety events suggests an opportunity to support improved patient outcomes, and this could be considered in future investigations.

Although it was discouraging to discern that staff perceive flexible visitation as negatively affecting their workloads, it is a realistic assessment. It may be that pressures created by orienting new staff (because of additional patient capacity) or unfamiliarity with the new environment contributed to the staff perception of flexible visitation. The authors do not know of any nursing workload measurement tools that account for visitor management. Note that nurses disagreed (although not strongly) with the statement, "I prefer when there are nonrestricted/open visiting hours." These data agreed with other reports in the literature indicating that an increased risk of job burden or burnout among ICU professionals is associated with increased visitor interactions.[5] Experts advocate for organizational infrastructure to support family presence. Despite best efforts, change agents need to be prepared to overcome both obstacles in changing behavior and challenges imposed by the built environment. We continue to support flexible visitation in our MICU by orienting new staff to this practice and recently adopting bedside hand-off reports to allow family/visitor input.

Limitations

This article is the report of a single site and may not be generalizable to all MICUs or ICUs. The surveys were all investigator initiated. However, this MICU resembles the reports of other academic MICUs. Visitors in an ICU are more likely to have commonalities than differences, such as heightened emotional states, a need to be close to the family member, and the desire to communicate regularly with staff about their loved ones.[19] The common needs of family and visitors during a loved one's ICU hospitalization may override the unique setting.

We did not keep counts of visitors at any phase of the project. Measuring this variable would help quantify the impact on outcomes. We recommend adding this measure to future projects about visitation. We did not have sufficient institutional patient experience scores to link data to our project. Patients are more likely to comment on their floor or outpatient experiences, perhaps because of limited recall of experiences in the ICU.[20] The authors suggest patients as a source of data to investigate visitation satisfaction in future studies, when patients are able to recall their ICU experience and are verbal.

SUMMARY

Integration of flexible visitation in critical care settings can be challenging, but the authors continue to believe that it benefits patients and families and supports a healing environment. This article reports a transition to flexible visitation and sustaining flexible visitation following a move to a newly built, expanded space in an MICU. Specific training and simulation for health care staff to promote family presence was a useful tool for successful integration of policy into practice in the new ICU building. A unique experience was offered using actors to portray family members during a simulated cardiac arrest to help staff identify issues and solutions to family presence and participation in care in the newly built MICU space. The transition to flexible visitation did not adversely alter patient safety events, although additional research is needed to explore causal and temporal relationships. We continue to support flexible visitation as essential to patient-centered care and urge future investigations into how visitation affects nursing workload and patient outcomes.

DISCLOSURE

Phase 2 data collection was supported by The PCOR-ICU collaborative through a Patient-Centered Outcomes Research Institute (PCORI, 2015) Eugene Washington PCORI Engagement Award, offered by SCCM. https://www.pcori.org/research-results/2015/improving-carecritically-ill-patients-families-through-research.

REFERENCES

1. Davidson JE, Aslakson RA, Long AC, et al. Guidelines for family-centered care in the neonatal, pediatric, and adult ICU. Crit Care Med 2017;45(1):103–28.
2. American Association of Critical-Care Nurses. Family visitation in the adult intensive care unit. Crit Care Nurse 2016;36(1):e15–9.
3. The Joint Commission. Requirements related to CMS patient visitation rights conditions of participation (CoPs). 2011. 2019. Available at: https://www.jointcommission.org/assets/1/6/20110701_Visitation_Rights_HAP.pdf. Accessed January 10, 2019.
4. Centers for Medicare & Medicaid Services, HHS. Changes to the hospital and critical access hospital conditions of participation to ensure visitation rights for all patients. Fed Regist 2010;75(223):70831–44.
5. Nassar Junior AP, Besen B, Robinson CC, et al. Flexible versus restrictive visiting policies in ICUs: a systematic review and meta-analysis. Crit Care Med 2018; 46(7):1175–80.
6. Rosa RG, Tonietto TF, da Silva DB, et al. Effectiveness and safety of an extended ICU visitation model for delirium prevention: a before and after study. Crit Care Med 2017;45(10):1660–7.
7. Garrouste-Orgeas M, Philippart F, Timsit JF, et al. Perceptions of a 24-hour visiting policy in the intensive care unit. Crit Care Med 2008;36(1):30–5.
8. Liu V, Read JL, Scruth E, et al. Visitation policies and practices in US ICUs. Crit Care 2013;17(2):R71.
9. Kleinpell R, Heyland DK, Lipman J, et al. Patient and family engagement in the ICU: report from the task force of the World Federation of Societies of intensive and critical care medicine. J Crit Care 2018;48:251–6.
10. Sir MY, Dundar B, Barker Steege LM, et al. Nurse-patient assignment models considering patient acuity metrics and nurses' perceived workload. J Biomed Inform 2015;55:237–48.
11. QuadraMed. Available at: https://www.quadramed.com/. Accessed December 4, 2019.
12. Monroe M, Wofford L. Open visitation and nurse job satisfaction: an integrative review. J Clin Nurs 2017;26(23–24):4868–76.

13. Schmitz CC, Chipman JG, Luxenberg MG, et al. Professionalism and communication in the intensive care unit: reliability and validity of a simulated family conference. Simul Healthc 2008;3(4):224–38.
14. Harris PA, Taylor R, Thielke R, et al. Research electronic data capture (REDCap)– a metadata-driven methodology and workflow process for providing translational research informatics support. J Biomed Inform 2009;42(2):377–81.
15. Kleinpell R, Zimmerman J, Vermoch KL, et al. Promoting family engagement in the ICU: experience from a national collaborative of 63 ICUs. Crit Care Med 2019;47(12):1692–8.
16. Davidson JE, Zisook S. Implementing family-centered care through facilitated sensemaking. AACN Adv Crit Care 2017;28(2):200–9.
17. Maben J, Griffiths P, Penfold C, et al. Health services and delivery research. In: Maben J, Griffiths P, Penfold C, et al, editors. Evaluating a major innovation in hospital design: workforce implications and impact on patient and staff experiences of all single room hospital accommodation, vol. 3.3. Southampton (United Kingdom): NIHR Journals Library; 2015.
18. Bates V. 'Humanizing' healthcare environments: architecture, art and design in modern hospitals. Design Health (Abingdon) 2018;2(1):5–19.
19. Carlson EB, Spain DA, Muhtadie L, et al. Care and caring in the intensive care unit: family members' distress and perceptions about staff skills, communication, and emotional support. J Crit Care 2015;30(3):557–61.
20. Moult D, Breeze R, Molokhia A. A family-based survey on the ICU. Critical Care BMC 2012;16(Supple1):493.

The Critical Care Nurse Communicator Program

An Integrated Primary Palliative Care Intervention

Andrew O'Donnell, DNP, RN, AGPCNP-BC[a],*, April Buffo, BSN, RN[b],
Toby C. Campbell, MD, MS[c], William J. Ehlenbach, MD, MSc[d]

KEYWORDS

- Shared decision making • Palliative care • Intensive care unit • Family support
- Communication

KEY POINTS

- In the intensive care unit (ICU), surrogate decision makers are often required to make complex, high-stakes decisions for their loved one under immense stress.
- Communication among patients, families, and clinicians in the ICU if often delayed and inefficient, particularly at the end of life.
- A nurse-led, primary palliative care intervention to improve communication and surrogate decision-maker support in the ICU is feasible and strongly supported by staff.
- The program improves the quality and consistency of communication, augments support for patients, families, and staff, and contributes to a decrease in resource utilization at the end of life.

INTRODUCTION

Although most Americans express a preference to die at home, approximately 20% die in an intensive care unit (ICU), often incapacitated and dependent on surrogates for decision making.[1] Surrogate decision makers, under immense psychological, emotional, and physical stress, are often required to make urgent, complex, high-stakes decisions for their loved one.[2] To compound their challenge, evidence suggests that communication among patients, families, and clinicians in the ICU is often

[a] Trauma Life Support Center, UW Health, 600 Highland Avenue, Madison, WI 53792, USA;
[b] Critical Care Nurse Communicator Program, UW Health, 600 Highland Avenue, Madison, WI 53792, USA; [c] Division of Hem/Onc/Pall Care, University of Wisconsin School of Medicine and School of Nursing, 1111 Highland Avenue, Madison, WI 53711, USA; [d] University of Wisconsin School of Medicine Public Health, 1685 Highland Avenue, Madison, WI 53705, USA
* Corresponding author.
E-mail address: aodonnell@uwhealth.org

Crit Care Nurs Clin N Am 32 (2020) 265–279
https://doi.org/10.1016/j.cnc.2020.02.008
0899-5885/20/© 2020 Elsevier Inc. All rights reserved.
ccnursing.theclinics.com

delayed and inefficient, with frequent missed opportunities to support the emotional needs of patients and surrogates, particularly at the end of life.[3] Poor communication, inadequate emotional support, and a failure to focus on the patient's goals, values, and treatment preferences contributes to the use of unwanted life-sustaining therapies at the end of life.[3,4] Integration of a communication specialist or family navigator within the ICU team has been shown to improve the quality and consistency of communication and augment support for surrogate decision makers while simultaneously reducing both the length of stay and cost of care in patients who die, without changing the mortality rate.[1,3] The Critical Care Nurse Communicator (CCNC) program is a primary palliative care ICU intervention at an academic, quaternary referral center designed to augment support for patients and surrogate decision makers facing serious, life-limiting illness.

BACKGROUND

Family meetings serve as a critical forum for family and health care team members to discuss a patient's diagnosis, clinical course, prognosis, treatment preferences, and goals of care.[5] These crucial conversations have been shown to improve the quality of communication and reduce family distress, particularly at the end of life.[6] However, although 90% of ICU directors support interdisciplinary meetings for critically ill patients, they consistently occur in only 35% to 40% of intensive care units.[7] The Trauma Life Support Center (TLC) at the University of Wisconsin has invested significant time and resources into improving patient and family communication and surrogate decision-maker support. Two key quality improvement initiatives preceded the implementation of the CCNC program with the goal of improving the frequency, quality, and consistency of communication in the ICU: (1) a palliative care intervention on daily ICU rounds and (2) a family meeting protocol and communication skills training for ICU nurses.[8]

Braus and colleagues[8] conducted a prospective, pre/postintervention study to improve the timeliness and consistency of family meetings in ICU patients at high risk for death. The intervention included the addition of a palliative care nurse on daily ICU rounds tasked with identifying patients at high risk for morbidity, mortality, or unmet palliative care needs. For all patients who met criteria, the clinician suggested an interdisciplinary family meeting to the attending ICU physician. Rates of family meetings were 63% higher in the intervention group and time from ICU admission to the first family meeting was 41% shorter. In those patients who died, ICU length of stay was 19% shorter, and hospital length of stay was 26% shorter without any difference in the overall proportion of patients who died.[8] The intervention ended, but administrators and program leaders used this work to inform the development of the CCNC program.

To build on the success of this intervention, the ICU launched an interdisciplinary quality improvement effort to implement protocolized family meetings for all ICU patients. This effort was paired with communication skills training for all 90 ICU nurses, and all attending physicians and fellows. The nursing course included a brief didactic on empathic communication and a role-playing exercise to practice the skills during a simulated challenging family interaction. The physicians' course was a 6-hour training program focused on breaking bad news and serious illness communication. The training and family meeting protocol led to an increase in the number of patients who had a family meeting by ICU day 4 (69% preintervention, 89% postintervention) and a significant decrease in moral distress in ICU nurses. The family meeting protocol continued, although family meeting rates declined after the initial data collection period because of challenges with sustainability, such as staff turnover and competing priorities.

These efforts addressed some of the communication challenges patients, families, and clinicians face in the ICU but fell short of identifying and holistically addressing the complex informational and emotional barriers surrogate decision makers face through the shared decision-making process. Evidence suggests that the addition of a "family navigator" or "communication facilitator" might more comprehensively address these challenges.[1,3]

White and colleagues[9] conducted a single-center, single-arm interventional study to assess the feasibility, acceptability, and clinician perceptions of a nurse-led support intervention to improve surrogate decision making in the ICU. The nurse-led intervention focused on 4 areas of surrogate decision-maker support: (1) emotional support, (2) communication support, (3) decision support, and (4) anticipatory grief support. All participants reported they would recommend the role to others, and 90% of physicians and surrogates "felt the role (1) improved the quality and timeliness of care, (2) facilitated discussion of the patient's values and treatment preferences, and (3) improved the patient-centeredness of care."[9]

Curtis and colleagues[1] conducted a 2-center randomized trial to evaluate the impact of a trained communication facilitator on family distress and intensity of care at the end of life in the ICU. Two facilitators, a nurse and a social worker, received training on (1) the existing evidence on patient-family communication in the ICU, (2) understanding attachment styles and communication approaches tailored to supporting the surrogate within each attachment style, and (3) the 6 steps of mediation. Communication facilitator activities included (1) interviews with family to understand their concerns, needs, and communication characteristics; (2) meetings with clinicians to share family concerns, needs, and communication characteristics; (3) delivery of communication and emotional support adapted to the individuals' attachment style; (4) facilitation of and participation in family conferences; and (5) follow-up with family 24 hours after discharge from the ICU. The intervention was associated with decreased depressive symptoms in families at 6 months and a significant decrease in cost and length of stay among decedents.

With this supporting evidence, an interdisciplinary team of key strategic leaders from palliative care, critical care, ICU nursing, and the chief nurse executive successfully secured 2 full-time positions to design and implement the CCNC program. Their vision, leadership, and strategic ability to promote this intervention as a win for patients, families, providers, and the health system made this program possible. The nurse communicators (NCs) were tasked with leading the design, implementation, and evaluation of a program to improve the quality and consistency of family meetings, facilitate timely goals-of-care conversations and palliative care consultation, apply best practices in surrogate decision-maker support, and deliver anticipatory grief support.

Setting

The TLC is a 24-bed medical/surgical ICU at a large academic health center in the Midwest. Three interdisciplinary teams (2 medical, 1 surgical) serve a diverse population of critically ill medical and preoperative and postoperative surgical patients. Each interdisciplinary team includes an attending physician, fellow physician, 2 resident physicians, an advanced practice provider, and a pharmacist. A social worker and case manager provide supportive services to all 3 ICU teams. Most ICU nurses work full-time (three 12-hour shifts per week) with a nurse-to-patient ratio of no more than 2 patients to every 1 nurse. The ICU serves an average of 2230 patients per year, and approximately 11.7% of these patients die during their ICU stay.

METHODS

Before program implementation, the NCs were allocated 3 months of protected time to complete advanced training, meet with key stakeholders throughout the organization, conduct a comprehensive needs assessment and literature review, and design an evidence-based program to address the challenges identified. The program was launched in February 2017.

Nurse Communicator Training

Both NCs had bachelor of science degrees in nursing, with a combined 12 years of ICU experience before hire. Both were also simultaneously pursuing a doctorate in nursing practice. They were identified as well-respected ICU nurses who possessed strong communication skills and a solid understanding of the quality improvement process, although neither had received advanced training in palliative care or serious illness communication before this role transition. It was crucial these individuals possess the ability to think creatively, tolerate uncertainty, and be self-directed to both create and implement a plan.

Training for the NC role included a 20-hour workshop and 40 hours of immersive training with the inpatient specialty palliative care team. PalliTalk, a 2-day simulation-based workshop, is "designed to help practicing clinicians increase their comfort and confidence in common and challenging clinical situations with seriously ill patients and families."[10] The workshop included content on sharing difficult news, reading and responding to emotion, dealing with conflict, high-risk shared decision making, and conducting family meetings. The content was then applied in a series of simulated patient/family interactions with professional actors and included real-time feedback and debriefing with experienced palliative care clinicians.[11] The NCs returned to their home institution with new skills and a clearer understanding of personal strengths and opportunities for growth. These skills were then applied and refined through 40 hours of immersive training with the inpatient specialty palliative care team.

Needs Assessment

The needs assessment included one-on-one interviews with ICU clinicians, an organizational inventory of existing supportive resources, and administration of an evidence-based survey to measure staff perceptions of the quality of palliative care in the ICU.

One-on-one interviews were conducted with both medical and surgical ICU physicians (n = 20), ICU nurses (n = 20), and other key stakeholders (n = 22), including social work, case management, patient and family advisors, spiritual care, health psychology, and palliative care team members. The purpose of the interviews was to identify current successes and challenges regarding interdisciplinary communication and communication with patients and families in the ICU. The program implementation team (NCs, chief of palliative care, intensivist) designed a question prompt to guide the interviews. The prompt asked interviewees to consider 3 different "types" of ICU patients and the unique challenges each presents (**Box 1**). Interview notes were recorded and then analyzed to identify major themes (**Table 1**).

To complement the needs assessment interviews, the team administered the ICU Palliative Care Quality Assessment Tool developed at the University of Washington.[12] The survey was administered to ICU physicians (n = 14), advanced practice providers (n = 2), and nurses (n = 48). Survey results identified strengths and opportunities to improve the quality of palliative care in the ICU (**Table 2**).

Box 1
Intensive care unit physician and nurse question prompt

Question: Think of a fairly typical patient and family you recently cared for. To help guide our conversation, you might think about patients falling into 3 categories:

1. Patients who are doing well and we anticipate a good outcome

2. Patients who are doing poorly and we anticipate they might die

3. Acute-on-chronic patients who are going to survive but are dealing with sequelae of an underlying illness, which is an indicator of progression of their underlying disease

For each patient, or each category, consider the challenges you face in creating a shared vision for the care plan within the intensive care unit team, and communicating and collaborating on that vision with the patient and family.

With these patients in mind, and with our current communication structure,

1. What are we doing well?

2. What can we improve on?
   a. What are the barriers?
   b. What are the challenges?

3. What do you see your role being in overcoming these barriers?

Program Description

The CCNC program was designed and implemented in collaboration with the chief of palliative care and a medical intensivist. The program delivers supportive interventions focused on 4 domains: (1) surrogate decision-maker support, (2) structured interdisciplinary and patient/family communication, (3) transitional care coordination, and (4) grief support. The program's mission is to address the informational and emotional needs of patients and families and achieve outcomes that matter most to the patient through thoughtful questioning, compassionate listening, high-quality communication, and seamless care coordination.

Target Patients

The program focuses on ICU patients at high risk for morbidity and mortality, unmet palliative care needs, and patients and families predicted to face complex care decisions during their hospital stay. The following trigger criteria are used to identify patients who may benefit from the CCNC program. These criteria were developed through appraisal of evidence suggesting which patients in the ICU may benefit from palliative care consultation (**Box 2**).[8,13–15]

In addition to these criteria, the NC uses the sequential organ failure assessment (SOFA) score to triage patients. The SOFA score is a morbidity severity score and mortality estimation tool calculated daily based on physiologic data available in the electronic health record (EHR). The NC targets patients with an SOFA-estimated 40% or greater ICU mortality. Each morning the nurse meets with social work, case management, charge nurses, and advanced practice providers from each ICU team to discuss patients and collaboratively assess appropriateness for the program.

Program Activities

The following section describes detailed activities within each of the 4 program supportive domains.

Table 1 Challenges identified through staff interviews	
Competing priorities	• "Understanding the patient/family perspective, I think that's missing. It's hard for me to find time to do that." -ICU physician • "When these patients are so sick, it is hard to sit down and have a conversation. I would rather sit down and talk rather than chart. There is always something else I could be doing." -ICU nurse • "Time is a big barrier. We talk about all the pathophysiology and now we don't have time to talk about emotions or patient preferences." -ICU physician
Failure to discuss the "big picture"	• "I think we focus on the here and now and not the future, of what life will look like after the ICU. We get lost in trying to be aggressive with treatment because that is what we do in the hospital." -ICU nurse • "We don't always have 'big picture' meetings. We talk to family about treating the infection but don't talk about the patient's leukemia." -ICU physician
Inconsistent messaging	• "Any environment where there are so many providers, especially in the ICU, is particularly challenging for patients and families. The signal-to-noise ratio is high. There is a lot of noise, but the signal is lost. The physician might come in and tell the family something. Or the resident physician, who is not versed in critical care, will tell the family something, and it's inconsistent or inaccurate. There are a lot of cooks in the kitchen and details will be different." -ICU physician • "I feel like we are not communicating early enough, poor communication between services. Some services paint a pretty picture for patients and families and other services say they are doing poorly." -ICU nurse
Lack of education and training	• "It would help to have more education regarding goals-of-care conversations. Sometimes it is difficult to know when to have these conversations. Sometimes I feel it is my place to start that conversation, many times I do not feel comfortable starting this conversation." -ICU nurse • "Residents don't get as much practice having EOL discussions with family here. This is much more faculty driven here, which is probably good for families, but leaves a bit of a gap in the residents' education." -ICU physician

Abbreviations: EOL, end of life; ICU, intensive care unit.

Surrogate decision-maker support

The NC operates as a fully integrated member of the ICU team and staffs the ICU 7 days per week. Within the first 24 to 48 hours of ICU admission, the NC conducts an initial visit with the patient and/or their surrogate decision makers. More than 90% of patients enrolled in the CCNC program are incapacitated at the time of this initial visit. Subsequently, this conversation most often occurs with the patient's surrogate decision-maker and other members of the primary support system. During this visit, the NC introduces the NC role and conducts a palliative-focused visit (**Box 3**).

This visit serves as an opportunity to gather important information, address informational and emotional needs, and begin to establish a trusting, therapeutic relationship with the patient's support system. Information gathered is documented in a

Table 2
Quality of palliative care in the intensive care unit survey results

Strengths	Opportunities for Improvement
• Management of symptoms and provision of comfort care • Attention to the emotional and practical needs of dying patients and their families • Communication with patients and families about goals of care and treatment • Communication with members of the clinical team to clarify goals of care • Eliciting and respecting patient and/or family preferences regarding goals of care and treatment	• Provision of education about palliative care • Provision of emotional support for clinicians caring for dying patients • Assessment of the spiritual/religious needs of the patients and families • Communication about goals of care to the next caregivers • Communication with colleagues about the patients' and/or families' emotional needs

comprehensive note in the electronic medical record and questions, concerns, gaps in understanding, or misalignment between the patient's stated preferences and the treatment plan are communicated to the treatment team. After the initial visit, the NC conducts daily visits to address informational and emotional needs, discuss interval changes in the context of the "big picture," coordinates timely initial and ongoing family meetings, and offers decision-making support when indicated. The NC identifies needs out of their scope of practice and refers to others. Consultation most often occurs with spiritual care, health psychology, social work, and specialty palliative care (**Box 4**).

Structured interdisciplinary and patient/family communication

The NC manages a family meeting protocol with a goal to hold an interdisciplinary family meeting by ICU day 4 for all patients anticipated to have a prolonged ICU stay or those likely to face complex care decisions. The NC schedules, coordinates, and attends all family meetings. The NC coordinates with family and consulting services to ensure all important support people can attend and crucial consulting perspectives are represented at the meeting. A series of activities occurs before, during, and after the family meeting to support the family and ensure the medical team is prepared to

Box 2
Critical Care Nurse Communicator patient trigger criteria

- Metastatic, incurable malignancy
- Hospital length of stay greater than 10 days before intensive care unit (ICU) transfer
- ≥80 years old with 2 significant chronic diseases (chronic obstructive pulmonary disease [COPD] on home oxygen, chronic kidney disease on dialysis, end-stage liver disease, congestive heart failure (CHF), advanced dementia, advanced cancer)
- Cardiac arrest
- ICU transfer from long-term acute care hospital
- Multiple ICU admissions or multiple recent hospital admissions related to sequelae of an underlying chronic health condition (eg, COPD, CHF, pulmonary fibrosis)
- Multiple recent hospital admissions
- Concern for significant brain injury

Box 3
Initial visit

- Describe the nurse communicator role and ICU communication structure (daily bedside rounds, family meetings)
- Establish rapport with the family and understand the patient's primary support system
- Understand the patient as a person: prehospital state of health, what brings the patient joy, what does the patient value most, how would support persons describe the patient?
- Address emotional symptoms through compassionate listening and empathic communication
- Assess for spiritual needs and address through coordination with spiritual care
- Assess the family's understanding of the medical situation: patient's current condition, expected course; address questions and clarify misinformation/misunderstandings
- Understand the patient's/family's short-term and long-term goals with ICU care
- Identify and address major concerns, worries
- Evaluate previously stated treatment preferences: does the patient have a medical power of attorney, living will? Has the surrogate had conversations with the patient about treatment preferences in the past? Do the patient's stated wishes align with the treatment plan?

---

deliver a clear and consistent message tailored to the patient's and family's unique needs (**Fig. 1**).

Before the family meeting, the NC meets with the patient and/or surrogate decision-maker to share the medical team's meeting goal, elicit the patient and family's meeting goal, and collect questions and concerns the patient and family would like to address. This information is brought back to the ICU team and shared during an interdisciplinary family meeting pre-huddle. The pre-huddle is a brief conversation (under 5 minutes) involving all meeting participants from the treatment team. The NC completes an evidence-based pre-huddle checklist to make certain the medical team is prepared to address family questions and concerns and communicate a clear and consistent message (**Box 5**).

During the meeting, the NC serves as a patient advocate and family support person. The NC clarifies medical jargon, addresses family emotion, orients the conversation around the patient as a person, and fosters best-practice content and flow of the meeting. Although these supportive activities are consistently delivered across all family meetings, attending physicians, consultants, and advanced practice providers differ in their preferred communication style and comfort level during difficult conversations. The NC is able to adapt to this variability to provide consistent, high-quality

---

Box 4
Criteria for specialty palliative care consultation

- Complex goals of care
- Unclear goals of care, particularly in the patient facing multiple care transitions who is at high risk for ICU readmission
- Complex symptom management
- Significant patient, family, or clinician distress

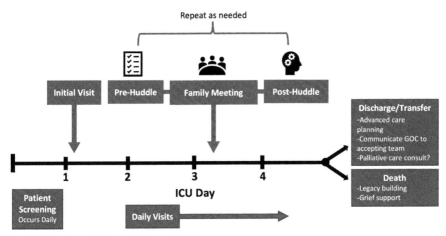

Fig. 1. NC role activities. GOC, goals of care.

communication and patient and family support. After the family meeting, a post-huddle occurs with both the medical team and the family. During the medical team post-huddle, the NC clarifies who will document the conversation in the EHR and leads a short debriefing on how the meeting went, opportunities for improvement, and checks in with clinicians if it was a difficult meeting. During the postmeeting debriefing with the family, the NC prepares meeting summary notes for the family and reviews this document with meeting participants (Appendix 1). This postmeeting debrief also serves as an opportunity to address unanswered questions, clarify misunderstandings, and offer additional emotional and decision-making support. If the meeting is a goals-of-care conversation in which 2 distinct treatment options are presented, the NC collaborates with the attending physician to complete a best case/worst case decision aide for the patient and family.[16] This tool translates benefit/risk prognostic information into a best case, worst case, and most likely case scenario narrative to assist in decision making (Appendix 2). The NC reviews the best case/worst case decision aid tool with family and supports the surrogate as they process how each path does or does not align with their loved one's values and treatment preferences.

Box 5
Family meeting pre-huddle checklist

- Are all meeting participants present?
- What is our goal for this meeting?
- Are there any test results pending that will influence the patient's trajectory or this conversation?
- Will we address code status during this meeting?
- What is the family's understanding of the medical situation?
- Are there important family dynamics to be aware of?
- Will the power of attorney or surrogate decision-maker be present?
- Who will lead this meeting?

Transitional care coordination

Approximately 45% (n = 131) of patients enrolled in the CCNC program survive their ICU stay. Most transition from the ICU to a variety of post-ICU care settings, such as a step-down hospital unit, long-term acute care hospital, or skilled nursing facility. As care transitions to a new interdisciplinary team, the NC facilitates communication with the accepting team regarding ongoing goals-of-care discussions and advanced care planning needs. For patients who have not completed a power of attorney for health care, the NC coordinates with social work and chaplaincy to assist the patient in completing this or creating a plan to do so in the future. In the patient with acute-on-chronic illness whose ICU admission was related to sequelae from an underlying chronic health condition (eg, chronic obstructive pulmonary disease, heart failure, pulmonary fibrosis), the NC provides the patient and family with resources to start a conversation about treatment preferences and end-of-life wishes (The Honoring Choices Conversation Starter Kit). This is also an opportunity to assess the need for specialty inpatient or outpatient palliative care.

Grief support

More than half of patients enrolled in the CCNC program die during their ICU stay. For these patients and families, the NC helps facilitate legacy building activities, such as plaster and ink handprints and teddy bears for children, with an audio recording of their loved one's heartbeat. The NC coordinates with social work to support children through memory-making projects and anticipatory grief support, and counsels parents on how to best support their children through this difficult time. The NC provides family grief support resources, addresses questions about the post-death transition, and sends a condolence card to families 2 to 4 weeks after death.

RESULTS

Evaluation of the NC Program reveals that 74.6% of all ICU patients have an interdisciplinary family meeting by day 4 of ICU stay (n = 134). In addition, there have been improvements in family meeting preparedness (team pre-huddle occurs before 87.9% of meetings, n = 348), and consistent interdisciplinary participation in family meetings (NC present 94.9%, nurse present 89.5%, physician/nurse practitioner present 100%, n = 352). All families surveyed would recommend the NC role to other patients and families (n = 14), and more than 85% of physicians and nurses agree or strongly agree the NC role has improved the care we deliver to patients and families and believe the role has been a valuable addition to the ICU team (n = 32). Nurse and physician feedback illustrates how the NC role improves patient, family, and staff outcomes (**Table 3**). The NCs conducted a pre/post comparison of ICU and hospital length of stay in those patients who die in the hospital. The program has been associated with an 8.4% decrease in average ICU length of stay (95% confidence interval [CI] 2.4% decrease to 14.1% decrease, $P<.001$) and 7.1% decrease in hospital length of stay (95% CI 3.1% decrease to 11.0% decrease, $P<.001$) in Poisson regression models adjusting for severity of illness using APACHE IV. Ongoing program evaluation includes patient and family outcomes (ICU satisfaction, quality of communication, post-ICU distress) and cost of care.

Discussion

With an aging population and an increasing number of individuals living with chronic disease, demand for quality care and health care costs will continue to rise. Furthermore, given that approximately 20% of Americans die in ICUs and critical care costs account for an estimated 13% of inpatient hospital costs, the ICU represents an

Table 3
Physician and nurse perceived benefits of the NC role

Perceived Benefit	Nurse or Physician Statement
Increased emphasis on patient-centered care	"I have noticed increased emphasis on family communication and knowledge of our patients' lives and wishes for care—we all profit from the time and effort that they [the NCs] dedicate."
Timely, structured communication	"Communication between family, providers, and nurses is carried out in a structured and consistent manner, which otherwise was often delayed, inconsistent, and/or missing prior. The NC has bridged a gap in health care where patients and families were left to make uninformed or underinformed decisions despite provider and nurse efforts."
Job satisfaction	"I cannot imagine working here without having the NC role." -ICU nurse
Continuity	"The attendings may change every week, or sometimes every day, but they do not. They are able to provide very valuable consistency for patient care and planning." "It provides patients and their family/friends a consistent 'go to' person when RNs and MDs are always changing.
Support nurses in difficult situations	"In situations that are especially complex and difficult, they help the RN facilitate conversations between the primary team and the family."
Families are less stressed, anxious: enable nurse to be more efficient and effective	"Families seem more relaxed and less anxious when they are working with the NC. Staff nurses have more time to attend to medical concerns of patients."
Better-informed families	"They are better informed and not blind-sided by patient prognosis or discharge needs."
"Big picture" conversations	"The communication helps patients and families understand best, worst, and most likely outcomes in a setting where they are comfortable and can ask questions."
Facilitates communication to achieve patient-centered care	"The NC facilitates patient and family, as well as provider and nurse communication prior, during, and after the meeting in order to best meet the needs of the patient and ensure the best and most appropriate patient-centered outcome."
Helps staff develop communication skills	"The NCs are able to help staff work through how to address difficult situations with patients and families, helping staff develop these skills."
Enables nurse to care for the patient without neglecting the family	"They allow me to be able to focus on the patient and the medical side of care. Meanwhile, I know that the family is being supported and getting the care that they need too."
Consistent communication, focus on patients' wishes	"It helps increase communication between patients/families and the medical team, which alleviates stress on their part, decreases their anxiety, and helps keep patients' wishes at the forefront of our care."

Abbreviations: ICU, intensive care unit; MD, medical doctor; NC, nurse communicator; RN, registered nurse.

important opportunity to improve the quality of care delivered and simultaneously reduce costs.[1,4] It is widely recognized that palliative care for patients with serious illness can simultaneously improve quality of life and support for patients and families, while reducing health care costs.[14] However, although demand for specialty palliative care continues to rise, there is a critical shortage of specialty palliative care providers. To meet this growing demand, clinicians working with patients facing a life-limiting illness should possess certain primary palliative care skills; however, there is no clear consensus on how to best facilitate this in the ICU setting.

The CCNC program has proven to be a successful and innovative subspecialized palliative care intervention in the ICU setting. As experienced ICU nurses with additional intensive palliative care training, the NCs are fully integrated into both the ICU and palliative care teams. They staff the ICU 7 days per week to promote continuity, and outcomes suggest the program has improved communication; augmented support for patients, families, and staff; and may have an impact on resource utilization and cost of care.

Although daily operations occur within the ICU setting with ICU physicians and nurses, the NCs maintain a close collaborative relationship with the inpatient and outpatient palliative care teams. This helps facilitate appropriate and timely palliative care consultation, as well as ongoing knowledge and skills development opportunities. This unique hybrid ICU/palliative nurse role is an innovative means to meet the growing demand for primary palliative care in the ICU setting while reserving the specialty palliative care team for refractory cases.[17]

Effective workflows and standardized communication processes are crucial to achieving high-quality shared decision making in the ICU. Although most clinicians recognize the importance of timely goals-of-care conversations with patients and families, many lack the training, resources, and time to have these conversations, and significant barriers exist to scheduling and coordinating family meetings in a busy ICU setting.[5,18] Integration of an NC in the ICU has yielded an efficient workflow and consistent structure around these conversations. It has raised the ICU team's collective consciousness of the importance of sitting down with patients and families to ensure the treatment plan aligns with what matters most to the patient. Subsequently, our ICU team is having better conversations and earlier conversations for more patients.

The CCNC program not only improves the quality and consistency of family meetings, but also improves support for surrogate decision makers. Decision science suggests that complex medical decision making is much more than just a cognitive exercise. Emotional stress has a strong influence on a surrogate's ability to make sound, rational decisions. Subsequently, interventions that improve communication and information sharing but fail to address the emotional stress associated with making a difficult medical decision may not be adequate.[19] The CCNC program strives to address both the cognitive and emotional aspects of medical decision making through compassionate listening, empathic communication, and reassurance.

The program also augments support for nurses and physicians and improves nurses' confidence in their own communication skills. We believe more consistent, high-quality goals-of-care conversations and better support for surrogate decision makers has led to a decrease in inappropriate medical care at the end of life. Reduction in potentially inappropriate medical care has not been directly measured and could be a topic of future study. In addition, nurses caring for critically ill patients are better able to attend to the physiologic needs of the patient without feeling as though they are neglecting the needs of the family. One concern before implementation was that the NC would displace the nurse as the primary family support person and rob the nurse of opportunities to improve their primary palliative care skills. Instead, what we have observed is an improvement in nurses' confidence in their own communication skills. Often, the NC is conducting crucial conversations at the bedside in the presence of the primary nurse, serving as an informal mentor. Primary nurses are then continuing these conversations with their patients and families, adding new skills to their communication toolbox and improving their confidence in difficult situations. The NC does not replace but adds support and serves as an informal "communication mentor" for the bedside nurse. The role has added value to every aspect of patient care, with benefits experienced by the nurses, doctors, patients/families, and health system.

SUMMARY

Integration of an NC in the ICU is feasible and benefits patients, families, the health system, and frontline clinicians. The program is strongly supported by families, physicians and staff, and is associated with an increased frequency of early family meetings, improved quality of communication, and a decrease in resource utilization in patients who die. The program addresses unmet palliative care needs, improves communication and shared decision making, and bolsters support for patients, families, and staff in the ICU.

DISCLOSURE

The authors have nothing to disclose.

REFERENCES

1. Curtis JR, Treece PD, Nielsen EL, et al. Randomized trial of communication facilitators to reduce family distress and intensity of end-of-life care. Am J Respir Crit Care Med 2016;193(2):154–62.
2. McAdam JL, Dracup KA, White DB, et al. Symptom experiences of family members of intensive care unit patients at high risk for dying. Crit Care Med 2010;38(4):1078–85.
3. White DB, Angus DC, Shields AM, et al. A randomized trial of a family-support intervention in intensive care units. N Engl J Med 2018;378(25):2365–75.
4. Khandelwal N, Curtis JR. Economic implications of end-of-life care in the ICU. Curr Opin Crit Care 2014;20(6):656–61.
5. Gay EB, Pronovost PJ, Bassett RD, et al. The intensive care unit family meeting: making it happen. J Crit Care 2009;24(4):629.e1-12.
6. Sullivan SS, da Rosa Silva CF, Meeker MA. Family meetings at end of life. J Hosp Palliat Nurs 2015;17(3):196–205.
7. Nelson JE, Angus DC, Weissfeld LA, et al. End-of-life care for the critically ill: a national intensive care unit survey. Crit Care Med 2006;34(10):2547–53.
8. Braus N, Campbell TC, Kwekkeboom KL, et al. Prospective study of a proactive palliative care rounding intervention in a medical ICU. Intensive Care Med 2016;42(1):54–62.
9. White DB, Martin Cua S, Walk R, et al. Nurse-led intervention to improve surrogate decision making for patients with advanced critical illness. Am J Crit Care 2012;21(6):396–409.
10. PalliTalk communication workshop. 2019. Available at: https://www.medicine.wisc.edu/hematology-oncology/pallitalk. Accessed September 3, 2019.
11. Arnold RM, Back AL, Baile WF, et al. The oncotalk/vitaltalk model. In: Kissane DW, Bultz BD, Butow PN, et al, editors. Oxford textbook of communication in oncology and palliative care. Oxford: Oxford University Press; 2017. p. 363.
12. Ho LA, Engelberg RA, Curtis JR, et al. Comparing clinician ratings of the quality of palliative care in the intensive care unit. Crit Care Med 2011;39(5):975–83.
13. Huffines M, Johnson KL, Smitz Naranjo LL, et al. Improving family satisfaction and participation in decision making in an intensive care unit. Crit Care Nurse 2013;33(5):56–69.

14. Khandelwal N, Benkeser DC, Coe NB, et al. Potential influence of advance care planning and palliative care consultation on ICU costs for patients with chronic and serious illness. Crit Care Med 2016;44(8):1474–81.

15. Weissman DE, Meier DE. Identifying patients in need of a palliative care assessment in the hospital setting: a consensus report from the Center to Advance Palliative Care. J Palliat Med 2011;14(1):17–23.

16. Kruser JM, Nabozny MJ, Steffens NM, et al. "Best case/worst case": qualitative evaluation of a novel communication tool for difficult in-the-moment surgical decisions. J Am Geriatr Soc 2015;63(9):1805–11.

17. Mun E, Umbarger L, Ceria-Ulep C, et al. Palliative care processes embedded in the ICU workflow may reserve palliative care teams for refractory cases. Am J Hosp Palliat Care 2018;35(1):60–5.

18. Scheunemann LP, Ernecoff NC, Buddadhumaruk P, et al. Clinician-family communication about patients' values and preferences in intensive care units. JAMA Intern Med 2019;179(5):676–84.

19. Power TE, Swartzman LC, Robinson JW. Cognitive-emotional decision making (CEDM): a framework of patient medical decision making. Patient Educ Couns 2011;83(2):163–9.

APPENDIX 1: FAMILY MEETING SUMMARY EXAMPLE

Date: 1/13/18
Time: 11 am
Medical Team Members Present: MD, RN, NP, SW
Family Present: Husband, Daughter, Son, Brother

PROBLEM	OPTIONS	POSSIBLE OUTCOMES	NEXT STEPS
1. Respiratory Failure -Patient is requiring support from the breathing machine to provide oxygen and protect her airway. She is too weak to breathe without the machine due to pneumonia	-We will continue trying to remove fluid and help patient's kidneys to pee more fluid out so she can breathe better. We will test he ability to breathe without the machine each morning. She is not quire ready for the tube to be removed. She is also on antibiotics to treat the lung infection.		-Continue antibiotics to treat Patient's lung infection (pneumonia) -Remove fluid so Patient is better able to breathe on her own. Possibly remove breathing tube in the next 1–2 d -Monitor Patient's kidney function closely. Will need dialysis support for at least the next 1–2 wk.
2. Kidney Injury -Patient's kidneys have been injured from infection and low blood pressure.	-Patient is on dialysis, which is a life support machine for the kidneys when they have failed. We are hopeful her kidney function will return over the next few weeks.	See next page for **Best Case/Worst Case** Diagram	-When Patient is more awake and able to participate in therapy, will have PT/OT see her three times per week to start work on regaining strength.
3. Profound Weakness -Patient has been in a hospital bed for 2 wk, she has lost considerable muscle strength.	-When her critical illness has resolved, patient will require weeks to short months of physical therapy and rehabilitation to regain strength.		-Continue antiarrhythmic medication per cardiology's recommendation. -Continue to support each other and take care of yourself through
4. Atrial Fibrillation (abnormal heart rhythm) -Patient's heart is in an abnormal rhythm which is causing her blood pressure to be low.	-We will continue the anti-arrhythmic medicine to try to convert Patient's heart rhythm to a normal rhythm.		this difficult time. Eat, drink, sleep, try to get home if able – Patient needs you to stay healthy through this difficult time!

APPENDIX 2: BEST CASE/WORST CASE DECISION AID EXAMPLE

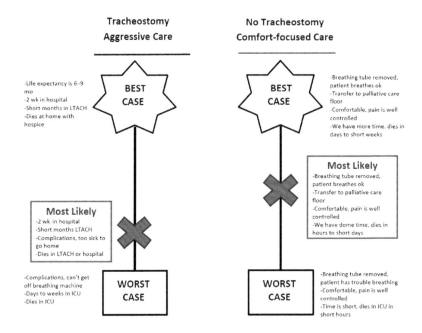

Tracheostomy
Aggressive Care

No Tracheostomy
Comfort-focused Care

BEST CASE

-Life expectancy is 6–9 mo
-2 wk in hospital
-Short months in LTACH
-Dies at home with hospice

BEST CASE

-Breathing tube removed, patient breathes ok
-Transfer to palliative care floor
-Comfortable, pain is well controlled
-We have more time, dies in days to short weeks

Most Likely
-2 wk in hospital
-Short months LTACH
-Complications, too sick to go home
-Dies in LTACH or hospital

Most Likely
-Breathing tube removed, patient breathes ok
-Transfer to palliative care floor
-Comfortable, pain is well controlled
-We have dome time, dies in hours to short days

WORST CASE

-Complications, can't get off breathing machine
-Days to weeks in ICU
-Dies in ICU

WORST CASE

-Breathing tube removed, patient has trouble breathing
-Comfortable, pain is well controlled
-Time is short, dies in ICU in short hours

Bereavement Care in the Adult Intensive Care Unit

Directions for Practice

Alyssa Erikson, RN, PhD[a],*, Jennifer McAdam, RN, PhD[b]

KEYWORDS

- Bereavement • Grief • Adult critical care • Family-centered care • Nursing

KEY POINTS

- Family-centered care guidelines recommend providing bereavement support to surviving ICU family members.
- Bereavement is an individual experience so a one-size-fits-all bereavement program may not work for all ICU families.
- There are many components that ICUs can include in their bereavement programs, including brochures, sympathy cards, and follow-up meetings.
- Using a bereavement risk assessment tool could be 1 strategy for ICU staff to tailor follow-up to at-risk families.
- ICUs developing a bereavement program need to consider factors such as how many components to include, resources, and potential barriers.

INTRODUCTION

Mortality rates in adult critical care settings can range from 10% to 29%.[1] This leaves a contingent of family members enduring the impact of a loved one's death in the intensive care unit (ICU). Family-centered care (FCC) guidelines in critical care advocate for addressing both the patients' and families' needs and values, which includes bereavement care.[2] Therefore, the purpose of this literature review is to provide direction for bereavement care through evaluating common components of bereavement programs and help guide ICU professionals in bereavement program planning and development.

DEFINITIONS OF KEY TERMS

Critical care nurses must understand the universality of grief and its enduring impact on families' lives.[3] Definitions for key concepts around bereavement, loss, grief, and

[a] Department of Nursing, California State University Monterey Bay, 100 Campus Center Drive, Seaside, CA 93955, USA; [b] School of Nursing, Samuel Merritt University, 3100 Telegraph Avenue, Oakland, CA 94609, USA
* Corresponding author.
E-mail address: aerikson@csumb.edu

Crit Care Nurs Clin N Am 32 (2020) 281–294
https://doi.org/10.1016/j.cnc.2020.02.009
0899-5885/20/© 2020 Elsevier Inc. All rights reserved.
ccnursing.theclinics.com

mourning can be found in **Box 1**.[4] Supporting the family is an expected component of critical care nursing. Critical care nurses who have a clear understanding of these concepts will better appreciate the family bereavement experience and provide appropriate bereavement care.

WHY ARE INTENSIVE CARE UNIT FAMILIES AT RISK?

The death of a loved one forces the family to reconstruct their lives. Death disrupts the normal flow of family life and reshapes family communication.[4] Death has financial implications for the family and affects social patterns within the family.[4] In addition, ICU family members have an increased risk of negative physical and psychological sequelae after a patient's death, when they may experience significantly higher levels of complicated grief, posttraumatic stress, and depressive symptoms.[5–9]

Critical care consensus groups support providing bereavement care to surviving family members to help alleviate these issues.[2] Yet, it is not fully understood the extent of how bereavement services affect surviving family members' grief or the magnitude of difference it makes in their lives. As one researcher stressed, conducting more empirical research is necessary to root practice in evidence so that we can serve families in the best ways possible.[10]

THE CURRENT STATUS OF INTENSIVE CARE UNIT BEREAVEMENT SUPPORT

ICU bereavement support varies widely across global locations.[11–15] The types of support ranged from sending a sympathy card to holding formal family support groups. In most of these studies, bereavement support was delivered either by ICU nurses or social workers. In addition, most bereavement programs had little to no formal evaluation of their effectiveness on family bereavement outcomes. See **Table 1** for the current status of ICU bereavement support.[11–15] See **Table 2** for examples of specific bereavement programs along with the evaluation of their outcomes.[16–19]

FAMILY PERSPECTIVES—PREPARATION AND COMMUNICATION

What factors influence bereavement intensity for families? One variable is how prepared a family feels for the death. Although no one is ever fully prepared for death, preparation intersects with good communication. Understanding the circumstances

---

Box 1
Definitions of key concepts

Bereavement	The state of having experienced the death of a significant other; confers obligations (such as disposition of the body, ritual ceremonies) as a temporary halt from life's activities (such as work or school).
Loss	A general term representing the absence of something valued (such as a person, a pet, a position or status, a prized object, or an attribute).
Grief	One's emotional response; influenced by age, sex, cultural mores, ethnic background, educational preparation, socioeconomic conditions, and the physical/mental health of the bereaved person or family.
Mourning	The social and cultural customs and practices that follow a death or loss; the purpose is an outward and public expression of loss, to incorporate the loss into the fabric of ongoing life.

From Jenko M, Short NM. A systems approach to improving care for all bereaved families. Dimens Crit Care Nurs. 2016;35(6):315–22, with permission.

Table 1
Intensive care units by country and percent of bereavement components offered

Country	Adult ICU Responses (n)	% that Offered Bereavement Follow-up and % of Each Individual Bereavement Component
United States	237	Offered bereavement follow-up (37.6%) Condolence card (62.9%) Bereavement brochure (43.8%) Follow-up telephone call to the family (36%) Memorial service (11%)
England	113	Information provided about follow-up support (76%)
New Zealand Australia	153	Offered bereavement follow-up (31.9%) Phone call to family (89%) Meeting with medical staff (45.7%) Sympathy card (26.2%)
Denmark	46	Offered bereavement follow-up (59%) ICU visit for family (41%) Meeting with medical staff by request (30%) Condolence letters (28%) Follow-up telephone call to the family (26%) Referral to priest or clergyman (24%) Routine meeting with medical staff (24%) Referral to counseling (11%)
European ICUs	85	Offered bereavement follow-up (41.1%) Viewing the deceased (90.6%) Providing follow-up information (79.8%) Sympathy letter (20%) Calling family to arrange meeting (31%)

Data from Refs.[11–15]

around the death (eg, violent death, unexpected death, prolonged death) and the preparedness of the death is important aspect for families' psychological adjustment during bereavement.

One group of researchers found that being more prepared was associated with higher coping skills and less bereavement intensity in family members 6 months after the ICU death.[20] Similarly, a study on the suddenly bereaved ICU family member found that both verbal and written information was helpful in their bereavement process.[21] Whereas others reported that family satisfaction with the ICU was low when they received poor communication and a lack of information.[22] Whether or not an ICU has a formal bereavement support program for families, ICU health care professionals' actions during the time they are in ICU can make a difference in how families cope with the death.[18] This includes clear, compassionate communication that assists in keeping the family prepared.[23,24]

FAMILY PERSPECTIVES—SUPPORT AND EXPERIENCES

There is strong evidence that ICU families want and need bereavement support.[18,22,25,26] The following quote from an ICU family member highlights this point:

> After he died, they just came in there and pronounced him dead, and started covering him up and moving him, and pulling out all these things.... They did not give me a minute to just kind of get up and grab my stuff and get out. So, I just left. I would have appreciated some follow-up or grief *support* or social

Table 2
Examples of bereavement programs and evaluation of outcomes

Site	Bereavement Components	Evaluation
Cardiac ICU	• A bereavement packet mailed to families at 4 wk with a list of support groups in the area and 7 brochures with information on grief • A sympathy card (in English or Spanish) at 2 wk • A telephone call at 6 wk • Two handwritten condolence letters (at 6 mo and at the 1 y anniversary of the patient death)	Informally evaluated with qualitative statements from family and staff Families reported that they felt cared for through these interventions and staff responded positively to the bereavement program
24 Bed Medical-Surgical ICU at a University Hospital	• "After a Loved One Has Died" bereavement brochure was given by a chaplain or a bedside nurse to the family • A sympathy card signed by nursing staff was sent 10 d postdeath • A telephone call at 3 wk was provided by a social worker • An invitation to a quarterly hospital memorial service developed by the Spiritual Care Department	No formal evaluation of the program but found that it was feasible to implement but did not have enough data to determine its effectiveness or helpfulness for families
32 Medical-Surgical ICU at a Tertiary Academic Hospital	• A bereavement brochure provided to families when the patient died • A condolence card signed by staff sent to families 1 wk after the death • A practical tasks resource packet with information and resources to grief support groups sent 1–2 wk after the patient death • A follow-up telephone call made 4 to 5 wk after the patient death and then again at 6 mo postdeath to assess how families were coping • A card sent to families acknowledging the patient's birthday	Qualitatively and quantitatively evaluated One family member reported finding the bereavement follow-up helpful: "You can't ever know which particular thing is going to help the most. I think just reaching out and making an attempt, that might help people the most." p315 Researchers compared the group that received the bereavement follow-up with another group that did not and found higher overall posttraumatic stress scores and prolonged grief in the nonbereavement group, but no difference in anxiety, depression, or satisfaction of care scores

Data from Refs.[16–19]

work or anything. Because I did not cry at all, until 2 months ago, I finally had myself a good little fit. I did not know that I was messed up. I wished that I had spoken with someone. Or someone had reached out to me in some way.[26(p815)]

Below is an additional list of what ICU families have shared regarding their needs and experiences around bereavement care:[18,27]

- Bereavement is an individual experience for families and a one-size-fits-all bereavement program may not work
- Situations that occurred during the ICU experience remained significant for families beyond a year after the patient's death (this included both positive and negative experiences with ICU staff)
- Social, cultural, spiritual, and religious events after the death held extreme importance for ICU families
- Timely bereavement support is important to families
- Reliable information on financial issues is needed
- Follow-up with a bereavement counselor is beneficial
- Connections to people who have experienced similar bereavement issues is appreciated

DEVELOPING AN INTENSIVE CARE UNIT BEREAVEMENT PROGRAM

For ICUs that are considering adding bereavement support, it is important to consider the following: (1) what components to include, (2) is a bereavement risk screening tool necessary, and (3) how to develop a plan to ensure the program is successful and sustainable. The remainder of this paper discusses these aspects in more detail.

WHAT COMPONENTS TO INCLUDE?

Common components found in bereavement programs include such items as bereavement brochures, sympathy cards, and counseling services. These common components, along with their positives and considerations, are highlighted below.

BEREAVEMENT PACKET

FCC guidelines recommend providing families with a packet of bereavement materials addressing families' multiple emotional, psychosocial, and financial needs.[2] A bereavement packet is typically a collection of information, including an index for community resources (eg, therapists, support groups, funeral homes), directions for completing practical tasks after a death (eg, planning a funeral or obtaining a death certificate), and a description of the grief process. Some ICU staff provide this packet to family right after a patient's death when the family is still in the hospital, although others have described mailing the packet in the weeks after the death.[17]

Positives

Families have described a bereavement brochure as useful because they could access the information on their own time and had guidance on how to complete post-death tasks.[16,28] In addition, this packet provided information on grief that normalized the experience for many families.[28] Finally, families stated they could share the packet of information with others (eg, family or friends) who may go through a similar experience.[4,28]

Considerations

One consideration regarding a bereavement packet is the timing of when to deliver it to families. Some families are in a state of shock at the time of death. Therefore, if the packet was given to them at that time, they may forget they received it.[28] In 2008, Ross[17] also found that families often did not read the bereavement information at the time of the patient's death. Because of this, they sent the bereavement packet via mail 4 weeks after the patient's death and checked in by phone with the family 2 weeks later. Another consideration is that some families may find that the resources listed are not applicable or accessible to them.[28] A final concern is that the packet would require ongoing updates by staff. Even with all these considerations, a bereavement packet is a low-cost, minimal risk intervention for ICUs that may help families' cope with their loss. ICUs could consider offering a follow-up phone call to check in with families about the packet, answer any questions, provide referrals, and reinforce any important information.

SYMPATHY CARD OR LETTER

A sympathy card is an intervention to recognize a family's loss. It is typically sent to families within a few weeks after a patient's death and is usually signed by ICU staff who cared for the patient. This can be standardized or it can be personalized to the family as a condolence letter.

Positives

In general, ICU families appreciate receiving a sympathy card and regard it as a meaningful gesture.[28,29] Even if families could not remember when they received it, or who signed it, they accepted it as a token of compassion and remembrance of their loved one.[19,28] In 1 study, families appreciated the high-touch, personal aspect of a condolence letter, which is more individualized than a signed sympathy card, and reported that it was something tangible they could hold onto.[29]

Considerations

A randomized trial reported a potential negative outcome of a condolence letter.[30] In this study, a physician or nurse handwrote the letter in the following format: (1) recognition of the death and the name of the deceased, (2) mention of the deceased, (3) recognition of the family members, (4) an offer to help, and (5) an expression of sympathy. Researchers found higher levels of complicated grief in the families who received the letter versus those who did not. Researchers also interviewed families who participated in the study and surmised that this finding may be due to families feeling suspicious of why the medical team would send a personalized, handwritten letter.[30] Even though sympathy cards require staff's time to organize and implement, in general, they are a low-cost bereavement follow-up service. In addition, many families seem to appreciate the sentiment of a sympathy card. However, given the 1 report of harm, more research is needed to identify the best method of sending a personalized sympathy letter to families.

FOLLOW-UP PHONE CALL OR MEETING

A follow-up phone call or meeting from the ICU staff is another component of a bereavement program that may benefit some families. This is usually offered anywhere within a few weeks or months after the ICU death. The follow-up call or meeting can provide information about the events that led up to the death and the cause of death. A meeting also can be used to assess how the family is coping and if they need any additional support or referrals. These are usually conducted by ICU nurses, physicians, or chaplains.[31–33]

Positives

Most family members appreciated the option of having a follow-up phone call and/or meeting.[28,31] However, families who may benefit the most from this bereavement component are the ones who had unresolved questions about a patient's death. These families expressed that they would have appreciated a follow-up phone call to help them process the emotions and unanswered questions surrounding their experience in the ICU and to provide closure.[28]

Considerations

Follow-up meetings may not be necessary for every bereaved ICU family. In general, only about 7% to 10% of families reported that they needed this and it was usually to get answers regarding the cause of death.[32] In addition, families felt this should be offered by someone who knew the medical history of the patient (eg, physician).[28] Also, this component could be time consuming and staff may require additional training to conduct the calls or meetings. Therefore, 1 approach may be to screen families for bereavement risks to assess who may benefit most from this component.

COUNSELING SERVICES

Families will have a variety of reactions to loss and providing psychological interventions that assist with coping can be beneficial. Because of this, counseling services are an important component for ICUs to consider offering to families. Therapy can be a useful intervention in helping families deal with troubling emotions, thoughts, and behaviors after the loss of a loved one. These services usually include a trained mental health care professional and can be delivered in individual, family, or group settings.[34]

Positives

In a recent study on bereavement, most families found counseling on their own and were in favor of ICUs offering it.[28] These families reacted positively toward counseling during the grief process. All the families who attended therapy thought it should be a routine component in bereavement support.[28] This finding is supported by others who found individual counseling and support groups to be one of the bereavement services that were the most helpful in processing family grief.[35]

Considerations

Again, as with other components, timing is an important factor to consider when recommending counseling. Families have reported that within 2 weeks immediately after the death is too soon for counseling. During this period they are still suffering from information overload.[28] Most families suggested that the optimal timing of offering counseling should be 3 to 4 weeks after death.[28] An additional factor to consider is where the family lives. If the ICU staff provides recommendations close to the hospital, yet serves families from a wide geographic region, many families may not be able to use these services. One suggestion for ICUs to consider is to provide information on how to find counseling services in the families' local geographic region in either a bereavement packet or during follow-up communication.

MEMORY-MAKING INTERVENTIONS

Memory-making interventions include items, such as a memory box, ICU diaries, storytelling, and an ECG Memento©. A memory box typically contains a physical reminder of the patient (eg, a lock of hair, handprint, or photograph) and is created immediately after the patient's death.[16,36] An ICU diary is written by family members and nurses when the patient is critically ill (eg, sedated and ventilated) and is read at a later time to help understand the events in the ICU.[37] Storytelling includes the ICU families sharing their experience before, during, and after the patient's illness and death.[38] Finally, the ECG Memento© is composed of a 3-inch strip of the patient's heart rhythm mounted on a card, which is signed by the health care staff (see **Fig. 1** for an example).[39]

Positives

Memory-making interventions can provide a tangible, physical presence for bereaved families to feel closer to their loved one by providing comfort during the grieving process.[39–41] For example, in 1 study, when asked about a memory box, a family member's response was:

> I think going home there is just this void. You know you miss the physical presence of that person being there. Just to have something to hold onto and hold in your hands. I think that would have been really helpful.[28(p215)]

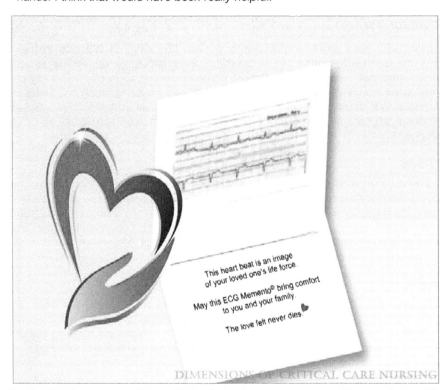

Fig. 1. ECG Memento©. A 7.5-cm ECG strip laminated and mounted in a card signed by nursing staff. (*From* Beiermann M, Kalowes P, Dyo M, Mondor A. Family members' and intensive care unit nurses' response to the ECG Memento© during the bereavement period. Dimens Crit Care Nurs. 2017;36(6):320, with permission.)

ICU diaries are recommended by FCC guidelines[2] because they may decrease anxiety and depression in ICU families and increase health-related quality of life.[42] ICU diaries can help bereaved families understand the events leading to a patient's death and answer potential questions about their experience. Families described ICU diaries as a bridge between the past (the ICU) and the future (the postdeath bereavement period)[43] and may help bereaved families construct a coherent narrative about their loved one's death. In addition, storytelling was found to be a feasible and helpful intervention for those families who suffered from a traumatic or unexpected death in the ICU.[38] In 2017, Beiermann and colleagues[39] found that families positively evaluated the ECG Memento© because they had a visible reminder of their loved one that they found comforting. They also reported that this intervention demonstrated caring by the ICU staff as recognition of the heartbreaking situation.[39]

Considerations

The concept of memory-making interventions can be off-putting to some families.[28] When offered by critical care nurses, these interventions need to be handled in a sensitive, caring way. These interventions should not be forced on grieving family members. In 1 study when families were asked about a memory box, they were clear that this needed to be discussed delicately and at the right time. Most families suggested offering the memory box right before the death as something to think about.[28] Contrary to this, families who received the ECG Memento© remarked that it was best to offer this after the patient dies and not during the active phase of dying.[39] The authors shared the revised script they use when approaching families:

> I don't know if you've heard of this really special thing we do here. We capture the heartbeat of your loved one and put it in a laminated card. Some families find it really helpful, especially if someone can't be here at this time. It's free as a gift to you and your loved ones. Our goal of care is patient and family comfort. We hope it brings comfort to you.[39(p324)]

The idea of memory making has been used in neonatal ICUs[36] and has potential to be valuable in adult ICUs. However, continued research is needed to understand the impact these memory-making interventions have on families' grief and bereavement.

MEMORIAL SERVICES

A memorial service is a way to ceremoniously remember and honor the families' loved one. Families often regard it as a ritual that facilitates accepting the reality of the death. The service also provides a vehicle for expressing feelings, stimulating memories, and providing support to the family and friends of the deceased. Memorial services can be offered by a hospital or specific units within a hospital on an annual or biannual basis.

Positives

Memorial services may be helpful to some bereaved ICU families.[35] In 1 study of 12 families, 25% of the ICU families reported that attending a memorial service would be beneficial in their grieving process.[28] In another study, most ICU families wanted a memorial service to be offered.[27] Benefits of a memorial service may include allowing families to reconnect with other families they met in the ICU and provide an opportunity to acknowledge and thank ICU staff. Families even thought it might be helpful for the ICU staff's own grieving.[28,44]

Considerations

Families have reported that attending a memorial service from the ICU or hospital may be redundant because they held their own personalized memorial for their loved one.[19,28] Other identified barriers for not attending a memorial service included feeling distressed returning to the place where their loved one died, living too far away from the hospital, parking concerns, a lack of time, and feeling like a memorial service would prevent them from moving forward in their grieving process.[28] The literature on hospital-based memorial services is limited and inconclusive on the effectiveness to ICU families. However, if the hospital or the ICU has the resources, offering a memorial service could serve as a shared experience for both families and health care professionals to honor those that died.

IS BEREAVEMENT RISK SCREENING NECESSARY?

Another aspect for ICUs to consider regarding bereavement support is if they should routinely screen families for bereavement risk factors. Families in 1 study described their bereavement experience as highly individualized.[18] By screening ICU families, this would allow ICUs to assess who would benefit most from bereavement services. Ideally, screening should occur in 3 phases.[45]

1. On admission to the ICU to allow staff to respond to mental health issues or bereavement support needs in a timely manner
2. Within 3 to 6 weeks after the patient death to ascertain any trauma related to the death
3. At 12 weeks postdeath to determine whether additional assessment or support is needed

Screening is also important because universal preventative therapy does not seem to be beneficial for all bereaved individuals.[46] In 1 study, over half of the family members believed routine bereavement screening should be a standard of care in the ICU. In addition, most professionals reported they would support and participate in bereavement screening.[22]

If an ICU decides to screen families, use of a reliable and valid risk screening tool is essential. The selected tool should be useful in assessing the effectiveness of bereavement interventions and identify areas where improvement may be needed.[47] Screening tools that have potential to be effective for use in the ICU are the Bereavement Risk Inventory and Screening Questionnaire, which may help identify families early on that need support,[48] and the CAESAR tool, which assists in tailoring support specifically for ICU family members.[47] Please see Sealey and colleagues'[45] scoping review on other potential bereavement risk screening tools that may be appropriate based on an individual ICUs family population.

HOW TO DEVELOP A SUCCESSFUL AND SUSTAINABLE PROGRAM

The final aspect for ICUs to consider is developing a solid plan to ensure that the bereavement program is successful and sustainable. **Box 2** suggests 8 questions ICU professionals can ask to guide the planning stages and address common barriers. First, ICUs need to consider identifying who will lead the program (eg, nurse, social worker, chaplain). Second, ICUs need to select what interventions may best address families' bereavement while a family is still in the ICU and in the weeks to months after the death. They can decide to offer a single intervention or develop a formal bereavement program with multiple interventions and determine the timing of when to offer

---

Box 2
Questions to ask in planning bereavement follow-up

1. Who will take the lead?
2. What interventions are needed? What supplies are needed?
3. What is the best timing to provide services?
4. How much will it cost to support bereavement follow-up services?
5. What is the funding source?
6. Will staff receive release time to lead the program?
7. What training or education will staff receive?
8. What is the evaluation plan to determine if follow-up was effective?

---

these interventions. Third, the ICU needs to consider the financial sustainability of the program, which includes how professionals will be compensated for training and leading the program and the annual budget for delivering the program along with continuous funding sources (eg, donations). Fourth, providing end-of-life and bereavement training for ICU staff will be necessary. Finally, evaluating outcomes through interviews and surveys is a necessary aspect of any program implementation. Potential outcomes may include family satisfaction of care, anxiety, depression, and complicated or prolonged grief.[16,30,49]

ICUs do not have to be overly ambitious because even 1 new intervention can be helpful. As 1 family member stated, just receiving a sympathy card from the ICU helped them feel recognized, *"We weren't just another sad little family coming through..."*[28(p212)] In addition, authors of a systematic review on bereavement care in the ICU strongly advise involving families in planning a formal bereavement care program.[50] **Table 2** provides examples of bereavement programs that ICUs can use as inspiration for their own plans.[16–19]

SUMMARY

FCC in the ICU does not end when the patient dies. Providing bereavement support is necessary and needed. Directions for practice can include:

- Offering bereavement components
- Screening families for bereavement risk factors and
- Developing sustainable bereavement programs.

DISCLOSURE

The authors have nothing to disclose.

REFERENCES

1. SCCM SoCCM. Critical care statistics: morbidity and mortality website. 2019. Available at: https://www.sccm.org/Communications/Critical-Care-Statistics. Accessed February 7, 2019.
2. Davidson JE, Aslakson RA, Long AC, et al. Guidelines for family-centered care in the neonatal, pediatric, and adult ICU. Crit Care Med 2017;45(1):103–28.
3. Switzer D. The dynamics of grief. Nashville (TN): Abingdon Press; 1970.

4. Jenko M, Short NM. A systems approach to improving care for all bereaved families. Dimens Crit Care Nurs 2016;35(6):315–22.

5. Anderson WG, Arnold RM, Angus DC, et al. Posttraumatic stress and complicated grief in family members of patients in the intensive care unit. J Gen Intern Med 2008;23(11):1871–6.

6. Gries CJ, Engelberg RA, Kross EK, et al. Predictors of symptoms of posttraumatic stress and depression in family members after patient death in the ICU. Chest 2010;137(2):280–7.

7. Kentish-Barnes N, Chaize M, Seegers V, et al. Complicated grief after death of a relative in the intensive care unit. Eur Respir J 2015;45(5):1341–52.

8. Kross EK, Engelberg RA, Gries CJ, et al. ICU care associated with symptoms of depression and posttraumatic stress disorder among family members of patients who die in the ICU. Chest 2011;139(4):795–801.

9. Probst DR, Gustin JL, Goodman LF, et al. ICU versus non-ICU hospital death: family member complicated grief, posttraumatic stress, and depressive symptoms. J Palliat Med 2016;19(4):387–93.

10. Buckley T. End of life and bereavement care in the intensive care unit: a need for more quality empirical research. Aust Crit Care 2017;30(3):137–8.

11. Berry M, Brink E, Metaxa V. Time for change? A national audit on bereavement care in intensive care units. J Intensive Care Soc 2017;18(1):11–6.

12. Egerod I, Kaldan G, Albarran J, et al. Elements of intensive care bereavement follow-up services: a European survey. Nurs Crit Care 2019;24(4):201–8.

13. Egerod I, Kaldan G, Coombs M, et al. Family-centered bereavement practices in Danish intensive care units: a cross-sectional national survey. Intensive Crit Care Nurs 2018;45:52–7.

14. McAdam JL, Erikson A. Bereavement services offered in adult intensive care units in the United States. Am J Crit Care 2016;25(2):110–7.

15. Mitchell M, Coombs M, Wetzig K. The provision of family-centred intensive care bereavement support in Australia and New Zealand: results of a cross sectional explorative descriptive survey. Aust Crit Care 2017;30(3):139–44.

16. McAdam JL, Puntillo K. Pilot study assessing the impact of bereavement support on families of deceased intensive care unit patients. Am J Crit Care 2018;27(5): 372–80.

17. Ross MW. Implementing a bereavement program. Crit Care Nurse 2008;28(6): 88, 87.

18. Jones C, Puntillo K, Donesky D, et al. Family members' experiences with bereavement in the intensive care unit. Am J Crit Care 2018;27(4):312–21.

19. Santiago C, Lee C, Piacentino R, et al. A pilot study of an interprofessional, multicomponent bereavement follow-up program in the intensive care unit. Can J Crit Care Nurs 2017;28(3):18–24.

20. Buckley T, Spinaze M, Bartrop R, et al. The nature of death, coping response and intensity of bereavement following death in the critical care environment. Aust Crit Care 2015;28(2):64–70.

21. Walker W, Deacon K. Nurses' experiences of caring for the suddenly bereaved in adult acute and critical care settings, and the provision of person-centred care: a qualitative study. Intensive Crit Care Nurs 2016;33:39–47.

22. Downar J, Barua R, Sinuff T. The desirability of an Intensive Care Unit (ICU) clinician-led bereavement screening and support program for family members of ICU Decedents (ICU Bereave). J Crit Care 2014;29(2):311.e9-16.

23. Curtis JR, Treece PD, Nielsen EL, et al. Randomized trial of communication facilitators to reduce family distress and intensity of end-of-life care. Am J Respir Crit Care Med 2016;193(2):154–62.
24. White DB, Angus DC, Shields AM, et al. A randomized trial of a family-support intervention in intensive care units. N Engl J Med 2018;378(25):2365–75.
25. van der Klink MA, Heijboer L, Hofhuis JG, et al. Survey into bereavement of family members of patients who died in the intensive care unit. Intensive Crit Care Nurs 2010;26(4):215–25.
26. Nelson JE, Puntillo KA, Pronovost PJ, et al. In their own words: patients and families define high-quality palliative care in the intensive care unit. Crit Care Med 2010;38(3):808–18.
27. Donnelly S, Prizeman G, Coimin DO, et al. Voices that matter: end-of-life care in two acute hospitals from the perspective of bereaved relatives. BMC Palliat Care 2018;17(1):117.
28. Erikson A, Puntillo K, McAdam J. Family members' opinions about bereavement care after cardiac intensive care unit patients' deaths. Nurs Crit Care 2019;24(4):209–21.
29. Kentish-Barnes N, Cohen-Solal Z, Souppart V, et al. "It was the only thing I could hold onto, but…": receiving a letter of condolence after loss of a loved one in the ICU: a qualitative study of bereaved relatives' experience. Crit Care Med 2017;45(12):1965–71.
30. Kentish-Barnes N, Chevret S, Champigneulle B, et al. Effect of a condolence letter on grief symptoms among relatives of patients who died in the ICU: a randomized clinical trial. Intensive Care Med 2017;43(4):473–84.
31. Kock M, Berntsson C, Bengtsson A. A follow-up meeting post death is appreciated by family members of deceased patients. Acta Anaesthesiol Scand 2014;58(7):891–6.
32. Lebus C, Parker RA, Morrison K, et al. Families' concerns after bereavement in hospital: what can we learn? J Palliat Med 2014;17(6):712–7.
33. Moi AL, Storli SL, Gjengedal E, et al. The provision of nurse-led follow-up at Norwegian intensive care units. J Clin Nurs 2018;27(13–14):2877–86.
34. NIMH. Psychotherapies. 2016. Available at: https://www.nimh.nih.gov/health/topics/psychotherapies/index.shtml. Accessed October 12, 2019.
35. Banyasz A, Weiskittle R, Lorenz A, et al. Bereavement service preferences of surviving family members: variation among next of kin with depression and complicated grief. J Palliat Med 2017;20(10):1091–7.
36. Kenner C, Press J, Ryan D. Recommendations for palliative and bereavement care in the NICU: a family-centered integrative approach. J perinatology 2015;35(Suppl 1):S19–23.
37. Garrouste-Orgeas M, Perier A, Mouricou P, et al. Writing in and reading ICU diaries: qualitative study of families' experience in the ICU. PLoS One 2014;9(10):e110146.
38. Schenker Y, Dew MA, Reynolds CF, et al. Development of a post-intensive care unit storytelling intervention for surrogates involved in decisions to limit life-sustaining treatment. Palliat Support Care 2015;13(3):451–63.
39. Beiermann M, Kalowes P, Dyo M, et al. Family members' and intensive care unit nurses' response to the ECG Memento© during the bereavement period. Dimens Crit Care Nurs 2017;36(6):317–26.
40. Coombs M, Mitchell M, James S, et al. Intensive care bereavement practices across New Zealand and Australian intensive care units: a qualitative content analysis. J Clin Nurs 2017;26(19–20):2944–52.

41. Hockey J, Kellaher L, Prendergast D. Of grief and well-being: competing conceptions of restorative ritualization. Anthropol Med 2007;14(1):1–14.
42. McIlroy PA, King RS, Garrouste-Orgeas M, et al. The effect of ICU diaries on psychological outcomes and quality of life of survivors of critical illness and their relatives: a systematic review and meta-analysis. Crit Care Med 2019;47(2):273–9.
43. Johansson M, Wahlin I, Magnusson L, et al. Family members' experiences with intensive care unit diaries when the patient does not survive. Scand J Caring Sci 2018;32(1):233–40.
44. Muta R, Sanjo M, Miyashita M, et al. What bereavement follow-up does family members request in Japanese palliative care units? A qualitative study. Am J Hosp Palliat Care 2014;31(5):485–94.
45. Sealey M, Breen LJ, O'Connor M, et al. A scoping review of bereavement risk assessment measures: implications for palliative care. Palliat Med 2015;29(7):577–89.
46. Mancini AD, Griffin P, Bonanno GA. Recent trends in the treatment of prolonged grief. Curr Opin Psychiatry 2012;25(1):46–51.
47. Kentish-Barnes N, Seegers V, Legriel S, et al. CAESAR: a new tool to assess relatives' experience of dying and death in the ICU. Intensive Care Med 2016;42(6):995–1002.
48. Roberts K, Holland J, Prigerson HG, et al. Development of the Bereavement Risk Inventory and Screening Questionnaire (BRISQ): item generation and expert panel feedback. Palliat Support Care 2017;15(1):57–66.
49. Wilson DM, Dhanji N, Playfair R, et al. A scoping review of bereavement service outcomes. Palliat Support Care 2017;15(2):242–59.
50. Efstathiou N, Walker W, Metcalfe A, et al. The state of bereavement support in adult intensive care: a systematic review and narrative synthesis. J Crit Care 2019;50:177–87.

Enhancing Family-Centered Care in Cardiothoracic Surgery

Kelly A. Thompson-Brazill, DNP, ACNP-BC, CCRN-CSC, FCCM[a],*,
Catherine C. Tierney, DNP, ACNP-BC[a,b,1], Lori Brien, DNP, ACNP-BC[a,b,1],
Jeremy W. Wininger, MSN, AGACNP-BC[a,c,2],
Judson B. Williams, MD, MHS[d]

KEYWORDS

- Cardiothoracic surgery • Family-centered care
- Enhanced recovery after surgery (ERAS) cardiac • Perioperative education
- Patient engagement • Electronic patient portals

KEY POINTS

- Over the past 2 decades, professional groups and patient safety organizations have crafted family-centered care (FCC) models that support both hospitalized patients and their families.
- Although cardiac surgery procedures are common, there are few data on use and outcomes of FCC in cardiothoracic intensive care units.
- Novel ways of increasing patient and family engagement in care include both bedside nursing change-of-shift handoff and the use of electronic patient portals and decision support tools.
- Enhanced Recovery after Surgery (ERAS) Cardiac Surgery embraces nurse-led education, placing the patient and family at its center. Through the use of multimedia patient engagement tools, preoperative patients and their families are provided with the evidence-based data that support the ERAS initiative, which spans their entire hospitalization.
- Family presence during resuscitation is becoming more accepted throughout the United States. This may not be appropriate for cardiac surgery patients who require bedside resternotomy. Research is needed to determine best approaches to FCC in this population.

[a] Adult Gerontology Acute Care Nurse Practitioner Program, Georgetown University School of Nursing & Health Studies, Washington, DC, USA; [b] Cardiovascular and Thoracic Surgery, Virginia Hospital Center, 1625 North George Mason Dr., Arlington, VA, 22205 USA; [c] Pulmonology and Critical Care Medicine, Wake Med Health & Hospitals, Raleigh, NC, USA; [d] Cardiovascular and Thoracic Surgery, Wake Med Health & Hospitals, 3000 New Bern Avenue, Suite 1100, Raleigh, NC 27610, USA
[1] Present address: 3700 Reservoir Road Northwest, Washington, DC 20057.
[2] Present address: 3000 New Bern Avenue Suite, Raleigh, NC 27610.
* Corresponding author. Georgetown University School of Nursing & Health Studies, 3700 Reservoir Road Northwest, Saint Mary's Hall #421, Washington, DC 20057.
E-mail address: Kelly.thompsonbrazill@georgetown.edu

Crit Care Nurs Clin N Am 32 (2020) 295–311
https://doi.org/10.1016/j.cnc.2020.02.010
0899-5885/20/© 2020 Elsevier Inc. All rights reserved.
ccnursing.theclinics.com

INTRODUCTION

The psychological impact of critical illness is far reaching, affecting both patients and their loved ones.[1] For some, the duration is short, but for others it may last months or years.[1] Family members face a multitude of stressors beginning at admission.[1] They range from concerns about the possibility of death or permanent disability to financial anxiety over health care costs and lost wages.[2–4] Some may encounter legal issues, such as obtaining power of attorney, in order to pay a patient's bills or gain guardianship to care for minor children, all of which pose significant emotional and financial strain.[2] Without intervention, loved ones may themselves suffer posttraumatic stress disorder (PTSD), anxiety, and depression. Patients who survive critical illness are at risk for developing post–intensive care syndrome (PICS).[5–10] PICS can have long-term negative effects on employment and quality of life.[4,7,9,11] Approximately 1 out of 5 critical care survivors is at risk for developing PTSD.[12] Families also can develop PICS, including the children of critically ill adults.[13,14] This is referred to as PICS-family (PICS-F).[5,7,8,10,15,16] Over the past 2 decades, professional groups and patient safety organizations have crafted family-centered care (FCC) models, which support both hospitalized patients and their families.[5,10,17–20] This article describes the principles of FCC and why they are beneficial to the unique needs of families of postoperative cardiothoracic surgery patients and includes novel ways of increasing patient and family engagement (**Fig. 1**).

This new paradigm gained traction when the Society for Critical Care Medicine (SCCM) introduced its first FCC guidelines in 2007.[5,17] This seminal work stimulated a large number of studies evaluating the benefits of FCC.[21] Moreover, it brought the concept of providing attentive, supportive care to the family to a larger national audience.[5,17,20,22] In 2011, the Institute for Healthcare Improvement released the white paper, *Achieving an Exceptional Patient and Family Experience of Inpatient Hospital Care*.[18] This paper is important because it debunked myths associated with FCC while promoting FCC ideals, such as increasing access to information (eg, medical record access) and partnering with patients and families to achieve the best outcomes.[18] Moreover, it was authored by a large, nationally respected organization to which medical center executives and policy leaders look for quality guidance, it was hoped that the information would spur adoption of FCC by more health systems.

Multiple studies have shown the positive benefits of implementing FCC in a variety of intensive care units (ICUs), ranging from neonatal and pediatric to adult general medical/surgical and specialty ICUs.[21,22] Although cardiac surgery procedures are

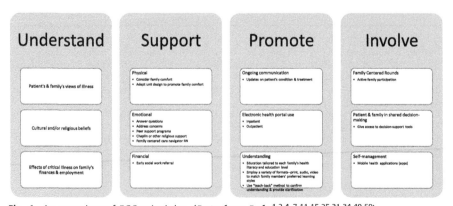

Fig. 1. An overview of FCC principles. (*Data from* Refs.[1,2,4–7,11,15,25,31,34,49,50])

common, with more than 400,000 performed in the United States annually,[23] there are few data on the use and outcomes of FCC in cardiothoracic ICUs (CTICUs).

For many patients, the need for cardiothoracic surgery develops insidiously over several years: thoracic aneurysms enlarge, coronary artery disease worsens, valves become more stenotic, and lung tumor cells proliferate. For others, the need for surgery arises quickly: a patient who presents with a stroke is found to have emboli from an atrial myxoma whereas another presents with sepsis and is found to have infective endocarditis.[23] Regardless of the duration of the illness and whether or not the procedure is curative or palliative, the notion of major surgery is frightening for patients and their loved ones.[14,24,25] The risks of uncontrolled pain, perioperative complications, death, disability, and functional status are just a few of the myriad factors that cause worry.[24,26–28]

PRINCIPLES OF FAMILY-CENTERED CARE

According to the SCCM FCC guidelines, "family" is defined by each individual.[5] The family unit may comprise individuals who are or are not genetically related to the person.[5,20] Family presence in the ICU, family support, and family-provider communication are key to providing effective care for families.[5,7,20,29,30] Many families prefer to stay at the bedside to comfort their loved ones.[31] Being near a patient also may decrease feelings of anxiety that are exacerbated by physical separation.[8,10,32] Open visitation helps decrease apprehension while improving families' satisfaction and communication with members of the care team.[33] Families of patients in the ICU have a need to understand the setting where their loved will recover and their role in this environment. In the CTICU, in particular, the array of medications and assistive devices can be particularly intimidating for families.[34] Facilitated sense-making is the deliberate practice of guiding family members through the experience of having a loved one in the ICU.[34]

A recent study evaluating the use of strategic facilitated sense-making introduced families of cardiac surgery to the structure and schedule of the CTICU environment.[34] Families' need for information was met by frequent updates about the patient's medical condition and the facilitation of communication between families and providers.[34] Family members were allowed to participate in nonmedical patient care to decrease their sense of helplessness and instructed in self-care and patient advocacy.[34] In essence, they were given the skills they need to navigate this alien environment. As a result, their situational anxiety significantly decreased.[34]

EDUCATION

Cardiac surgery patients and their families' journey starts with the surgical consultation. They have many questions about the procedure itself, the estimated postoperative length of stay in the CTICU and hospital, and what to expect during the perioperative period.[34] Trained nurse educators are integral members of the multiprofessional surgical team.[30,35,36] Families and patients who receive an orientation to the CTICU routines and education outlining cardiac surgery patients' care goals may participate more in their family member's care.[36] This can have both short-term and long-term benefits. Understanding patient care goals allows family members to encourage patients to move along care pathways acting in concert with the care team rather than in opposition.[30,36]

An important tenet in preoperative teaching is to evaluate each patient's health literacy and tailor education strategies according to the specific needs of patients and their families.[37] Patients should feel that they are receiving empathetic, nonjudgmental teaching in an understandable way.[18] As with other adult learners, patients who find the information taught pertinent and useful are more likely to integrate it and participate in their recovery.[18] When there is trust in the person delivering the information and the patient and family feel respect and support, they are more apt to view their hospital experience as positive.[18]

Trained nurse educators' interactions with patients and families also have positive effects on outcomes.[38] A quasi-experimental study by Kalogianni and coworkers[38] evaluated the effect of preoperative teaching by nurses trained in patient-centered care on patient outcomes. The nurses used interactive methodologies while delivering preoperative education.[38] Patients who had the specialty-trained, nurse-led teaching showed increased patient satisfaction, decreased ICU length of stay, and fewer arrhythmias than patients who received nonstructured information from the nursing staff who had not received the training.[38]

A systematic review of preoperative education programs and their effect on postoperative outcomes also identified that the skills, experience, and knowledge of the nurse educator had an impact on the confidence of the patients and their families.[25] Prior to cardiac surgery, a preoperative nurse educator visits, engages, and imparts knowledge to patients and their families.[25] This intervention allows for questions and clarification of complex information as well as for learning nonclinical information about the patient and family and their unique situation.[35,36] Individualizing teaching to meet learning needs along with providing material, such as booklets or leaflets, is paramount for optimal postoperative self-care.[25] Additionally, this interaction may lower anxiety and positively affect a the patient's and family's perceptions of the health care team.[18,24,25,39]

Preoperative instruction enhances the informed consent process.[39] Many patients and families are overwhelmed when urgent or emergent surgery is recommended.[24] Despite thorough descriptions of the procedure, along with the risks and benefits provided by surgeons, lay people may not remember or truly comprehend unfamiliar, complex information.[40] The nurse educator ensures patients and families time to ask questions and clarify their understanding, which augments their ability to make informed decisions about care.[40] The Agency for Healthcare Research and Quality recommends using the teach-back method to ensure patients comprehend a procedure before they give consent.[40]

There are multiple opportunities for patient and family education throughout the hospitalization. In addition to in-person nurse educator visits, videos, online education, and printed booklets and leaflets also are beneficial sources of information.[39,41,42] Not surprisingly, educational tools that employ audiovisual modalities improve knowledge retention compared with other types of media alone.[39] Combining these resources as part of a cohesive educational strategy should improve self-care.[41]

COMMUNICATION

Effective communication forms the basis for a solid relationship between providers and patients.[31] It is essential in establishing rapport and trust with patients' families.[21,31] Traditional communication has occurred in person during provider visits with the patients in their own hospital rooms and during telephone conversations. Historically, handoff at change of nursing shifts has occurred at the nurses' station away from patients and families.[43] During these exchanges, crucial information may not be communicated to the oncoming nurse, which may jeopardize patient safety.[43] The Joint Commission and World Health Organization have developed alternative methods to ensure patient safety at these critical junctures.[44] As a result, some medical centers have instituted bedside nursing change-of-shift rounds to reduce care errors.[43] This paradigm shift also has improved patient engagement.[43,44] A recent study of bedside change-of-shift report demonstrated 54% of patients actively participated during handoff.[45]

Most families want to participate in critical care rounds.[7,31,46] Family presence during rounds is referred to as family-centered rounds (FCRs).[5,29,31] Multiple professional organizations, such as the SCCM, the American College of Critical Care Medicine, the American Association of Critical-Care Nurses, and the National Academy of Medicine, support family presence during rounds.[5,19,20,36] Although the American Academy of Pediatrics deemed FCR a standard of care in 2003, it has gained traction slowly in adult critical care.[47] FCR is a real-time information exchange.[31] It promotes discussion of a patient's condition, treatment plan, and goals of care.[29,31] It has been shown to alleviate stress and anxiety and improve their satisfaction with the health care team.[6,9,31,32] It also allows the family to hear correct information at one time with input from members of a multidisciplinary team.[48] FCR prevents clinicians from giving contradictory reports to families, which ultimately leads to discontentment as families doubt the veracity of staff.[41] Conversely, dissatisfaction may lead to a breakdown in patient support systems and lead families to mistrust members of the care group.[32,41,42]

Providers often are reticent of implementing FCR due to the possibility of lengthening the duration of morning rounds and the potential for breeches patient confidentiality.[31,47,49] Faculty at teaching hospitals may worry about diminished opportunities for learners to participate in rounds.[6,49] Residents and students are concerned about appearing to have inadequate knowledge in front of families.[46,47,49] Fortunately, studies have shown that implementing FCR does not significantly increase rounding times and that teaching opportunities may be improved with family involvement.[21,31,47,49] Prior to leaving the room, a provider, such as the attending physician, acute care nurse practitioner, or physician assistant, recapping the salient points made in lay terms, may improve family members' understanding of the discussion.[46,48] As a result, FCR may improve the workflows of nurses and providers by decreasing the number of phone calls or in-person requests for information on a patient's status or plan of care.[31] Moreover, FCR may affect families' medical decision making positively by allowing them to share in the medical decision making (shared decision making [SDM]).[29,50]

Health care leadership also should institute proactive plans to mitigate accidental disclosure of patients' private information. This could occur if the team discusses the treatment of a disease, which the patient has not shared with the family,[51] such as human immunodeficiency virus (HIV). Maintaining patient confidentiality may be difficult if rounds occur in shared patient rooms or confined spaces with little privacy.[49] Davidson[46] recommends first asking families if they have any privacy concerns. If they do, suggest alternative arrangements, such as meeting in private, and then ask the family if the proposed changes are acceptable.[46] Providers along with medical center leadership should evaluate potential pitfalls fully and remedy them with policy changes.[49]

Communication is evolving with the development of newer technologies. An example of this is digital communication between patients and providers via electronic patient portals.[52–54] Medical centers using electronic health record (EHR) systems often have electronic patient portals that allow patients to view their medications, immunization records, and laboratory results.[52] Several companies offer more advanced portals that allow 2-way communication between patients and providers, request prescription refills, and contain educational videos specific to a patient's diagnoses, among other features that are particularly useful to outpatients.[52] The portals facilitate patient engagement by increasing dialogue between patients and providers and can improve self-management of chronic diseases. Although their use in primary care settings is expanding, particularly among whites, women, and those with higher education and income levels, their adoption in acute care has been less robust.[52–54]

There are a multitude of reasons supporting broadening the use of portals in the acute care settings.[53] The benefits of inpatient portal use include enhancing patient engagement, augmenting SDM, and improving patient satisfaction while decreasing anxiety (**Box 1**).[52,53,55] Some inpatient EHR portals show photos and names of caregivers and their roles and display upcoming diagnostic testing, such as a chest radiograph scheduled for 6:00 AM the following day.[56,57] Additionally, they have the capability to bolster patient education by employing audio and visual modules, which patients and families can access and re-review at any time. Reinforcing learning throughout a patient's hospitalization is found more effective than a single teaching session.[58–60] Portals also may aid patients and families deal with a potentially overwhelming amount of information at the time of discharge.[55]

DECISION SUPPORT TOOLS

Decision support tools (DSTs) increasingly are used by providers in the acute care setting to help clinicians by alleviating information overload when determining the

---

Box 1
Factors affecting electronic patient portal use in acute care

Benefits of inpatient portal use
• Increased communication
• Enhanced patent engagement
• Decreased patient anxiety
• Augmented SDM
• Improved patient satisfaction

Barriers to patient use
• Delirium, sedation, immobility, and neurologic disorders
• May have poorly designed interfaces
• Password loss
• Patient concerns about data privacy
• Patients not believing the portals are useful
• Patient anxiety about reading their own health information
• Providers' lack of encouragement surrounding portal use

Barriers to hospital adoption
• Cost
• Staff resistant to the idea

Reasons for hospitals to promote portal use by patients
• Improved patient-provider communication
• Allowing patients to easily access their health information
• Patients able to keep better track of their health information

Ways to improve inpatient portal use
• Provide patient-friendly training videos on portal use
• Include disease-specific educational videos and information
• Have providers encourage patients to use the portal
• Garner strong support from hospital leadership to promote portal use

(*Data from* Refs.[2,5,8,9,11,35,36,52])

appropriate course of action for a patient.[61–63] For example, artificial intelligence algorithms may identify disease processes, such as sepsis, before clinicians become aware of the diagnosis.[64] EHR-based DSTs can improve adherence to guidelines and best practices,[64] such as prompts to remind providers to order anticoagulation education when prescribing new oral anticoagulants. These tools also can decrease the costs of providing care while reducing human errors and improving patient outcomes.[61,65]

DSTs typically are embedded into EHR software, which employs artificial intelligence and algorithms to analyze patient-specific information.[63] Some organizations, such as the Canadian Cardiovascular Society, have DSTs as part of their smartphone applications.[61] Evidenced-based DSTs are available to assist acutely and critically ill patients and their families make choices regarding treatment options and goals of care.[61,63] Tools are available in a variety of formats, such as booklets and Web-based resources, such as videos.[20,63]

A family may have difficulty deciding which therapies to pursue and which to avoid if their loved one did not leave advance directives and/or health care power of attorney.[66,67] Researchers also are investigating how to best incorporate the use of hospital-provided tablet computers with Internet access at the bedside to increase patient engagement, decision making, and education.[54,68] A growing number of professional societies offer DSTs for patients and families on their Web sites. The American College of Cardiology CardioSmart site https://www.cardiosmart.org/SDM/Decision-Aids/Find-Decision-Aids has DSTs that range from booklets and infographics to videos to assist patients in deciding what treatment(s) would be best for them for common conditions and treatments.[69] Examples of these include videos regarding surgical or transcatheter aortic valve replacement versus medical management for people living with aortic stenosis[70] and booklets and videos regarding left ventricular assist device (LVAD) implantation for severe heart failure that is refractory to medical management.[69,71]

ENHANCED RECOVERY AFTER SURGERY PROGRAMS FOR CARDIAC PATIENTS

Enhanced Recovery after Surgery (ERAS) programs initially were applied to abdominal surgery patients.[72–74] An ERAS program involves the use of an interprofessional team implementing evidence-based practice guidelines to improve outcomes and decreases complications throughout the entire perioperative period.[75] The preadmission phase of ERAS engages the surgeon, the anesthesiologist, and the nurse to advance preoperative wellness through comprehensive preoperative education.[74,75]

ERAS cardiac surgery programs have been adapted to fit this unique patient population with the addition of a frailty assessment coupled with a pre-habilitation component that promotes preoperative exercise to improve improve functionality.[74] Nutritional supplementation is initiated preoperatively if indicated.[74] Alcohol and tobacco cessation, tight glycemic control, and pulmonary exercise through incentive spirometry reduce perioperative risk and accelerate a patient's return to normal function after surgery.[73,74,76,77]

In the postoperative phase, patients are quickly weaned from mechanical ventilation and mobilized to prevent delirium as well as pulmonary and vascular complications. Opioids are minimized through multimodal pain management.[73,74,76,77] This standardized prescription for recovery is shared with all members of the health care team, including the patient and family.[73,74,76,77]

THE EDUCATIONAL COMPONENT OF ENHANCED RECOVERY AFTER SURGERY

ERAS Cardiac Surgery embraces nurse-led education, which places patient and family at its center. Through the use of multimedia patient engagement tools, preoperative patients and their families are provided with the evidence-based data that support the ERAS initiative, which spans their entire hospitalization.[73,74,76,77] Patients participate in their own preoperative optimization by increasing their physical activity and caloric intake, improving their pulmonary function and altering unhealthy habits.[74,78] Families participate in these prehabilitation efforts, such as smoking cessation or a walking program, creating a sense of shared responsibility.[78]

Prior to surgery, explaining the progression of events during the perioperative period may comfort patients and families.[34] Understanding the importance of early mobilization and pulmonary rehabilitation leads to improved patient participation and reduced anxiety.[74,78] By providing patients with a pathway for surgical success, they share in the accountability and become partners with the health care team working toward the best surgical outcome.[76,77]

FAMILY-CENTERED CARE DURING PROLONGED CRITICAL ILLNESS AND MECHANICAL CIRCULATORY SUPPORT

Although a majority of patients move through the intensive care within 24 hours after cardiac surgery, approximately 5% to 10% experience ICU stays longer than 48 hours.[79] These longer ICU stays often are unexpected and responsible for increased family burden and are associated with higher levels of PTSD in both patients and families.[79,80] Providers should understand that there is a correlation between the severity of the patient's illness and the likelihood of a family member developing PTSD after a loved one's lengthy ICU stay.[80]

Extubation within 6 hours of cardiac surgery is expected for most patients. Extubation greater than 24 hours postoperatively is termed, *prolonged mechanical ventilation*. Patients who remain intubated experience frustration trying to communicate with their families and care providers. This impaired communication may leave patients fearful and anxious.[81] Risk factors predictive of prolonged intubation include a history of chronic obstructive pulmonary disease, smoking, low left ventricular ejection fraction, and blood and fresh frozen plasma infusion during surgery.[82] Both patients and families express the desire to have family members at the bedside during weaning.[81] Before surgery, providers should prepare at-risk patients and their families about the possibility of prolonged intubation. Expanded visiting hours that allow family member presence during weaning and extubation should decrease both patient and family anxiety.[5]

Postcardiotomy cardiogenic shock (PCCS) that is refractory to inotropic intervention is a life-threatening condition.[83] Mechanical circulatory support (MCS) is introduced to improve blood pressure, cardiac output, and tissue oxygenation.[83,84] MCS interventions include venoarterial extracorporeal membrane oxygenation (ECMO), ventricular assist devices (VADs), and intra-aortic balloon pump insertion.[84] Depending on the degree of hemodynamic instability and whether or not cardiac surgical intervention is considered urgent or emergent, MCS devices may be placed percutaneously in the cardiac catheterization laboratory or intraoperatively at the time of the index operation.[85] If a patient develops PCCS postoperatively in the CTICU, MCS may be initiated at the bedside, cardiac catheterization laboratory, or operating room (OR).[85]

Venoarterial ECMO oxygenates blood and provides the highest level of circulatory support (biventricular support).[84–86] ECMO carries the risks of bleeding, hemolysis, left ventricular distention, acute kidney injury, upper body hypoxia (peripheral cannulation), infection, and embolic events, such as stroke or limb ischemia.[84] Survival rates to hospital discharge range between 30.8% and 44% survival to hospital discharge.[83,87] A multicenter study showed survival rate of 60.5% of patients with an ECMO duration greater than 7 days.[88]

VADs most commonly are inserted on the left (LVAD) may be used to wean a patient off ECMO.[84,85] Some patients require placement of right-sided VAD alone or in combination with an LVAD for biventricular support.[86] Percutaneous or open left ventricular support in the form of LVAD to augment cardiac output is the most common configuration. The length of LVAD use varies based patient recovery. Patients with temporary LVADs may need long-term support, some of which may carry several of the same risks as ECMO, such as bleeding, infection, and hemolysis.[85,86] Those inserted peripherally (pVAD) also may cause limb ischemia due to the large cannula sizes.[85] Patients may recover fully and have their LVADs removed. Unfortunately, others may need pVADs exchanged for those approved for longer-term use. pVADs in this scenario are considered a bridge to a bridge.[86] Surgically implanted LVADs can be used as destination therapy or as a bridge to transplantation.[86] For patients who are not candidates for heart transplant or destination therapy LVADs, temporary LVADs are referred to as a bridge to recovery.[84,86] Palliative care consultation to discuss goals of care, withdrawal of mechanical support, and/or initiation of comfort care is paramount for those patients for whom myocardial recovery or candidacy for durable support are not likely.[84]

The families of patients treated with these invasive devices are abruptly faced with the reality of a loved one's mortality and must make difficult decisions, often rapidly.[83] For this reason, these families are at a heightened risk for ICU-related psychological sequelae. The level of acuity, the likelihood of mortality, and the increased length of time in the ICU all have a positive correlation to post-ICU PTSD.[79,80] Families should be evaluated for symptoms of PTSD. Interventions should be put in place to support coping strategies.[80]

The principles of FCC are imperative in this setting. Communication provides a basis for trust and assists families in staying current with the frequently changing patient status. By participating in rounds, families hear the presentation of and rationalization for the complete plan of care.[31] When communication includes sharing patient information, providing emotional support for families and minimizing uncertainty, it decreases family members' levels of stress.[89] Decision-making support tools allow providers to clearly explain the care plan and promote SDM with families. This eases the family decision-making burden while allowing participation.[63]

As patients are weaned from MCS and recover from PCCS, both patients and their family members experience the cumulative stress of the prolonged ICU stay, which can have an impact on their quality of life.[84] Fatigue and insecurity surrounding a patient's predicted level of function can result in depression.[80] During this phase, both caregiver and patient propensity toward anxiety and PTSD can have an impact on each other, because a positive correlation between patient and family symptoms has been shown. Qualitative data describe the importance of acute care nurse practitioners and clinical registered nurses (RNs) providing emotional support for both patients and families.[90] RNs were shown to be important in promoting SDM.[90] Because the strength of the patient-caregiver relationship can be protective to both parties, nurses and providers need to support dyad coping strategies.[80]

FAMILY PRESENCE DURING RESUSCITATION OF CARDIAC SURGERY PATIENTS

Despite data suggesting family presence during resuscitation (FPDR) is beneficial for family members, it may not be appropriate for those whose loved ones require resuscitation after cardiac surgery.[51] Common causes of cardiac arrest in postoperative patients are tamponade, bleeding, ventricular arrhythmias, and heart blocks associated with conduction problems.[91–95] The unique physiology of post–cardiac surgery patients requires a different approach to resuscitation compared with other groups.[93,95] Advanced cardiac life support (ACLS) recommends chest compressions (external cardiac massage) and administration of epinephrine for a majority of causes of cardiac arrest.[96] External cardiac massage is ineffective in cases that require surgical intervention, such as postpericardiotomy hemorrhage or pericardial tamponade.[92–95] Even though these methods are widely used, they can pose risks to cardiac surgery patients. Internal cardiac massage not only is more effective than external cardiac massage but also it mitigates the risk of myocardial/pericardial damage.[92–94] The proliferation of MCS and ECMO poses additional challenges during cardiac arrest resuscitation.[93]

Cardiac surgery advanced life support (CSU-ALS) addresses the unique challenges of managing of cardiac arrest in these postsurgical patients.[92–95] CSU-ALS recommends resternotomy after 3 unsuccessful defibrillation attempts to remedy etiologies, such as cardiac tamponade and hypovolemic shock.[92–95] Resternotomy also is indicated for pulseless electrical activity arrests when nonsurgical causes cannot be identified.[92,95] Research shows that some physicians often are reticent to allow FPDR due to the potential of putting extra pressure on staff, causing alterations in their level of performance.[19,51] They also worry about a heightened risk of litigation.[29,51]

At present, there is a paucity of literature regarding family presence during open chest resuscitation. This may be due to the relatively low volume of these events (approximately 0.7%–8.0% of cardiac patient develop cardiac arrest postsurgery) compared with closed chest resuscitation.[92] A recent study evaluated FPDR in trauma patients and showed a reduction in family anxiety in the FPDR group.[32] Unfortunately, cardiac trauma patients' families were excluded from the study.[32] There are several reasons surgeons may be reticent about FDRP during resternotomy. The Society of Thoracic Surgeons Task Force on Resuscitation After Cardiac Surgery recommends "aseptic technique" for resternotomy procedures.[92] Staff may be concerned that distraught family members may contaminate surgical instruments or the surgical field itself. Providers also may want to shield family members from the psychological trauma of such an invasive and likely bloody procedure, combined with health care professionals' discomfort with family presence during surgical procedures.[32,51] As discussed in multiple articles, staff may worry about their safety if a patient's family member becomes disruptive or violent.[32] Although this notion has not been validated during standard cardiopulmonary resuscitation, there are no data in resternotomy patients. A study evaluating parental presence during anesthesia induction for pediatric neurosurgery showed parents had mixed feelings about the experience, but most felt it was positive.[97] There is a case report demonstrating family presence during extubation in the OR prior to donation after cardiac death organ procurement.[98] There also is some literature regarding the initiation of FDRP in ORs,[99] but scant information on the outcomes of such programs. None of these reports included family visualizing an open chest. Research is needed to determine the risk/benefit to family members involved with FDRP during resternotomy.

PATIENT AND FAMILY-CENTERED CARE FOLLOW-UP

Readmissions increase costs and interfere with patients' quality of life. Most of the causes of post–cardiac surgery readmissions are clinical complications, such as congestive heart failure, arrhythmia, and infection.[100] Interventions that focus on patient discharge education, supporting the caregiver in the home environment, have been found to make some impact on these rates.[58]

The successful discharge of a postoperative patient depends on a patient's continued medical adherence and continued relationship with a health care provider.[101] These require a smooth transition from the surgery team to the primary care team and cardiologist. Implementing strategies, such as video-recorded teaching and telephone follow-up, can be used to bridge patients from one level of care to the next, to decrease readmissions and support patients and caregivers in their transition from hospital to home after cardiovascular surgery.[58] Other patients may benefit from referral to ICU aftercare programs, which include debriefing of the ICU experience with a qualified provider, such as an advanced-practice RN.[11] Post-ICU care delivery varies across health systems. Some may provide a 1-time follow-up whereas others focus on connecting patients with rehabilitation specialists while offering more regular and long-term monitoring.[11]

RECOMMENDATIONS FOR FUTURE STUDIES

There are significant opportunities for translational research regarding FCC in cardiothoracic surgery. Studies evaluating barriers to FCC and best practice strategies to overcoming barriers are vital in augmenting FCC adoption. In order for FCC to gain wider traction in CTICUs across the country, more data are needed regarding which FCC interventions improve patient and family outcomes. Quantifiably measuring the impact of family engagement on patient outcomes is an area of needed research. Assessing cost-effectiveness and impact on reducing resource utilization (eg, unnecessary diagnostic tests and/or specialist consultations) as well as data that gauge FCC's effects on length of stay (ICU and hospital) and readmission rates will be key to garnering widespread adoption of FCC in the cardiothoracic community.[21]

SUMMARY

Multiple studies have shown the positive benefits of implementing FCC in a variety of ICUs, ranging from neonatal and pediatric to adult general medical/surgical and specialty ICUs.[21,22] FCC principles, such as FDR, improve satisfaction and lower anxiety levels in family members. PICS-F may be prevented by implementing FCC in CTICUs.[5,6] FCC may be of particular importance to families of patients with prolonged CTICU stays and those receiving MCS, because they are at higher risk of developing PTSD.[79,80] FCR not only facilitates communication but also builds trust between families and health care teams.[31] FPDR is becoming more accepted in ICUs throughout the United States.[5] Family presence during resternotomy is a complex topic. Best practices for balancing the needs and wants of patient and family with imperatives of maintaining sterility during resternotomy and rapid restoration of spontaneous circulation are not yet delineated. More data are needed to determine best approaches to FCC during open chest resuscitation.

DISCLOSURE

The authors have nothing to disclose.

REFERENCES

1. Cairns PL, Buck HG, Kip KE, et al. Stress management intervention to prevent post-intensive care syndrome-family in patients' spouses. Am J Crit Care 2019;28(6):471–6.
2. Hageman SA, Tarzian AJ, Cagle J. Challenges of dealing with financial concerns during life-threatening illness: perspectives of health care practitioners. J Soc Work End Life Palliat Care 2018;14(1):28–43.
3. Dzau VJ, McClellan MB, McGinnis JM, et al. Vital directions for health and health care: priorities from a National Academy of Medicine Initiative. Jama 2017; 317(14):1461–70.
4. McPeake J, Mikkelsen ME, Quasim T, et al. Return to employment after critical illness and its association with psychosocial outcomes. A systematic review and meta-analysis. Ann Am Thorac Soc 2019;16(10):1304–11.
5. Davidson JE, Aslakson RA, Long AC, et al. Guidelines for family-centered care in the neonatal, pediatric, and adult ICU. Crit Care Med 2017;45(1):103–28.
6. Harvey MA, Davidson JE. Postintensive care syndrome: right care, right now...- and later. Crit Care Med 2016;44(2):381–5.
7. Davidson JE, Harvey MA. Patient and family post-intensive care syndrome. AACN Adv Crit Care 2016;27(2):184–6.
8. Davidson J, Stutzer K. The ethics of post–intensive care syndrome. AACN Adv Crit Care 2016;27(2):236–40.
9. Davidson JE, Harvey MA, Bemis-Dougherty A, et al. Implementation of the pain, agitation, and delirium clinical practice guidelines and promoting patient mobility to prevent post-intensive care syndrome. Crit Care Med 2013;41(9 Suppl 1):S136–45.
10. Liu V, Read JL, Scruth E, et al. Visitation policies and practices in US ICUs. Crit Care 2013;17(2):R71.
11. Eaton TL, McPeake J, Rogan J, et al. Caring for survivors of critical illness: current practices and the role of the nurse in intensive care unit aftercare. Am J Crit Care 2019;28(6):481–5.
12. Righy C, Rosa RG, da Silva RTA, et al. Prevalence of post-traumatic stress disorder symptoms in adult critical care survivors: a systematic review and meta-analysis. Crit Care 2019;23(1):213.
13. Bharadwaj P, Sandesara N, Sternberg SE, et al. Talking with children about a parent's serious illness. Am Fam Physician 2013;88(9):571–2.
14. Ferge JL, Le Terrier C, Banydeen R, et al. Prevalence of anxiety and depression symptomatology in adolescents faced with the hospitalization of a loved one in the ICU. Crit Care Med 2018;46(4):e330–3.
15. Davidson JE, Jones C, Bienvenu OJ. Family response to critical illness: postintensive care syndrome-family. Crit Care Med 2012;40(2):618–24.
16. Serrano P, Kheir YNP, Wang S, et al. Aging and postintensive care syndrome-family: a critical need for geriatric psychiatry. Am J Geriatr Psychiatry 2019; 27(4):446–54.
17. Davidson JE, Powers K, Hedayat KM, et al. Clinical practice guidelines for support of the family in the patient-centered intensive care unit: American College of Critical Care Medicine Task Force 2004-2005. Crit Care Med 2007;35(2):605–22.
18. Balik B, Conway J, Zipperer L, et al. Achieving an Exceptional Patient and Family Experience of Inpatient Hospital Care. IHI Innovation Series white paper. Cambridge, Massachusetts: Institute for Healthcare Improvement; 2011. Available at: www.IHI.org.

19. AACN. Practice alert: family presence during resuscitation and invasive procedures. Crit Care Nurse 2016;36(1):e11–4.

20. Hwang DY, El-Kareh R, Davidson JE. Implementing intensive care unit family-centered care: resources to identify and address gaps. AACN Adv Crit Care 2017;28(2):148–54.

21. Goldfarb MJ, Bibas L, Bartlett V, et al. Outcomes of patient- and family-centered care interventions in the ICU: a systematic review and meta-analysis. Crit Care Med 2017;45(10):1751–61.

22. Long AC, Kross EK, Curtis JR. Family-centered outcomes during and after critical illness: current outcomes and opportunities for future investigation. Curr Opin Crit Care 2016;22(6):613–20.

23. Fernandez FG, Shahian DM, Kormos R, et al. The society of thoracic surgeons national database 2019 annual report. Ann Thorac Surg 2019;108(6):1625–32.

24. Williams JB, Alexander KP, Morin JF, et al. Preoperative anxiety as a predictor of mortality and major morbidity in patients aged >70 years undergoing cardiac surgery. Am J Cardiol 2013;111(1):137–42.

25. Guo P. Preoperative education interventions to reduce anxiety and improve recovery among cardiac surgery patients: a review of randomised controlled trials. J Clin Nurs 2015;24(1–2):34–46.

26. Thompson-Brazill KA. Pain control in the cardiothoracic surgery patient. Crit Care Nurs Clin North Am 2019;31(3):389–405.

27. Holmes SD, Fornaresio LM, Miller CE, et al. Development of the cardiac surgery patient expectations questionnaire (C-SPEQ). Qual Life Res 2016;25(8): 2077–86.

28. Freeman RK, Arevalo G, Ascioti AJ, et al. An assessment of the frequency of palliative procedures in thoracic surgery. J Surg Educ 2017;74(5):878–82.

29. Coombs M, Puntillo KA, Franck LS, et al. Implementing the SCCM family-centered care guidelines in critical care nursing practice. AACN Adv Crit Care 2017;28(2):138–47.

30. Davidson JE. Family-centered care. AACN Adv Crit Care 2017;28(2):136–7.

31. Strathdee SA, Hellyar M, Montesa C, et al. The power of family engagement in rounds: an exemplar with global outcomes. Crit Care Nurse 2019;39(5):14–20.

32. Leske JS, McAndrew NS, Brasel KJ, et al. Family presence during resuscitation after trauma. J Trauma Nurs 2017;24(2):85–96.

33. Owens RL, Huynh TG, Netzer G. Sleep in the intensive care unit in a model of family-centered care. AACN Adv Crit Care 2017;28(2):171–8.

34. Skoog M, Milner KA, Gatti-Petito J, et al. The impact of family engagement on anxiety levels in a cardiothoracic intensive care unit. Crit Care Nurse 2016; 36(2):84–9.

35. Crawford TC, Conte JV, Sanchez JA. Team-based care: the changing face of cardiothoracic surgery. Surg Clin North Am 2017;97(4):801–10.

36. Balas MC, Pun BT, Pasero C, et al. Common challenges to effective ABCDEF bundle implementation: the ICU liberation campaign experience. Crit Care Nurse 2019;39(1):46–60.

37. Maniar H. Hospital readmissions after cardiac surgery: is it a game worth playing? maniarh@wudosis.wustl.edu. J Thorac Cardiovasc Surg 2015;149(3):858.

38. Kalogianni A, Almpani P, Vastardis L, et al. Can nurse-led preoperative education reduce anxiety and postoperative complications of patients undergoing cardiac surgery? Eur J Cardiovasc Nurs 2016;15(6):447–58.

39. Villanueva C, Talwar A, Doyle M. Improving informed consent in cardiac surgery by enhancing preoperative education. Patient Educ Couns 2018;101(12): 2047–53.

40. Agency for Healthcare Research and Quality. Making informed consent an informed choice: training for healthcare leaders - training-for-health-care-leaders.pdf. 2019. Available at: https://www.ahrq.gov/sites/default/files/wysiwyg/professionals/systems/hospital/training-for-health-care-leaders.pdf. Accessed October 3, 2019.

41. Lai VK, Lee A, Leung P, et al. Patient and family satisfaction levels in the intensive care unit after elective cardiac surgery: study protocol for a randomised controlled trial of a preoperative patient education intervention. BMJ Open 2016;6(6):e011341.

42. Ramesh C, Nayak BS, Pai VB, et al. Effect of Preoperative education on postoperative outcomes among patients undergoing cardiac surgery: a systematic review and meta-analysis. J Perianesth Nurs 2017;32(6):518–29.e2.

43. White-Trevino K, Dearmon V. Transitioning nurse handoff to the bedside: engaging staff and patients. Nurs Adm Q 2018;42(3):261–8.

44. Ford Y, Heyman A. Patients' perceptions of bedside handoff: further evidence to support a culture of always. J Nurs Care Qual 2017;32(1):15–24.

45. Chou R, Gordon DB, de Leon-Casasola OA, et al. Management of postoperative pain: a clinical practice guideline from the American pain Society, the American Society of Regional Anesthesia and Pain Medicine, and the American Society of Anesthesiologists' Committee on Regional Anesthesia, Executive Committee, and Administrative Council. J Pain 2016;17(2):131–57.

46. Davidson JE. Family presence on rounds in neonatal, pediatric, and adult intensive care units. Ann Am Thorac Soc 2013;10(2):152–6.

47. Stanski N, Patel A. Improving trainee education during family-centered rounds: a resident's perspective. Pediatrics 2016;137(1):e20153679. Available at: pediatrics.aappublications.org.content/pediatrics/137/1/e20153679.full.pdf.

48. Freiman DB, Freiman AO, Meyer N, et al. A most irritating awakening. Ann Am Thorac Soc 2013;10(2):175–7.

49. Mittal V. Family-centered rounds. Pediatr Clin North Am 2014;61(4):663–70.

50. Kon AA, Davidson JE, Morrison W, et al. Shared decision making in ICUs: an American College of Critical Care Medicine and American Thoracic Society Policy Statement. Crit Care Med 2016;44(1):188–201.

51. Brasel KJ, Entwistle JW 3rd, Sade RM. Should family presence be allowed during cardiopulmonary resuscitation? Ann Thorac Surg 2016;102(5):1438–43.

52. Griffin A, Skinner A, Thornhill J, et al. Patient portals: who uses them? What features do they use? And do they reduce hospital readmissions? Appl Clin Inform 2016;7(2):489–501.

53. Dendere R, Slade C, Burton-Jones A, et al. Patient portals facilitating engagement with inpatient electronic medical records: a systematic review. J Med Internet Res 2019;21(4):e12779.

54. Baldwin JL, Singh H, Sittig DF, et al. Patient portals and health apps: pitfalls, promises, and what one might learn from the other. Healthc (Amst) 2017; 5(3):81–5.

55. Dalal AK, Bates DW, Collins S. Opportunities and challenges for improving the patient experience in the acute and postacute care setting using patient portals: the patient's perspective. J Hosp Med 2017;12(12):1012–6.

56. Goyal AA, Tur K, Mann J, et al. Do bedside visual tools improve patient and caregiver satisfaction? A systematic review of the literature. J Hosp Med 2017;12(11):930–6.

57. Hefner JL, Sieck CJ, Walker DM, et al. System-wide inpatient portal implementation: survey of health care team perceptions. JMIR Med Inform 2017;5(3):e31.

58. Annapoorna M. Prevention of 30-day readmission after coronary artery bypass surgery. Home Healthc Now 2017;35(6):326–34.

59. Coskun H, Senture C, Ustunsoz A. The effectiveness of discharge training for patients after cardiac surgery. Rehabil Nurs 2018;43(2):95–102.

60. O'Brien L, McKeough C, Abbasi R. Pre-surgery education for elective cardiac surgery patients: a survey from the patient's perspective. Aust Occup Ther J 2013;60(6):404–9.

61. Graham MM, James MT, Spertus JA. Decision support tools: realizing the potential to improve quality of care. Can J Cardiol 2018;34(7):821–6.

62. The Office of the National Coordinator for Health Information Technology. Clinical decision support/HealthIT.gov. 2019. Available at: https://www.healthit.gov/topic/safety/clinical-decision-support. Accessed October 3, 2019.

63. Austin CA, Mohottige D, Sudore RL, et al. Tools to promote shared decision making in serious illness: a systematic review. JAMA Intern Med 2015;175(7): 1213–21.

64. Miller DD, Brown EW. Artificial intelligence in medical practice: the question to the answer? Am J Med 2018;131(2):129–33.

65. Collins S, Dykes P, Bates DW, et al. An informatics research agenda to support patient and family empowerment and engagement in care and recovery during and after hospitalization. J Am Med Inform Assoc 2018;25(2):206–9.

66. Seaman JB, Arnold RM, Buddadhumaruk P, et al. Protocol and fidelity monitoring plan for four supports. A multicenter trial of an intervention to support surrogate decision makers in intensive care units. Ann Am Thorac Soc 2018;15(9): 1083–91.

67. Bute JJ, Petronio S, Torke AM. Surrogate decision makers and proxy ownership: challenges of privacy management in health care decision making. Health Commun 2015;30(8):799–809.

68. McAlearney AS, Sieck CJ, Hefner JL, et al. High Touch and High Tech (HT2) proposal: transforming patient engagement throughout the continuum of care by engaging patients with portal technology at the bedside. JMIR Res Protoc 2016;5(4):e221.

69. Cardiology ACo. Decision aids. 2019. Available at: https://www.cardiosmart.org/SDM/Decision-Aids/Find-Decision-Aids. Accessed October 3, 2019.

70. Cardiology ACo. Aortic stenosis: TAVR/SAVR. 2019. Available at: https://www.cardiosmart.org/SDM/Decision-Aids/Find-Decision-Aids/Aortic-Stenosis. Accessed October 3, 2019.

71. Patient Decision Aids. LVAD_Mahoney_December 2018 (Video).Vimeo. https://vimeo.com/304215151.

72. McConnell G, Woltz P, Bradford WT, et al. Enhanced recovery after cardiac surgery program to improve patient outcomes. Nursing 2018;48(11):24–31.

73. Williams JB, McConnell G, Allender JE, et al. One-year results from the first US-based enhanced recovery after cardiac surgery (ERAS Cardiac) program. J Thorac Cardiovasc Surg 2019;157(5):1881–8.

74. Engelman DT, Ben Ali W, Williams JB, et al. Guidelines for perioperative care in cardiac surgery: enhanced recovery after surgery society recommendations. JAMA Surg 2019;154(8):755–66.

75. Ljungqvist O, Hubner M. Enhanced recovery after surgery-ERAS-principles, practice and feasibility in the elderly. Aging Clin Exp Res 2018;30(3):249–52.
76. Coleman SR, Chen M, Patel S, et al. Enhanced recovery pathways for cardiac surgery. Curr Pain Headache Rep 2019;23(4):28.
77. Noss C, Prusinkiewicz C, Nelson G, et al. Enhanced recovery for cardiac surgery. J Cardiothorac Vasc Anesth 2018;32(6):2760–70.
78. Arora RC, Brown CHt, Sanjanwala RM, et al. "NEW" prehabilitation: a 3-way approach to improve postoperative survival and health-related quality of life in cardiac surgery patients. Can J Cardiol 2018;34(7):839–49.
79. Trivedi V, Bleeker H, Kantor N, et al. Survival, quality of life, and functional status following prolonged ICU stay in cardiac surgical patients: a systematic review. Crit Care Med 2019;47(1):e52–63.
80. Wintermann GB, Weidner K, Strauss B, et al. Predictors of posttraumatic stress and quality of life in family members of chronically critically ill patients after intensive care. Ann Intensive Care 2016;6(1):69.
81. Tingsvik C, Hammarskjold F, Martensson J, et al. Patients' lived experience of intensive care when being on mechanical ventilation during the weaning process: a hermeneutic phenomenological study. Intensive Crit Care Nurs 2018; 47:46–53.
82. Bartz RR, Ferreira RG, Schroder JN, et al. Prolonged pulmonary support after cardiac surgery: incidence, risk factors and outcomes: a retrospective cohort study. J Crit Care 2015;30(5):940–4.
83. Khorsandi M, Dougherty S, Bouamra O, et al. Extra-corporeal membrane oxygenation for refractory cardiogenic shock after adult cardiac surgery: a systematic review and meta-analysis. J Cardiothorac Surg 2017;12(1):55.
84. McGugan PL. The role of venoarterial extracorporeal membrane oxygenation in postcardiotomy cardiogenic shock. Crit Care Nurs Clin North America 2019; 31(3):419–36.
85. Miller PE, Solomon MA, McAreavey D. Advanced percutaneous mechanical circulatory support devices for cardiogenic shock. Crit Care Med 2017;45(11): 1922–9.
86. Rihal CS, Naidu SS, Givertz MM, et al. 2015 SCAI/ACC/HFSA/STS clinical expert consensus statement on the use of percutaneous mechanical circulatory support devices in cardiovascular care: endorsed by the American Heart Assocation, the Cardiological Society of India, and Sociedad Latino Americana de Cardiologia Intervencion; affirmation of value by the Canadian Association of Interventional Cardiology-Association Canadienne de Cardiologie d'intervention. J Am Coll Cardiol 2015;65(19):e7–26.
87. Fux T, Holm M, Corbascio M, et al. Venoarterial extracorporeal membrane oxygenation for postcardiotomy shock: risk factors for mortality. J Thorac Cardiovasc Surg 2018;156(5):1894–902.e3.
88. Biancari F, Dalen M, Fiore A, et al. Multicenter study on postcardiotomy venoarterial extracorporeal membrane oxygenation. J Thorac Cardiovasc Surg 2019. [Epub ahead of print]. https://doi.org/10.1016/j.jtcvs.2019.06.039.
89. Ganz FD, Yihye G, Beckman N. Family-centered communication and acute stress in israeli intensive care units. Am J Crit Care 2019;28(4):274–80.
90. Dillworth J, Dickson VV, Reyentovich A, et al. Patient decision-making regarding left ventricular assist devices : a multiple case study. Intensive Crit Care Nurs 2019;51:7–14.
91. Herrmann C. Cardiac advanced life support-surgical guideline: overview and implementation. AACN Adv Crit Care 2014;25(2):123–9.

92. Dunning J, Levine A, Ley J, et al. The Society of Thoracic Surgeons Expert Consensus for the resuscitation of patients who arrest after cardiac surgery. Ann Thorac Surg 2017;103(3):1005–20.

93. Ley SJ. Cardiac surgical resuscitation: state of the science. Crit Care Nurs Clin North Am 2019;31(3):437–52.

94. Ley SJ. Standards for resuscitation after cardiac surgery. Crit Care Nurse 2015; 35(2):30–7 [quiz: 38].

95. Michaelis P, Leone RJ. Cardiac arrest after cardiac surgery: an evidence-based resuscitation protocol. Crit Care Nurse 2019;39(1):15–25.

96. Link M, Berkow LC, Kudenchuk PJ, et al. Part 7: American Heart Association update for cardiopulmonary resuscitation an emergency cardiovascular care. Circulation 2015;132(18):S444–64.

97. Waseem H, Mazzamurro RS, Fisher AH, et al. Parental satisfaction with being present in the operating room during the induction of anesthesia prior to pediatric neurosurgical intervention: a qualitative analysis. J Neurosurg Pediatr 2018;21(5):528–34.

98. Reed CC, Gerhardt SD, Shaver K, et al. Case study: family presence in the OR for donation after cardiac death. AORN J 2012;96(1):34–44.

99. Balogh-Mitchell C. Is it time for family presence during resuscitation in the OR? AORN J 2012;96(1):14–25.

100. Redzek A, Mironicki M, Gvozdenovic A, et al. Predictors for hospital readmission after cardiac surgery. J Card Surg 2015;30(1):1–6.

101. Meslot C, Gauchet A, Hagger MS, et al. A randomised controlled trial to test the effectiveness of planning strategies to improve medication adherence in patients with cardiovascular disease. Appl Psychol Health Well Being 2017;9(1): 106–29.

Intensive Care Unit Patient Diaries
A Review Evaluating Implementation and Feasibility

Erica McCartney, BSN, RN, CCRN-CMC

KEYWORDS

- Intensive care unit • ICU • Diary • Post–intensive care syndrome • Family
- Patient support

KEY POINTS

- Patient selection is critical when implementing intensive care unit (ICU) diaries. Guidelines should be provided to staff, but there is room for individualization and nursing judgment for appropriateness.
- Diary content needs to be written in simple, nonmedical terms. No diagnoses or results should be included because the diary is not part of the official medical record.
- Family involvement benefits both the patient and family members. Diary use can help to increase their bond and show how important and meaningful their relationship is.
- Staff perceive diaries as being beneficial; however, education, practice, and time must be given to make diaries an effective and sustainable program.

INTRODUCTION

More than 5 million Americans are admitted to the intensive care unit (ICU) with a critical illness yearly.[1] Medical treatments have improved and advanced over the years, and mortality rates in the ICU are only 10% to 29%, depending on the severity of the disease. This means a majority of patients who have been admitted to the ICU survive, yet their journey to recovery does not end once discharged. Post–intensive care syndrome (PICS) is a cluster of symptoms that affects a person after surviving this critical illness.[1] PICS comprises mental and cognitive changes, including inability to concentrate and clouding of sensorium, along with anxiety, depression, posttraumatic stress disorder (PTSD), and muscle weakness and fatigue. The effects of PICS can be experienced for months to years and, in some people, have a lasting impact.

Critical Care Services, Swedish Edmonds Medical Center, Edmonds, WA, USA
E-mail address: erica.mccartney@swedish.org

Crit Care Nurs Clin N Am 32 (2020) 313–326
https://doi.org/10.1016/j.cnc.2020.02.011   ccnursing.theclinics.com

BACKGROUND

With approximately 70% of individuals surviving critical illness and being discharged, PICS could influence as many as 3.5 million Americans.[1] Although PICS is not necessarily experienced by all survivors of critical illness, cognitive changes associated with PICS has been reported in as many as 80% of survivors.[2] Depression, anxiety, and PTSD are common sequelae of critical illness survival and have been reported in as many as 60% of survivors. Physical impairments can have a large impact on survivors' quality of life after discharge; however, they are addressed more frequently using physical therapy and rehabilitation.

PICS is now considered more of a public health crisis, because as many as 50% of individuals who have survived a critical illness are not be able to return to their baseline functioning.[1] This means that previously functional and working adults no longer may be able to return to their jobs or care for themselves independently. The downstream consequence to society will place a higher burden on disability and other government and state resources. Mortality rates and risk of readmission are higher among survivors of a critical illness.[2] Mortality rates for survivors can be as high as 60% in the first year after discharge, and the risk of readmission has been reported as high as 40% over the first 2 years after the initial discharge.

Although PICS predominantly has impacts on the survivor, family members and caregivers also can experience PICS-family (PICS-F).[3] Family members also can experience psychological trauma from their loved one being hospitalized in the ICU. This stress, depression, and emotional distress have been reported in as many as 30% of family members who were hospitalized in the ICU. Poor sleep and poor sleep quality also are commonly reported symptoms of family members and caregivers.[4]

ICU patient diaries are a concept that has been used for more than 30 years in Scandinavian countries but now are beginning to be seen in the clinical setting in the United States. The ICU diary is used during a patient's stay in the critical care setting, and staff and family or friends write in lay terms about major events that have occurred during the stay.[5–7] Diaries help connect the memories the survivors and also family members may have during their hospitalization and help them recreate their timeline in the ICU. In creating memories, it is proposed that ICU patient diaries will help individuals by decreasing PICS or PICS-F by helping understand what happened in the ICU and that clinicians truly cared and connected during the process.[8,9]

SEARCH STRATEGY

A systematic search of the PubMed database was conducted from July 2019 to October 2019. Keywords [ICU AND Diary] were searched and a total of 113 articles resulted. Limiters of the English language, date range 2010 to 2019, and the adult population resulted in 41 articles. Further screening was performed to include literature addressing aspects of diary program implementation in the intensive care setting. Articles solely discussing patient outcomes were excluded because this article was focused on implementation and feasibility. Literature reviews also were excluded. A total of 15 articles ultimately was included for review (**Fig. 1**).

THEMES

In reviewing the literature, several themes began to emerge. Selection of patients appropriate for a diary and the content of the diary are pivotal aspects of a diary program.[7,9] Family involvement and teaching, along with staff education and buy-in, are instrumental in ensuring a sustainable program (**Table 1**).[8,10,11]

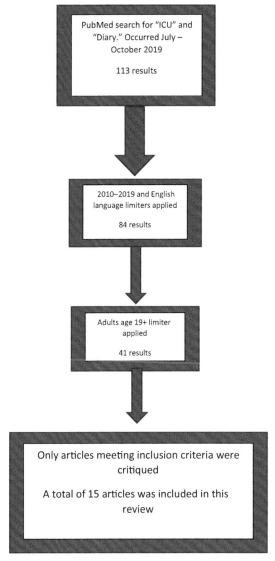

Fig. 1. Search strategy.

Selection of Patients

Appropriate patient selection is an essential component of ICU diary programs. An individualized approach is needed because some families may refuse to participate.[5,9] Patients who are receiving sedation, are mechanically ventilated, have a prolonged ICU stay, or are otherwise delirious after clinical assessment likely would benefit from the use of ICU diaries (**Box 1**). Individuals who are likely to have memory gaps about their hospitalization either due to medications or disease processes should be provided diaries.[6,9] Although this review focused only on an adult population, there is evidence supporting diary use in pediatric individuals as well.[12]

Table 1
Article summaries

Reference Number	Design Methodology	Number of Participants	Setting	Findings
Scruth et al,[16] 2017	Pilot project with qualitative methodology	No participants, discussed prototype development	ICUs in a 21-hospital health system in Northern California	It was feasible to develop and use an electronic ICU diary for patients during hospitalization. Families and staff expressed that it was easy to use and allowed for better communication.
Locke et al,[8] 2016	A mixed-methods evidence-based practice project	12 informal staff interviews were conducted	20-bed mixed medical-surgical ICU	17 diaries were initiated over a 3-month period of time, with 3–4 entries per day. Staff concluded that although it was an additional task, it was important for the patient and family members. Patient and families found it to be a useful resource both in the ICU and for the recovery once discharged

Aitken et al,[9] 2017	A mixed-methods exploratory study	57 patients and 22 family members participated	A tertiary metropolitan hospital in Brisbane, Australia	Several participant themes were encountered. The diary served as a useful tool, a way to fill in knowledge gaps, a way to differentiate reality from delusions, and a way for family to communicate with their loved one. Some individuals did not find it useful because they preferred not to dwell or think about the past. No statistically significant relationship was noted between psychological distress and diary preference.
Nielsen et al,[11] 2019	Hermeneutic-phenomenological study	10 patients and 13 family members	2 mixed medical-surgical ICUs in Denmark	The diaries were authored by family members during their loved one's hospitalization. Sharing this story with the patient led to a stronger relationship between the individuals.

(continued on next page)

Table 1
(continued)

Reference Number	Design Methodology	Number of Participants	Setting	Findings
Perier et al,[10] 2013	Phenomenological design	23 nurses, 4 nursing assistants, and 9 physicians were interviewed	10-bed ICU in a 460-bed tertiary hospital	Staff considered the diary to be beneficial for family members, like an outlet for their emotions during this difficult time. It was a way to communicate and give information to families, humanize the staff role, and help reconstruct the patient's journey. The theme of intrusion also was discovered, and staff considered it a violation of privacy to read family entries.
Nair et al,[19] 2015	A mixed-methods exploratory study	194 participants	Online Australian College of Critical Care Nurses survey	19% of participants already were using diaries on their units; 70% cited hesitancy with implementing a diary program. This hesitancy is attributed to a lack of policies and legal ambiguity of the use of diaries.

Pattison et al,[6] 2019	A mixed-methods 2-phase study	50 patients	ICU in the United Kingdom	95% of participants found the diaries to be helpful tools, and 90% reported that it assisted in filling in gaps about their hospitalization. The theme of the diary being a dynamic communication tool emerged from participants.
Gjengedal et al,[14] 2010	Qualitative descriptive design	30 participants	Phone interviews were conducted with experienced ICU nurses in Norway	Diaries were shown to serve 2 main purposes, 1 of caring, and another of therapy; 31 out of 70 ICUs had a diary program, and, although most had protocols or guidelines, the frequency of diary writing varied.
Johansson et al,[18] 2018	Hermeneutic study design	9 participants	Participants were from 3 different ICUs across Sweden	The main theme found was that the diary served as a bridge to connect to the past. The diaries helped to maintain a connection to the family member, even after they had passed, and they helped to bring about an emotional understanding of the situation.

(continued on next page)

Table 1
(continued)

Reference Number	Design Methodology	Number of Participants	Setting	Findings
Garrouste-Orgeas et al,[13] 2014	Qualitative study	32 family members	10-bed medical-surgical ICU in Paris, France	Several themes emerged. It was a communicative tool, was a way to document presence and allowed family members to maintain hope, humanized the experience, and also changed the perceptions of the family members toward staff. Family saw staff as more than just health care workers after they had written in the diaries; they were humanized.
Levine et al,[5] 2018	A descriptive qualitative study	26 participants recruited, 13 completed all phases	10-bed cardiac care unit in a large urban academic medical center	69% of participants found that the diaries helped to fill in the gaps during their hospitalization; 30.8% of participants were not ready to emotionally read the diary initially; and 23.1% found that the entries by the nursing staff showed caring and concern. There also was a desire to have more entries from nursing and other health care staff.

Nielsen & Angel,[17] 2016	Phenomenological-hermeneutic study	7 family members who had written in an ICU diary	ICU at a regional hospital in Denmark	Writing in the ICU diaries enabled the family member to influence the story of the hospitalization and critical illness. This was a large burden for some, and difficult family relationships had a negative impact on the diary and creation of the narrative.
Åkerman et al,[15] 2013	A mixed-methods descriptive, exploratory cohort design	115 patients responded to survey; 15 participants were interviewed	4 Swedish general ICUs	Photos, in addition to written entries, helped patients get the full picture of what occurred during their critical illness. It created and clarified visual memories.
Strandberg et al,[7] 2018	A qualitative empirical study	9 participants	ICU in Sweden	The diary was identified as a way to gain understanding. It allowed participants to gain understanding of their hospitalization, and it was important that they were able to return to their diary during their recovery after discharge.
Costa et al,[20] 2019	A mixed-methods quality-improvement project	55 individuals received diaries	9-bed ICU	Staff education and a plan-do-study-act format resulted in a diary provision increase, from 26.1% to 100%, during their 2-phase approach

---

Box 1
Suggested patient selection criteria

Consider ICU patient diary for the following:
- Mechanical ventilation greater than 24 hours
- ICU length of stay greater than 72 hours
- CAM +

Abbreviation: CAM, Confusion Assessment Method.

The use of the diary by survivors post-discharge helped fill in gaps and helped to connect and clarify the survivor's own memories.[5,6,9,13] This was a common theme identified throughout the literature and one to consider when selecting individuals appropriate for a diary. For this reason, preexisting neurologic deficits that prohibit a patient from complex thought and understanding prior to hospitalization likely would negate the usefulness of the diaries for that individual survivor. Diaries may not benefit individuals with advanced dementia, individuals with anoxic brain injury, some stroke patients, or individuals who are comatose. Family members may have benefits, however, not only of expressing their feelings and emotions about a critical illness but also in their ability to be able to go back and help process all the events that occurred after discharge.[13] Patients also should be able to read the native country location language, because this eases the burden on the staff. It is possible to have the entries translated; however, this extra burden may discourage nurses from completing diary entries.

Diary Content

Content of the diary is an extremely important concern. Several health care workers had concerns about legalities of writing in patient diaries because there are few guidelines or policies to help direct them.[5,7,10,14] It is important to remember that the diary is not part of the medical record, so confidentiality is key. Simple, nonmedical terms should be used when writing, and no medical diagnoses or test results are included (**Box 2**).

Box 2
Diary guide for staff

- Write in lay terms.
- Do not include diagnoses.
- Do not include test results.
- Write about the tone of the shift.
  - Were there any setbacks? Or progress?
- Consider confidentiality when writing.
  - Family members and friends will have access to this.
- Include people who have visited.
  - Encourage family participation.
- Include significant events that may be happening outside of the hospital.
  - Holidays
  - Sporting events
- Include date, time, and name with each entry.

The diary begins with a brief summary of what brought the patient into the ICU, and each subsequent day includes an excerpt about the events that have occurred.[5,7] Each entry in the diary includes a date and time and the name of the person completing the entry. The entry does not have to be long in length. Staff can write about any significant events that occurred during the shift, such as sitting in a chair and getting a tube or line removed. Messages of encouragement, healing, and presence also can be included. Staff can encourage the families to write about how they are feeling, about any significant events that may be occurring outside of the hospital, and about their visit.

Consider using other media in the diary also. Photographs were a helpful and visual way to clarify an individual's illness and events that occurred while hospitalized,[15] while paying attention to confidentiality and preserving a patient's dignity. Consent from the legal next of kin or health care proxy should be obtained prior to taking photographs of people. In addition to photos, drawings from loved ones not only can be an outlet for the family member but also help can visually create or make sense of memories the individual may experience on discharge.

The use of electronic diaries is another feasible option.[16] Electronic diaries are a more costly alternative to just paper and pen; however, they may connect more with technologically inclined individuals. Electronic diaries could be problematic for people who do not have a device to support its use because they likely require either a smartphone or tablet.

Family Involvement

Staff members should involve family throughout this process. It is important for families to help construct the story of the hospitalization. Storytelling through the diary can be an emotional outlet for families during their stay in the ICU.[9,11,13,17] Even if their loved one does not survive the hospitalization, it is a way to feel connected to them still and emotionally process what has happened.[18] Empower family and friends to write about their visit and what is happening outside of the hospital and also to include their feelings and concerns about what is occurring.[9,11,13,17] The diary is a place for the family to feel safe to truly express how they feel, including their fears, how much the person means to them, or how hopeful they are (**Box 3**).

Family members found that the use of the diaries helped give them a sense of support and a way to connect with their family member who was ill.[7,18] Using the diaries gave the family members a way to communicate with the patient and also helped them cope with the illness and situation. The diary was an outlet for the families, providing them an outlet to express their love, feelings, and emotions. Having the family members use the diaries also allowed survivors to see how the families were there for them during the hospitalization and allowed survivors insight into how the event had an impact on family as well.[9,11,13,17]

Families voiced how the diary was an essential tool and helped increase communication and build relationships with the health care team.[10,13] It helped humanize the health care members, and families saw them as more caring and relatable individuals. Increased trust and communication between the team and families have been shown to increase positive patient outcomes.

Staff Perceptions

Overall, many staff do see the value in using ICU diaries for their patients.[8,13] They are a way to communicate with family, tell a patient's story, and help humanize their role. Concerns about confidentiality, time, and what to include do persist.[10,19] Continuing

---

Box 3
Sample writing instructions

What it is?
  The ICU diary is used to give your family member an idea of all the events that occurred while they were in the ICU. It is a record of their day and activities. It includes excerpts from the ICU staff, mainly the nurses taking care of your family member, and we encourage you and any visitors to write in the diary as well. Research is supporting the use of these diaries to help reduce symptoms of anxiety, depression, and PTSD, which may occur after a prolonged stay in the ICU.

What to write?
• Write about your visit.
• Write about how your family member is doing in the hospital.
• Write about any significant events that are occurring outside of the hospital; this could be something in the news or a family event like a birthday.
• Write about your feelings about your family members illness.

You are just writing about you and your family members experiences in the ICU, so there is no wrong answer for what to write. Just try to include your name, the date, and time when completing the entry.

---

education and tip sheets seem to help bridge this gap between perceptions and practice.[8,20]

Concerns about having the time to write in the diaries is a major prohibitor for staff buy-in.[8,13,20] Nurses in particular are being loaded with an in increased number of tasks and responsibilities and often are having to do so with fewer resources available to them. Adding one more, nonessential task to their load at times can lead to a lack of completing it. Understanding why this actually is such an important part of holistic care and reinforcing the fact that brevity with entries is acceptable can increase compliance with this task. If this type of project is not well supported by staff, it is difficult to get enough data regarding the efficacy of it for patients. Staff buy-in and contribution are essential for this type of an intervention to be effective, and it is one of the challenges that could prevent the diaries from being used and ultimately being used correctly or as intended.[8,13,19]

Knowledge of what to include in the diary presented often in the literature.[13,19] There was a gap with staff, despite educational interventions. Like many skills in nursing, this one takes times to feel comfortable and competent with. Having practice sessions to write entries was a useful way to increase this skill as well as having clear and specific guidelines to follow (**Box 4**).[8,20]

The use of ICU patient diaries is supported mainly by qualitative evidence; patients often report that the diaries have helped with their recovery after the ICU.[5,6] Patients viewed their diary as a tool to understand what happened while they were in the ICU, because some did not have any real recollection of their hospitalization. It also was beneficial to family members while the patient was hospitalized. It gave family and friends an outlet to write to the patient, describe their fears and concerns, and fully express their feelings toward that individual.[11,13]

The critical care experience may result in PICS or PICS-F decreasing quality of life after discharge or death.[1,2] In using a diary during the ICU, adverse outcomes hopefully can be minimized, with a focus on a more holistic way to care for patients.[6,8] The use of the diaries also can help promote and strengthen the communication and relationship between the health care team and the patient and provide a more personalized approach to care.[10,13]

Box 4
Intensive care unit diary sample entries

10/01/2019 7:00 PM

You just came in to the hospital this morning. You were having trouble breathing at home, so your wife called 911. You had a tube put in to help you breathe, and you were given medication for pain and to make you sleepy. There was also a tube placed in your bladder to drain your urine, and the doctor placed a large catheter in your neck so we can give you medication. Soft ties were placed on both your wrists so that you didn't accidently pull anything. Your wife has been with you this whole time.

Mark (RN)

10/01/2019 9:00 PM

I am just going home for the night; I have been with you ever since you got to the hospital. I need to make sure the dog has food, I'm sure he is missing you a lot! I will be back first thing in the morning.

Love,

Cary (wife)

10/02/2019 7:00 AM

You had a pretty quiet night. I turned you every 2 hours to make sure you were comfortable and cleaned out your mouth with swabs. Your wife called asking about you.

Sam (RN)

10/02/2019 7:00 PM

You had quite the day! We turned down the medication that was keeping you sleepy and started trying to get the breathing tube out. You weren't quite ready, but we will try again tomorrow. Your wife and parents have been at the hospital most of the day.

Julia (RN)

10/02/2019 8:00 PM

We can't wait for you to wake up. We have the football game on for you, and we are about to go home for the night.

Tim (friend)

10/03/2019 7:00 AM

You had a busy night. We went down for a test and took pictures of your lungs. You still have the soft ties on your wrists. We will try to see how you do turning down the breathing tube settings again today. Your mom called overnight.

Carol (RN)

Abbreviation: RN, Registered Nurse.

DISCLOSURE

The author has nothing to disclose.

REFERENCES

1. Society of Critical Care Medicine. Post intensive care syndrome. 2013. Available at: https://www.sccm.org/MyICUCare/Thrive/Post-intensive-Care-Syndrome. Accessed July 29, 2019.
2. Howard AF, Currie L, Bungay V, et al. Health solutions to improve post-intensive care outcomes: a realist review protocol. Syst Rev 2019;8(1):11.

3. Rawal G, Yadav S, Kumar R. Post-intensive care syndrome: an overview. J Transl Int Med 2017;5(2):90–2.
4. Choi J, Tate JA, Donahoe MP, et al. Sleep in family caregivers of ICU survivors for two months post-ICU discharge. Intensive Crit Care Nurs 2016;37:11–8.
5. Levine SA, Reilly KM, Nedder MM, et al. The patient's perspective of the intensive care unit diary in the cardiac intensive care unit. Crit Care Nurse 2018;38(4): 28–36.
6. Pattison N, O'Gara G, Lucas C, et al. Filling the gaps: a mixed-methods study exploring the use of patient diaries in the critical care unit. Intensive Crit Care Nurs 2019;51:27–34.
7. Strandberg S, Vesterlund L, Engström Å. The contents of a patient diary and its significance for persons cared for in an ICU: a qualitative study. Intensive Crit Care Nurs 2018;45:31–6.
8. Locke M, Eccleston S, Ryan CN, et al. Developing a diary program to minimize patient and family post-intensive care syndrome. AACN Adv Crit Care 2016;(2):212.
9. Aitken LM, Rattray J, Kenardy J, et al. Perspectives of patients and family members regarding psychological support using intensive care diaries: an exploratory mixed methods study. J Crit Care 2017;38:263–8.
10. Perier A, Revah-Levy A, Bruel C, et al. Phenomenologic analysis of healthcare worker perceptions of intensive care unit diaries. Crit Care 2013;17(1):R13.
11. Nielsen AH, Egerod I, Hansen TB, et al. Intensive care unit diaries: developing a shared story strengthens relationships between critically ill patients and their relatives—a hermeneutic-phenomenological study. Int J Nurs Stud 2019. https://doi.org/10.1016/j.ijnurstu.2019.01.009.
12. Aitken LM, Rattray J, Hull A, et al. The use of diaries in psychological recovery from intensive care. Crit Care 2013;17:253.
13. Garrouste-Orgeas M, Périer A, Mouricou P, et al. Writing in and reading ICU diaries: qualitative study of families' experience in the ICU. PLoS One 2014; 9(10):e110146.
14. Gjengedal E, Storli SL, Holme AN, et al. An act of caring - patient diaries in Norwegian intensive care units. Nurs Crit Care 2010;15(4):176–84.
15. Åkerman E, Ersson A, Fridlund B, et al. Preferred content and usefulness of a photodiary as described by ICU-patients—a mixed method analysis. Aust Crit Care 2013;26(1):29–35.
16. Scruth EA, Oveisi N, Liu V. Innovation and technology: electronic intensive care unit diaries. AACN Adv Crit Care 2017;28(2):191–9.
17. Nielsen AH, Angel S. Consolation or confrontation when interacting through an ICU diary – a phenomenological–hermeneutical study. Intensive Crit Care Nurs 2016;37:4–10.
18. Johansson M, Wåhlin I, Magnusson L, et al. Family members' experiences with intensive care unit diaries when the patient does not survive. Scand J Caring Sci 2018;32(1):233–40.
19. Nair R, Mitchell M, Keogh S. The extent and application of patient diaries in Australian intensive care units: a national survey. Aust Crit Care 2015;28(2): 93–102.
20. Costa A, Padfield O, Elliot S, et al. Improving patient diary use in the intensive care unit: a quality improvement report. J Intensive Care Soc 2019;1–7. https://doi.org/10.1177/1751143719885295.

Nurses' Influence on Patient Wellbeing

Noise Reduction and Sunshine Therapy

Fiona A. Winterbottom, DNP, MSN, APRN, ACNS-BC, ACHPN, CCRN[a],*,
Karla LeBlanc-Lucas, BSN, RN, CPAN[b], Alexandra Boylan, BSN, CCRN[c]

KEYWORDS

• ICU • Noise • Sleep disruption • Family • Postintensive care syndrome

KEY POINTS

• Nurses are experts in creative and innovative solutions for patient care.
• Frontline nurses have the power to change factors that affect patient wellbeing.
• Bundles and protocols ease implementation and improve standardization of practices.

INTRODUCTION

Intensive care units (ICU) are noisy, busy places where patient's circadian rhythms are disrupted in a variety of ways. Stressors may be physiologic, pathophysiologic, psychological, or environmental.[1] Critically ill patients exhibit profound disruptions of circadian rhythmicity in critical care units. Mechanical ventilation, sedation, and ICU routines also cause noise, sleep disruption, and critical illness stressors. Exposure to bright light has alerting effects on the body. Studies show that light therapy can have a powerful influence on depression and may have a positive influence on patients and nursing staff.[2–4]

This article describes 2 nurse-driven programs that aimed to improve patient wellbeing and decrease ICU stressors to improve patients' experiences in the ICU. One program addresses noise reduction and the other describes Sunshine Therapy. Each program used evidence-based bundles and protocols to enhance patients' ICU experience with consideration of patient safety and ease of implementation.

[a] Critical Care Medicine, Ochsner Medical Center, 1514, Jefferson Highway, New Orleans, LA 70121, USA; [b] ICU Unit, 2626 Napoleon Avenue, New Orleans, LA 70115, USA; [c] CMICU, Ochsner Medical Center, 1514, Jefferson Highway, New Orleans, LA 70121, USA
* Corresponding author.
E-mail address: Fwinterbottom@ochsner.org

Crit Care Nurs Clin N Am 32 (2020) 327–334
https://doi.org/10.1016/j.cnc.2020.02.012
0899-5885/20/© 2020 Elsevier Inc. All rights reserved.

Noise Reduction: The Quiet Is Coming

Noise and sleep disruption can be particularly problematic for patients in the ICU. Invasive monitoring, x-rays, laboratory tests, and hygiene interventions make it difficult for patients to rest. Florence Nightingale stated that unnecessary noise is the most cruel absence of care which can be inflicted on the sick or well.[5] Nurses' are advocates for patients and inability to provide holistic patient care can compound burnout and staff engagement in work.

Studies show that sleep disturbance is a factor in the development of delirium, as well as producing specific effects on the respiratory, cardiovascular, and immunologic systems.[6] Patients with delirium have an increased risk of 6-month mortality and experience longer hospital stays even after adjusting for coma, sedatives, and analgesics in patients receiving mechanical ventilation.[7] Published clinical practice guidelines provide guidance to health care staff to mitigate physiologic, pathophysiologic, psychological, and environmental disruptions patients face in ICU.[1] The guidelines provide evidence-based strategies to reduce harm and improve the patient experience (**Table 1**).

In 2019, nurses in Ochsner Baptist ICU, New Orleans, decided to do something about noise in the ICU as it was affecting wellbeing and satisfaction of patients and staff. Nurses conducted a literature review and found that noise could negatively

Table 1	
Factors that patients report as disruptive to sleep	
Environmental	Physiologic and Pathophysiologic
Noise (447, 453, 454, 480, 483–488, 490, 491)	Pain (454, 483–486, 488, 490, 491)
Light (241, 453, 454, 480, 482–484, 486–488)	Discomfort (454, 483, 486, 488, 490)
Comfort of bed (483, 486–488)	Feeling too hot or too cold (484, 486, 488)
Activities at other bedsides (483, 486, 487)	Breathing difficulty (484, 491)
Visitors (clinician or family) (483)	Coughing (484, 491)
Room ventilation system (483)	Thirst (484, 486) and hunger (486, 488)
Hand washing by clinicians (483)	Nausea (484, 488)
Bad odor (486, 488)	Needing to use bedpan/urinal (486, 488)
Care Related	Psychological
Nursing care (447, 453, 480, 482–484, 486, 488, 491)	Anxiety/worry/stress (483, 484, 486, 489–491)
Patient procedures (447, 453, 480, 482, 483, 487, 488)	Fear (485, 486, 489)
Vital sign measurement (442, 448, 475, 477, 481, 483)	Unfamiliar environment (485, 488, 491)
Diagnostic tests (447, 453, 480, 483)	Disorientation to time (454, 486)
Medication administration (447, 453, 480, 482)	Loneliness (488, 491)
Restricted mobility from lines/catheters (454, 486, 488)	Lack of privacy (485, 488)
Monitoring equipment (454, 486, 488)	Hospital attire (486, 488)
Oxygen mask (486, 488)	Missing bedtime routine (483)
Endotracheal tube (491)	Not knowing nurses' names (486)
Urinary catheters (486)	Not understanding medical terms (486)

From Devlin JW, Skrobik Y, Gélinas C, et al. Clinical practice guidelines for the prevention and management of pain, agitation/sedation, delirium, immobility, and sleep disruption in adult patients in the ICU. Crit Care Med 2018;46(9):e854; with permission.

impact patients and simple evidence-based nursing interventions could be implemented to decrease noise, positively influence delirium, reduce length of stay, and promote a peaceful and healing environment.

One nurse-initiated intervention was placement of noise monitors in the central nurses' station. The World Health Organization suggests that environmental noise in hospitals should not exceed 40 decibels.[8] The monitors did not give continuous feedback on noise decibels but did provide prevalence measurements at noon and midnight that provided a snapshot of noise levels at the central nurse station of greater than 70 decibels. The monitors provided red, yellow, or green indicators on noise levels as a visual cue to interprofessional staff in the unit. Rapid feedback from the monitors provided an instant effect on noise levels in the ICU (**Fig. 1**).

Nurses' implemented sleep kits with facemasks and earplugs, diffusers, and night lights to reduce noise reduction and facilitate a calming environment. The day and night shift nurses worked together to cluster care and reassign tasks to provide a more patient-centered approach to care. Standardized quiet times were implemented. The nurses asked for and received hospital executive approval to reduce alarm volume in patient rooms from the default setting of 100% to 10%. In addition, since the ICU was undergoing renovations during the time of this project, the nurses advocated for the patient room walls to be painted in a soothing blue color. Hospital leadership supported the initiative and ICU painting is in progress (**Fig. 2**).

This ICU team demonstrated that staff nurses have the power to influence positive change and create healthy, healing environments that benefit patients and staff.

Sunshine Therapy: The Power of Light

Critically ill patients exhibit profound disruptions of circadian rhythmicity in critical care units. Mechanical ventilation, sedation, and ICU routines also cause sleep disruption and critical illness stressors.[1] Light is important to the central circadian clock, which

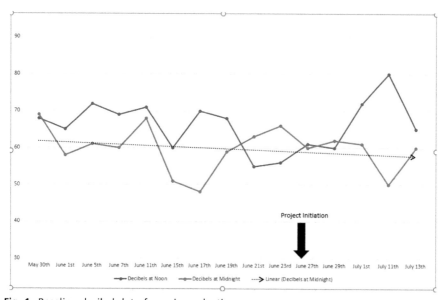

Fig. 1. Baseline decibel data for noise reduction program.

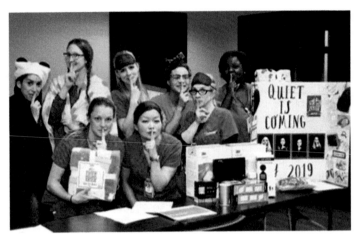

Fig. 2. Ochsner Baptist ICU nurses education.

provides a source of timing information to the rest of the body. Exposure to bright light has alerting effects on the body, mind, and soul. Studies show that light therapy can have a powerful influence on depression and may have a positive influence on ICU patients and nursing staff.[3,4] A nurse at Ochsner Medical Center Cardiac Medical ICU was concerned about the wellbeing of long-stay ICU patients. The nurse wanted to take patients outside into the sunshine and fresh air to make them feel better. She also did not want to burden other ICU staff with extra work that an excursion outside the building would incur.

I was inspired to create this group after taking care of a patient two summers ago. Due to hospitalization, he had been over 5 months since he had been outside. I brought him outside with help from charge nurses, It gave him so much hope and happiness just to breathe the fresh air. He ended up passing with us, so not only was that the first time he had been outside in 5 months, but it was the last time he was outside before he died.

There are patients that stay with us for so many months ...inside the same beige walls.

Their rooms are their kitchen, bedroom, bathroom, living room, and our work space.

Ultimately, I wanted to create this group so doing something nice doesn't feel like a burden. Sometimes I want to do something nice for patients, like bringing them outside but I can't because I have my hands full. By creating this group, that weight is lifted from me, the bedside nurse but the patients mind, body, and spirit is addressed giving the nurse and the team peace of mind. When all these areas are addressed that's when real progress is made.

The clinical nurse worked with the interprofessional Comprehensive Unit-based Safety Program team to create a protocol for long-stay ICU patients to receive Sunshine Therapy. The protocol provided a standardized algorithm to select and screen patients eligible for Sunshine Therapy in a safe and structured way.[9] The protocol included a safety screen, staffing plan, education, and implementation procedures to take patients outside into the sunshine. The protocol was approved by the unit leadership and the hospital's legal department. The protocol included a safety screen, checklist, staffing plan, education, and implementation procedures to take patients outside into the sunshine (**Fig. 3**).

Sunshine Therapy was planned so that safety, staffing, and plans of care could be organized. Staff volunteered to come in to take patients outside ensuring that unit staffing was not disrupted, and extra burden was not placed on the bedside nurse. The Sunshine Committee now has 18 ICU nurses and 6 respiratory therapists on the team. Approximately 15 patients have benefitted from Sunshine Therapy in the past 6 months. There have been subjective comments of wellbeing and liberation from patients, families, and staff. All groups have enjoyed the sunshine, wind, and freedom from the hospital room (**Box 1**, **Fig. 4**).

Sunshine Therapy

Why?
- To address patients' mind, body, and spirit

Who?
- US-Sunshine therapy committee, primary RN, & providers
- Multidisciplinary group who come in x1-2 mo (pre-planned dates) to bring appropriate patients outside for ~30 min

How?
- RN driven
- Providers will place in nx communication "ok for sunshine therapy" if appropriate
- 2 RNs: 1 patient—will travel with spectra link, number given to primary RN

Which patients are appropriate?
- **MOVE screen with criteria to pass:**
- Myocardial Stability—no dysrhythmia requiring new antiarrhythmic agent x24 H, no femoral cardiac devices
- Oxygenation—PEEP <10, FiO2 <=60%, SpO2 >88%, No continuous BIPAP/CPAP
- Vasopressors—<=1 low dose pressor, no new start in last 2 H, stable on current pressor over last 2 H at rest and with movement
- Engages to voice—RASS=0
- Plus primary RN judgment

Who is NOT appropriate?
- CRRT
- Nitric oxide
- cEEG
- Does not meet MOVE screen criteria
- RN judgment

When? + Where?
- Weather permitting
- Time not disruptive to POC
- Flagpoles—close to ED and elevators

Travel:
- 2 RNs: 1 patient
- RT—if patient not on RA or NC
- Portable monitor
- Ambu bag
- Travel kit—filled with emergency material, prn suctioning
- RNs participating will document after—similar to transfer notes

Fig. 3. Sunshine Therapy protocol.

Box 1
Comments on the Sunshine Therapy program

Patient Comments about Sunshine Therapy

After being in a comatose state for so long and scared... it was a God sent message for y'all to offer to take me outside to get fresh air.... I only knew those 4 walls and all the machines. Just going through the halls & then outside became familiar to me, and I began to feel happy and not so depressed. It was such a beautiful day outside and I felt like I was lifted with life again. It's a day that will always be a part of my happy times in the hospital. It gave me hope and encouragement... something that can't be done with medicine. Y'all became my angels of hope that day, and I will forever hold a special place in my heart for you guys.

Never in my life have I sat outside with a clear mind and just trusted God.... All of my fear and worries about my health, medicine, prognosis.... It all went away. I felt complete peace. I can never thank y'all enough...

Family Comments about Sunshine Therapy

He was getting so depressed in that room and I knew all he needed was some fresh air. Thank you so much.

Nurse Comments about Sunshine Therapy

There are no words to describe the peace that washes over our patients when the wind and sun touches them for the first time. It blows my mind how something so simple is so huge for someone else. The sun, the fresh air... it is liberating for our patients. It reminds them there is life and purpose.... And that gives them strength to keep fighting and pushing forward. These moments I get to witness and be a part of are the exact reason I chose nursing as my profession.

Mr. B was in literal heaven. You could see the anxiety and fear leave his body and an overwhelming sense of joy come over him. As he closed his eyes and breathed in the crisp, fall air, I couldn't't help but feel complete happiness within myself. This man sat in the same room for 33 days before he was able to experience sunshine therapy. The change you see in the patients during and after sunshine therapy is indescribable. Also, the way it makes you feel as a caregiver is priceless therapy in itself. The only thing I regret is not having offered this therapy years ago! I am so grateful to be part of such a great experience.

Sunshine Therapy not only brought life back to my patients, but back to me. It started with one patient that touched my heart and to see the smallest bit of joy and hope that we could give her just by simply taking her outside reignited a light for me that I felt was dimming with nursing. Sunshine therapy brings nursing full circle... it is what makes this career so much different than others. We have the opportunity to take care of the patient in every aspect and with sunshine therapy it's just another way that we can help improve outcomes for the patients and decrease burnout for the nurses. It brings back the reminder that these patients are people, not machines, and helps to bring fulfillment to the job on a high mortality unit. The joy that it brings these patients cannot be put into words.

SUMMARY

This article has described 2 nurse-driven programs that aimed to improve patient wellbeing and decrease ICU stressors to improve patients' experiences in the ICU. Both interventions were nurse-led and initiated by frontline clinical nurses as

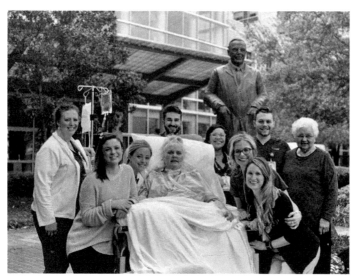

Fig. 4. Sunshine Therapy in action.

creative solutions to overcome patient problems and provide holistic approaches to care. These exemplars demonstrate that nurses have the power to influence wellbeing and create healing and healthy work environments for patients and staff.

DISCLOSURE

The authors have nothing to disclose.

REFERENCES

1. Devlin JW, Skrobik Y, Gélinas C, et al. Clinical practice guidelines for the prevention and management of pain, agitation/sedation, delirium, immobility, and sleep disruption in adult patients in the ICU. Crit Care Med 2018;46(9): e825–73.
2. Hodges S, Riley L, Dickson T, et al. A systematic literature review of noise and nurse stress levels in intensive care units. J Educ Soc Behav Sci 2018; 27(3):1–7.
3. Boeijen ER, Mertens MC, Rood P, et al. Effect of dynamic light application on cognitive performance and well-being of intensive care nurses. Am J Crit Care 2018;27(3):245–8.
4. Zhao X, Ma J, Wu S, et al. Light therapy for older patients with non-seasonal depression: a systematic review and meta-analysis. J Affect Disord 2018;232: 291–9.
5. Nightingale F. Notes on nursing: what it is, and what it is not (Commemorative Ed.). Philadelphia: Lippincott; 1992.
6. Xie H, Kang J, Mills G. Clinical review: the impact of noise on patients' sleep and the effectiveness of noise reduction strategies in intensive care unit. Crit Care 2009;13(2):208.

7. Ely EW, Shintani A, Truman B, et al. Delirium as a predictor of mortality in mechanically ventilated patients in the intensive care unit. JAMA 2004;291(14):1753–62.
8. Darbyshire JL, Young JD. An investigation of sound levels on intensive care units with reference to the WHO guidelines. Crit Care 2013;17(5):R187.
9. Bassett RD, Vollman KM, Brandwene L, et al. Integrating a multidisciplinary mobility programme into intensive care practice (IMMPTP): a multicentre collaborative. Intensive Crit Care Nurs 2012;28(2):88–97.

The Facilitated Sensemaking Model as a Framework for Family-Patient Communication During Mechanical Ventilation in the Intensive Care Unit

Ji Won Shin, PhD, RN*, Judith A. Tate, PhD, RN,
Mary Beth Happ, PhD, RN, FGSA

KEYWORDS

- Caregivers • Stress disorders • Posttraumatic • Depression • Anxiety
- Communication • Intensive care units • Critical care

KEY POINTS

- Family caregivers of nonvocal ICU patients are at high risk of developing psychological symptoms and further distressed with communication difficulty, but patient-family communication in the ICU is understudied.
- The Facilitated Sensemaking Model (FSM) is the first model to guide nursing interventions to help ICU family caregivers overcome and prevent the adverse psychological outcomes associated with post-intensive care syndrome-family (PICS-F).
- Applying and expanding the FSM, communication interventions delivered by critical care nurses may facilitate family caregiver bedside activities and a better understanding of the patient's feelings, symptoms, and needs, thereby reducing anxiety, depression, and PTSD.

INTRODUCTION

A stay in an intensive care unit (ICU) can be a highly stressful life event for both patients and their family caregivers. Family caregivers of ICU patients are at high risk of developing adverse psychological outcomes, such as anxiety, depression, and posttraumatic stress disorder (PTSD).[1] Post-intensive care syndrome-family (PICS-F) refers to the development of a cluster of common symptoms among family caregivers of ICU patients.[2] Family caregivers may experience psychological symptoms during

The Ohio State University College of Nursing, Newton Hall #352, 1585 Neil Avenue, Columbus, OH 43210, USA
* Corresponding author.
E-mail address: shin.527@osu.edu

Crit Care Nurs Clin N Am 32 (2020) 335–348
https://doi.org/10.1016/j.cnc.2020.02.013
0899-5885/20/© 2020 Elsevier Inc. All rights reserved.

ICU care and/or after ICU admission, and those symptoms can last for months to years after the ICU discharge.[2]

Approximately 40% of ICU patients in the United States need mechanical ventilation (MV) to assist or replace spontaneous breathing[3] rendering the patient unable to produce vocal speech. Patient communication is further limited by physical weakness and fluctuations in cognition. Communication difficulty is one of the most common burdens reported by mechanically ventilated patients in ICU.[4,5] Although communication difficulty during MV treatment is associated with negative feelings, such as frustration, fear, anxiety, and anger for patients,[4,6–9] family caregivers report emotional distress, feelings of loss, and frustration.[10–13] These negative feelings may induce or worsen adverse psychological outcomes, such as anxiety, depression, and PTSD, yet little is known about the impact of patient-family communication on psychological symptoms in ICU family caregivers.

Augmentative and alternative communication (AAC) methods, such as writing tools, communication boards, or electronic communication devices, may relieve or reduce communication challenges.[13] Despite a lack of evidence or support, clinicians report relying on family caregivers to provide interpretation of nonvocal communication when ICU patients are unable to speak.[10,14,15] Therefore, there is a need for effective strategies to facilitate communication between nonvocal ICU patients and family caregivers.

The Facilitated Sensemaking Model (FSM), a middle-range theory, provides a basis for how to care for family caregivers of ICU patients.[16] The FSM guides nursing interventions to prevent and/or reduce adverse psychological outcomes in family caregivers in the ICUs.[16] The purpose of this paper is to extend the FSM to promote an electronic intervention to aid patient-family communication in the ICU. In this paper, we present the scientific evidence and theoretic background for adding interventions to facilitate patient-family communication to prevent and/or alleviate adverse psychological outcomes in family caregivers of nonvocal ICU patients. An electronic tablet communication application is 1 example of an intervention to facilitate patient-family communication in the ICU.

LITERATURE REVIEW
Post-Intensive Care Syndrome-Family

Since investigators first recognized that family caregivers of ICU patients could have clinically diagnosable psychological problems in the early 1990s,[17] there has been growing interest in the impact of critical illness on family caregivers. There is a wide variation in reported prevalence of depression, anxiety, and PTSD-related symptoms among ICU family caregivers, which may be related to differences in study settings, time frames for symptom assessment, sample, and measurement tools.[18,19] For example, the reported short- and longer-term prevalence of post-ICU depressive symptoms in family caregivers ranged from 12% to 26% at 3 months and 23% to 44% at 1 year.[19] The prevalence of anxiety symptoms ranged between 24% and 63% at 3 months and the prevalence of PTSD-related symptoms was estimated between 32% and 80% at 1 year post-ICU.[18] Despite the wide variation of estimated prevalence, the findings still suggest that ICU family caregivers experience high levels of psychological symptoms considering that reported lifetime prevalence of depression in the general population ranged between 8% and 15%[20] and lifetime prevalence of PTSD among adult Americans is 6.8%.[21]

Clinical practice guidelines for support of family-centered care in the ICU[22,23] address the need for more structured family support interventions to reduce anxiety, depression, and posttraumatic stress in ICU family caregivers. However, few interventions have been developed and tested to improve adverse psychological outcomes in ICU family caregivers. An ICU diary is 1 strategy developed and implemented to reduce the psychological distress in ICU survivors and caregivers. ICU diaries are designed to provide a story of the patient's ICU stay,[24,25] and diaries are generally written by nurses, other hospital staff, or family caregivers during the ICU care. As a focus for family empowerment and family-centered care in the ICUs, several studies involving ICU diaries encouraged the participation of family caregivers, yet the impact of diaries on family caregivers' adverse psychological outcomes is inconclusive.[26–28]

The results on adverse psychological outcomes in ICU families were also mixed in other studies of information-related interventions, such as educational programs designed to inform family caregivers about care, diagnosis, or prognosis of the patient. Those programs can be delivered during the ICU admission[29–31] or after discharge as part of a post-ICU rehabilitation program.[32]

Communication Difficulty in Mechanical Ventilation Patients and Family Caregivers

Communication between ICU patients and family caregivers is seriously impaired during treatment with MV due to multiple factors, most prominently the placement of an oral endotracheal or tracheostomy tube, which prevents voice production and impedes communication with vocal speech.[33] Communication is essential to understand patients' needs and detect patients' symptoms, which may improve the quality of care and safety. MV patients generally use natural communication methods, such as gestures, head nods, mouthing words, and writing with paper and pen to communicate with nurses.[34] However, those natural methods are time-consuming and can be unreliable.

Communication impairment due to MV during ICU stay may add psychological distress, which can cause a new onset of psychological problems or worsen existing symptoms. A cross-sectional study conducted by Khalaila and colleagues[6] examined the correlation between communication characteristics and psycho-emotional distress in ICU patients. The study demonstrated a strong association between higher psychological distress and negative feelings, such as fear and anger, with perceived communication difficulty and indicated that perceived communication difficulty was the strongest predictor of psychological distress.[6] The results suggest possible associations between perceived communication difficulty and psychological symptoms in ICU family caregivers and support that providing effective communication strategies may help family caregivers alleviate their psychological symptoms.

AAC refers to all forms of communication used to supplement or replace oral speech, including all ways to express messages, such as facial expressions or gestures, body language, and aided low- and high-tech tools for those with speech or language impairment.[35] Alternative communication methods developed and tested to improve communication for MV patients in the ICUs include low-tech tools, such as communication boards and speaking valves for patients with tracheostomy, and high-tech tools, such as computerized communication tools. **Table 1** summarizes several low- and high-tech communication tools available and tested for nonvocal patients in the ICUs.[36]

Although there is a growing recognition that effective communication is essential to improve the quality of health care and multiple AAC tools are available for nonvocal patients in hospital settings, patient-family communication has received little to no attention in critical care research. The involvement of family caregivers in assisted communication strategies with nonvocal ICU patients and the use of AAC tools in patient-family communication in the ICU have not been systematically investigated.

Table 1
Summary of low- and high-tech communication tools for nonvocal patients

	Features
Low-tech tools	
Communication boards	• Usually consist of an arrangement of the alphabet, words/phrases, icons, or pictures. • Icons and pictures represent common messages in which patients can easily point with fingers.
Tracheostomy speaking valves	• Can be placed in the tracheostomy tube to allow phonation. • Facilitate verbal communication for tracheostomized patients.
High-tech tools	
Speech-generating devices (SGDs)	• Electronic AAC devices that produce prerecorded voice messages or computer-generated voice when touching specific locations on the device screen or keyboard. • SGDs can be simple, such as recorder devices or specialized computer systems.
Communication computer applications (apps)	• Communication apps may or may not be speech generating. • Several software apps for tablet computers or smartphones are commercially available. • Contain messages/icons, such as communication boards. • Most apps provide a keyboard feature that allows the user to create novel messages.
Eye tracking devices	• Can be used for paralyzed patients or others with restricted use of upper extremities. • Integrate the data by detecting eye movement and position to create a gaze point for selections on a computer screen. • Allow patients to use their eyes to operate a speech-generating device using eye-gaze control technology.

The role of family involvement in communication remains unknown. When evaluated through qualitative research, family caregivers expressed emotional distress, feelings of loss, and frustration with dysfunctional communication during MV treatment.[10–13,37] Families want to help patients and to protect their feelings by calming and encouraging them,[38,39] but they often do not know how to accomplish this. In previous research, patients described that a specific family member with exceptional ability to communicate took the time to understand their current condition, helped the patient to communicate, and made sure care providers understood the patient.[14,15] Family caregivers often served the role as interpreters for the nonvocal patients and nurses tended to rely on their interpretation to communicate with the patients.[10,14,15]

A retrospective descriptive study to identify communication methods and the content of communication with nonsurviving MV patients in the ICU showed that communication between patients and family caregivers often took the form of emotional expressions.[40] In a feasibility study of electronic speech-generating devices for MV patients, the primary content of speech-generating devices constructed messages was "I love you" and questions about home/family.[41] These findings suggest that communication between family caregivers and patients may be more complex and stressful than simple, standard yes or no questions. Broyles and colleagues[13] conducted a qualitative analysis of enrollment notes, intervention logs, and observation records from the Study of Patient-nurse Effectiveness with Assisted Communication Strategies study[42] to identify which AAC tools families used and to describe family caregivers' and nurses' perceptions of communication between family caregivers and MV patients. Family caregivers in this study were generally unprepared for the MV patient's inability to communicate. Family caregivers experienced negative feelings, such as frustration, with unsuccessful communication. Although family caregivers were not familiar with AAC tools and strategies, they expressed interest in learning about AAC strategies and desired the highest level of communication with their critically ill patients.[13]

Despite evidence of the communication difficulties expressed by family caregivers and their desire to improve communication, to date, families of MV patients typically have only simple and low-tech tools to overcome communication difficulties and these are not consistently available at the ICU bedside.[13] Information on the communication challenges between ICU patients and family caregivers is sparse and its impact on psychological outcomes family caregivers has not been addressed in previous studies.

THE FACILITATED SENSEMAKING MODEL

The FSM was developed by Davidson[16] to provide a basis for family-centered care in the ICU and guide interventions to prevent adverse psychological outcomes in ICU family caregivers. **Table 2** describes the theoretic underpinnings of the FSM. The FSM was also developed inductively through literature review, consultation with content experts and family members during the development of the intervention set, and input from doctoral students, professors, and clinical nurse specialists during the validating process.[16] The FSM has been tested for feasibility in the ICU setting.[43] A family engagement intervention based on the FSM was associated with decreased levels of anxiety in family caregivers of cardiac surgery patients.[44]

The primary goal of the FSM is to guide nursing interventions to prevent adverse psychological outcomes in family caregivers of ICU patients. The FSM assumes that exposure to critical illness can be a life crisis for family members of critically ill patients. The FSM proposes that nurses can provide a series of interventions to facilitate the sensemaking process with family caregivers. According to the model, family caregivers of an ICU patient experience life disruptions during the critical illness that may challenge their coping. In response to the disruption, family caregivers need a compensation period to overcome the challenges and adapt to the new situation. They need to make sense out of what has happened in the new situation and their new roles as ICU caregivers.[16,43] During this compensation period, the nurse can engage in and facilitate the sensemaking process with family caregivers through directed interventions.[16,44]

A facilitated sensemaking intervention has 2 main goals: (1) to help the family understand what is happening in the new situation and (2) to coach what the family should do as a caregiver of an ICU patient (**Fig. 1**). Sensemaking interventions include identifying the family caregivers' needs, providing information about the prognosis or care plan, providing family support, coaching the family on how to meet their own needs, and guiding bedside activities that they can perform while they visit their loved one in the ICUs.[44] As a result of nursing interventions, family caregivers may be able to adapt to the new situation in a more positive way through improved coping. The FSM provides suggestions on specific bedside activities in 2 categories: (1) personal

Table 2
Theoretic underpinnings of the Facilitated Sensemaking Model

		Central Propositions	Adaptation to the FSM
Combination of RAM and WOST by Davidson while developing the FSM	Roy Adaptation Model (RAM)	• The goal of nursing is to promote a person's adaptation whose life is disrupted, such as by illness. • Illness can cause a disruption in life, and adaptation occurs when people respond to the new environment in a positive way.	• The FSM follows the adaptation theory premise that family caregivers experience a life disruption that requires a compensatory process to adjust to the disruption and adapt to the new circumstances of a family member's critical illness and their role as ICU family caregivers.
	Weick's Organizational Sensemaking Theory (WOST)	• Leaders help others form a perception of a crisis event and make sense out of the situation. • Leaders can help others in the workplace with cue sorting to shape a positive impression of the situation.	• Nurses proactively take cues from the environment and help the family caregivers sort those cues appropriately to make sense of what is going on.
Sensemaking in psychology social and cognitive	Self-regulation theory	• Concrete, clear objective information facilitates coping by affecting the person's schema formation about stressful events, such as illness. • A schema based on concrete objective information can focus a person's attention away from the emotional dimensions of an impending experience leading to reduced emotional distress during the stressful experience.	• The FSM follows the self-regulation theory premise that facilitated sensemaking helps family caregivers reduce psychological symptoms by making sense out of what happened and their new roles as caregivers in the ICU environment.

care/healing and (2) *bringing normalcy into the room*. Personal care activities may include applying lip balm, giving a massage, assisting in passive range-of-motion exercises, praying, and engaging in cognitive exercises. The other group of activities includes reading aloud, talking about daily events, bringing in cards/pictures from home to *bring normalcy into the room*, which may help the patient feel relieved.[16] The sensemaking process will finally lead to adaptation that is described as lower adverse psychological outcomes, such as anxiety, depression, and PTSD.

APPLICATION OF THE FACILITATED SENSEMAKING MODEL TO A COMMUNICATION INTERVENTION

The communication column in the FSM model (see **Fig. 1**) is intended to focus on and guide communication between the clinicians and the family (Davidson, personal communication). The presence column refers to family bedside presence activities.

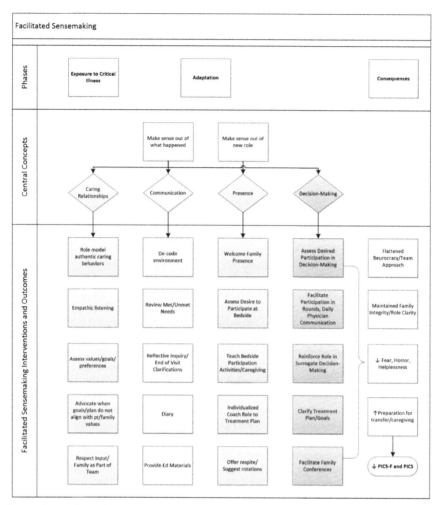

Fig. 1. The Facilitated Sensemaking Model. (*From* Davidson JE, McDuffie M, Kay M. Family-centered care. In: Goldsworthy S, Kleinpell R, Williams G, editors. International best practices in critical care nursing. 2nd edition. Dayboro, Australia: World Federation of Critical Care Nurses; 2018; with permission.)

We have, therefore, added patient-family communication interventions to that area of the model (see **Fig. 1**). Our application of the FSM to the problem of communication difficulty and impairment is depicted in a research model (**Fig. 2**).

The original FSM included low-tech communication tools, such as paper pad, pencil, and foam grip as one of the components in the family visiting kit to enhance patient-family communication.[43] This application of the FSM incorporates advances in technology not available at the time the model was originally constructed. We add an explicit assumption to the theory: Communication difficulty due to MV treatment is an unplanned and sudden event that seriously disrupts patient-family interactions and may cause or amplify psychological distress in family caregivers of nonvocal patients. Family-patient communication is an essential interaction for the family

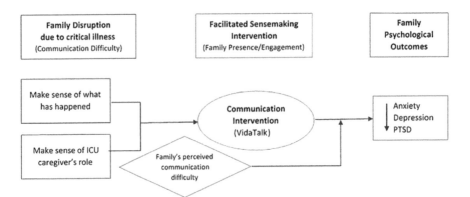

Fig. 2. Application of the Facilitated Sensemaking Model.

caregivers to interpret the experience of critical illness and understand the emotional reactions and thoughts of the patient. A communication intervention developed to improve communication between nonvocal patients and family caregivers may facilitate the family caregiver's sensemaking process to compensate for the disruption and adapt to the new situation. An electronic communication intervention in addition to traditional pen and paper techniques may help family caregivers meet their own needs for effective communication with the patient to understand the patient's situation, feelings/thoughts, and what they are experiencing. This will help family caregivers meet the first sensemaking goal: *to make sense of what has happened in the ICU.* More effective communication may also facilitate the family caregiver's bedside activities as they better understand the patient's expressed needs and allow the family caregivers to *bring normalcy into the room* by talking about daily events. Through these mechanisms, family caregivers would feel engaged and involved in the patient's care, instead of remaining as visitors, and meet the second sensemaking goal.

The results of previous studies exploring the communication experience between MV patients and their family caregivers support the need for a communication intervention to reduce family caregivers' psychological distress.[14,15] Although family members are usually familiar conversation partners, interpreting what the nonvocal MV patient is trying to say is typically a new role for a family caregiver, particularly in the context of serious and sudden illness or injuries and the ICU environment. The family caregiver needs to figure out how best to communicate with the nonvocal patient in a different way. We posit that more effective communication will help the family caregiver reduce the uncertainty and, therefore, alleviate their adverse psychological outcomes and may also decrease frustration and agitation in patients. The FSM has not been tested for the impact of patient-family caregiver communication on psychological outcomes in family caregivers. Communication distress is expected to be relieved in nonvocal ICU patients and family caregivers by providing strategies to allow the patients and their families to communicate with each other.

CLINICALLY APPLICABLE COMMUNICATION STRATEGY

To illustrate how the FSM can guide practice regarding patient-family communication in the ICU, we provide an example of a newly developed electronic patient communication application (app) as a potential intervention to facilitate making sense of the experience and performing in the role as ICU family caregiver. Newer technology-based communication tools, such as communication apps, may be beneficial because apps are easy to use and less expensive than other communication devices, such as specialized computer systems. Considering that approximately 50% of US adults possess tablet computers and 80% own smartphones,[45] and that the apps can be easily downloaded, using an electronic communication aid with nonvocal MV patients seems feasible. VidaTalk™ (Vidatak), an electronic patient communication board, is a tablet app designed to help patients who are unable to speak to communicate their needs to care providers and family caregivers. The communication app contains picture icons with words/phrases pertaining to needs and wellbeing, emotions, pain scales, pictures of the body to indicate needs in a certain area. Type and finger-drawing features allow the patient to generate novel messages. When a patient touches one of the icons, the message is produced audibly via digital speech and the text of the message is displayed on the screen, which enables 2-way communication between the patient and others.

As mentioned previously, there are 2 sensemaking goals to help family caregivers reduce their psychological symptoms in our theoretic framework (see **Fig. 2**): (1) make sense of what is happening in the new situation and (2) make sense of their new role as a caregiver of an ICU patient. Various preset messages that are commonly used by ICU patients and novel messages created by the patient using writing or typing within the VidaTalk™ app will facilitate more complex conversations between MV patient and family caregivers. Therefore, use of a communication app may help family caregivers to meet the first goal by assisting with understanding the patient's experience in the ICU and improving expressions of feelings/thoughts.

The second sensemaking goal incorporates the family's role as an ICU caregiver serving the bedside activities and bringing normalcy into the room.[16] More effective communication will help families understand the patient's expressed needs/requests, as well as help the patients express their wishes clearly. VidaTalk™ may help family caregivers to have clearer communication with the patient, which may promote family caregivers' bedside activities. For example, a family member may know, through the use of VidaTalk™, that the patient needs repositioning or pain medication, and would be able to provide or facilitate that bedside care assistance. This may further enhance the family caregiver's role as advocate for the patient in the ICU. Also, the ability to communicate a variety of messages, including conversations about everyday events outside of the hospital, such as home/family and patient's feelings/emotions may help families to bring normalcy into the room.

Happ and colleagues[46] (2007) described communication processes between patients and families that emphasized the importance of normalizing talk to distract patients during weaning from MV and included talking about everyday, nonillness-related events. Consistent with these findings, the FSM also suggests normalizing the ICU environment as an important component of the sensemaking process in family caregivers.[16] VidaTalk™ may help the families serve in the caregiver role by distracting patients from the stressful ICU environment with normalizing talk.

The keys to family-centered care are a beneficial relationship between family caregivers, patients, and care providers; and family presence, and family involvement in decision making and patient care.[47] Communication strategies to enhance patient-family communication in the ICU may increase family involvement and allow families serve more active roles as ICU caregivers, which may help them reduce psychological distress through sensemaking process. We present a clinical case exemplar of family caregiver's use of VidaTalk™ with the ICU patient to illustrate a family's communication experience with nonvocal patient, how a communication tool enables patient-family communication, and how families emotionally react to communication with their loved one in the ICU (**Box 1**).

Clinical Implications

The ICU environment can be unfamiliar to family caregivers. Many families are overwhelmed with the uncertainty associated with their loved one's serious illness. Families are typically not prepared for the patient's inability to communicate with MV.[13]

Critical care nurses have an opportunity to recognize the psychological and social importance of family caregivers' needs for effective communication with the MV patient. Assessment of family communication needs, perceived communication difficulty, and familiarity with AAC strategies can become standard care in the ICU. Nurses can further positively impact patient-family communication by encouraging

---

Box 1
Clinical case exemplar of a communication intervention in the Facilitated Sensemaking Model

Family disruption due to critical illness	Mr. Stone (pseudonym), a 65-year-old ICU patient was orally intubated, receiving mechanical ventilation, alert, and cognitively intact. His wife, a 62-year-old woman, stayed at the bedside in the ICU room for most of the day. They initially communicated with each other using hand gestures or writing with paper and pen. Because of developing hand and arm weaknesses from the illness and extended hospitalization, hand writing on a paper became difficult for Mr. Stone and his written messages became nearly uninterpretable to his wife. After tracheostomy placement, Mr. Stone was able to mouth words with his lips; however, lip reading was not always clear or successful. Family members, visitors, and staff often failed to understand his wishes or requests leaving them feeling frustrated and disappointed with these communication challenges. When Mr. Stone's wishes were not understood, he waved off any additional attempts to communicate.
Patient-family communication intervention	We introduced the VidaTalk™ communication app to Mr. and Ms. Stone on a hospital-issued android tablet. We provided a brief, 5-min demonstration of the communication app, including patient return demonstration, instruction on how to operate the tablet and an instruction sheet.
	The couple started using the app almost immediately. They used the app daily to communicate with each other during the rest of the hospitalization. Using the VidaTalk™ tablet app, Mr. Stone began asking a lot of questions, including questions about home or his children (bringing normalcy to the situation). He asked his wife about the treatment plan and insurance (making sense of what is happening) as well as about daily events outside of the hospital (bringing normalcy). Mr. Stone also said "I love you" to his wife almost every day, a normal, profound and meaningful expression between husband and wife. They continued to use hand gestures or mouthing words for simple messages, but used the VidaTalk™ app for conversations more complex than a simple request or when natural communication methods, such as gestures or lip reading did not work well.
Outcomes	With the communication app, Ms. Stone was able to clearly understand her husband's needs, thoughts, and feelings (making sense of the patient's experience). Clear communication with the app reduced the family's frustration and stress with inability to communicate and Ms. Stone described feeling "relieved" and "appreciated" (psycho-emotional outcomes) as a result of communication with the app.

MV patients and their family caregivers use AAC tools/strategies that are available in the unit. Nurses' awareness of and familiarity with available communication tools/devices in the unit is critical to facilitate use of the communication tools.

DISCUSSION

Although previous studies revealed the significance of adverse psychological outcomes in family caregivers,[19] the FSM is the only model that guides specific interventions to improve family caregivers' coping and adjustment to the challenging situation of a loved one's critical illness. Interventions to improve communication between family caregivers and patients might moderate or alleviate families' distress, and therefore prevent or reduce adverse psychological outcomes. By extending the FSM to address patient-family communicative interactions with electronic solutions, we propose that more effective communication will help the family caregivers make sense of what is happening. The VidaTalk™ application is an example of a communication intervention that may serve as a bedside activity and provide a means for bringing normalcy to the bedside.

The FSM provides a framework for understanding how critical care nurses can assist ICU family caregivers to overcome a disruptive situation and reduce adverse psychological outcomes through the sensemaking process. The FSM comprehensively considers a crisis, experience, interventions, and psychological outcomes specifically for the population of ICU family caregivers. The FSM, as a middle-range theory, is directly applicable to patient-family communication in the ICU. In our expanded version of the FSM, we added a new family communication intervention to the model to guide a communication intervention for ICU family caregivers. Because of its comprehensiveness, the FSM is useful to guide research on short- and long-term adverse psychological outcomes in family caregivers of ICU patients. The use of an electronic communication tool is one possible solution to reduce families' psychological distress by facilitating communication with the nonvocal ICU patient.

ACKNOWLEDGEMENTS

Case study from *"Improving Outcomes for Mechanically Ventilated Patients with the Digital EZ Board,"* funded by National Institutes of Health National Institute of Nursing Research, grant R42NR014087 (M Happ), and Sigma Theta Tau International Honor Society of Nursing, Epsilon Chapter Dissertation Grant (J Shin).

DISCLOSURE

The authors have nothing to disclose.

REFERENCES

1. Davidson JE, Hopkins RO, Louis D, et al. Post-intensive care syndrome. 2013. Available at: https://www.sccm.org/MyICUCare/THRIVE/Post-intensive-Care-Syndrome. Accessed April 29, 2019.

2. Davidson JE, Jones C, Bienvenu OJ. Family response to critical illness: postintensive care syndrome-family. Crit Care Med 2012;40(2):618–24.

3. Wunsch H, Wagner J, Herlim M, et al. ICU occupancy and mechanical ventilator use in the United States. Crit Care Med 2013;41(12):2712–9.

4. Rotondi AJ, Chelluri L, Sirio C, et al. Patients' recollections of stressful experiences while receiving prolonged mechanical ventilation in an intensive care unit. Crit Care Med 2002;30(4):746–52.

5. Nelson JE, Meier DE, Litke A, et al. The symptom burden of chronic critical illness. Crit Care Med 2004;32(7):1527–34.

6. Khalaila R, Zbidat W, Anwar K, et al. Communication difficulties and psychoemotional distress in patients receiving mechanical ventilation. Am J Crit Care 2011; 20(6):470–9.

7. Carroll SM. Nonvocal ventilated patients perceptions of being understood. West J Nurs Res 2004;26(1):85–103 [discussion: 104–12].

8. Patak L, Gawlinski A, Fung NI, et al. Patients' reports of health care practitioner interventions that are related to communication during mechanical ventilation. Heart Lung 2004;33(5):308–20.

9. Engström Å, Nyström N, Sundelin G, et al. People's experiences of being mechanically ventilated in an ICU: a qualitative study. Intensive Crit Care Nurs 2013;29(2):88–95.

10. Happ MB. Interpretation of nonvocal behavior and the meaning of voicelessness in critical care. Soc Sci Med 2000;50(9):1247–55.

11. Engström Å, Söderberg S. The experiences of partners of critically ill persons in an intensive care unit. Intensive Crit Care Nurs 2004;20(5):299–308.

12. Dreyer A, Nortvedt P. Sedation of ventilated patients in intensive care units: relatives' experiences. J Adv Nurs 2008;61(5):549–56.

13. Broyles LM, Tate JA, Happ MB. Use of augmentative and alternative communication strategies by family members in the intensive care unit. Am J Crit Care 2012; 21(2):e21–32.

14. Engström Å, Söderberg S. Receiving power through confirmation: the meaning of close relatives for people who have been critically ill. J Adv Nurs 2007;59(6): 569–76.

15. Magnus VS, Turkington L. Communication interaction in ICU–patient and staff experiences and perceptions. Intensive Crit Care Nurs 2006;22(3):167–80.

16. Davidson JE. Facilitated sensemaking: a strategy and new middle-range theory to support families of intensive care unit patients. Crit Care Nurse 2010;30(6): 28–39.

17. Pérez-San Gregorio MA, Blanco-Picabia A, Murillo-Cabezas F, et al. Psychological problems in the family members of gravely traumatised patients admitted into an intensive care unit. Intensive Care Med 1992;18(5):278–81.

18. Petrinec AB, Daly BJ. Post-traumatic stress symptoms in post-ICU family members: review and methodological challenges. West J Nurs Res 2016;38(1):57–78.

19. van Beusekom I, Bakhshi-Raiez F, de Keizer NF, et al. Reported burden on informal caregivers of ICU survivors: a literature review. Crit Care 2015;20(1):16.

20. Richards D. Prevalence and clinical course of depression: a review. Clin Psychol Rev 2011;31(7):1117–25.

21. Kessler RC, Berglund P, Demler O, et al. Lifetime prevalence and age-of-onset distributions of DSM-IV disorders in the National Comorbidity Survey Replication. Arch Gen Psychiatry 2005;62(6):593–602.

22. Davidson JE, Powers K, Hedayat KM, et al. Clinical practice guidelines for support of the family in the patient-centered intensive care unit: American College of Critical Care Medicine Task Force 2004–2005. Crit Care Med 2007;35(2):605–22.

23. Davidson JE, Aslakson RA, Long AC, et al. Guidelines for family-centered care in the neonatal, pediatric, and adult ICU. Crit Care Med 2017;45(1):103–28.

24. Egerod I, Schwartz Nielsen KH, Hansen GM, et al. The extent and application of patient diaries in Danish ICUs in 2006. Nurs Crit Care 2007;12(3):159–67.
25. Aitken LM, Rattray J, Hull A, et al. The use of diaries in psychological recovery from intensive care. Crit Care 2013;17(6):253.
26. Jones C, Bäckman C, Griffiths RD. Intensive care diaries and relatives' symptoms of posttraumatic stress disorder after critical illness: a pilot study. Am J Crit Care 2012;21(3):172–6.
27. Kloos JA, Daly BJ. Effect of a Family-Maintained Progress Journal on anxiety of families of critically ill patients. Crit Care Nurs Q 2008;31(2):96–107 [quiz: 108–9].
28. Garrouste-Orgeas M, Coquet I, Périer A, et al. Impact of an intensive care unit diary on psychological distress in patients and relatives. Crit Care Med 2012;40(7): 2033–40.
29. Garrouste-Orgeas M, Max A, Lerin T, et al. Impact of proactive nurse participation in ICU family conferences: a mixed-method study. Crit Care Med 2016;44(6): 1116–28.
30. Moreau D, Goldgran-Toledano D, Alberti C, et al. Junior versus senior physicians for informing families of intensive care unit patients. Am J Respir Crit Care Med 2004;169(4):512–7.
31. Curtis JR, Treece PD, Nielsen EL, et al. Randomized trial of communication facilitators to reduce family distress and intensity of end-of-life care. Am J Respir Crit Care Med 2016;193(2):154–62.
32. Jones C, Skirrow P, Griffiths RD, et al. Post-traumatic stress disorder-related symptoms in relatives of patients following intensive care. Intensive Care Med 2004;30(3):456–60.
33. MacAulay F, Judson A, Etchels M, et al. ICU-Talk, a communication aid for intubated intensive care patients. Proceedings of the fifth international ACM conference on Assistive technologies. Edinburgh, Scotland, July 2002.
34. Happ MB, Garrett K, Thomas DD, et al. Nurse-patient communication interactions in the intensive care unit. Am J Crit Care 2011;20(2):e28–40.
35. American Speech Language Hearing Association (ASHA). Augmentative and alternative communication 2018. 2018. Available at: https://www.asha.org/public/speech/disorders/AAC/. Accessed March 18, 2018.
36. Ten Hoorn S, Elbers PW, Girbes AR, et al. Communicating with conscious and mechanically ventilated critically ill patients: a systematic review. Crit Care 2016;20(1):333.
37. Alasad J, Ahmad M. Communication with critically ill patients. J Adv Nurs 2005; 50(4):356–62.
38. Hupcey JE, Penrod J. Going it alone: the experienes of spouses of critically ill patients. Dimens Crit Care Nurs 2000;19(3):44.
39. Ågård AS, Harder I. Relatives' experiences in intensive care—finding a place in a world of uncertainty. Intensive Crit Care Nurs 2007;23(3):170–7.
40. Happ MB, Tuite P, Dobbin K, et al. Communication ability, method, and content among nonspeaking nonsurviving patients treated with mechanical ventilation in the intensive care unit. Am J Crit Care 2004;13(3):210–8.
41. Happ MB, Roesch TK, Garrett K. Electronic voice-output communication aids for temporarily nonspeaking patients in a medical intensive care unit: a feasibility study. Heart Lung 2004;33(2):92–101.
42. Happ MB, Garrett KL, Tate JA, et al. Effect of a multi-level intervention on nurse-patient communication in the intensive care unit: results of the SPEACS trial. Heart & lung 2014;43(2):89–98.

43. Davidson JE, Daly BJ, Agan D, et al. Facilitated sensemaking: a feasibility study for the provision of a family support program in the intensive care unit. Crit Care Nurs Q 2010;33(2):177–89.

44. Skoog M, Milner KA, Gatti-Petito J, et al. The impact of family engagement on anxiety levels in a cardiothoracic intensive care unit. Crit Care Nurse 2016; 36(2):84–9.

45. Pew Research Center. Mobile fact sheet. 2019. Available at: https://www.pewresearch.org/internet/fact-sheet/mobile/. Accessed November 7, 2019.

46. Happ MB, Swigart VA, Tate JA, et al. Family presence and surveillance during weaning from prolonged mechanical ventilation. Heart Lung 2007;36(1):47–57.

47. Davidson JE, McDuffie M, Kay M. Family-centered care. In: Sandra Goldsworthy P, Kleinpell R, Williams G, editors. International best practices in critical care nursing. 2nd edition. Dayboro, Queensland: World Federation of Critical Care Nurses; 2018. Available at: http://wfccn.org/ebook/.

Moving?

Make sure your subscription moves with you!

To notify us of your new address, find your **Clinics Account Number** (located on your mailing label above your name), and contact customer service at:

Email: journalscustomerservice-usa@elsevier.com

800-654-2452 (subscribers in the U.S. & Canada)
314-447-8871 (subscribers outside of the U.S. & Canada)

Fax number: 314-447-8029

Elsevier Health Sciences Division
Subscription Customer Service
3251 Riverport Lane
Maryland Heights, MO 63043

*To ensure uninterrupted delivery of your subscription, please notify us at least 4 weeks in advance of move.